SONOGRAPHY

PRINCIPLES AND INSTRUMENTS

Eighth Edition
SONOGRAPHY
PRINCIPLES AND INSTRUMENTS

Frederick W. Kremkau, PhD
Professor of Radiologic Sciences
Director, Program for Medical Ultrasound
Center for Applied Learning
Wake Forest University School of Medicine
Winston-Salem, North Carolina

With contributions by:

Flemming Forsberg, PhD
Professor of Radiology
Jefferson Medical College
Thomas Jefferson University
Philadelphia, Pennsylvania

ELSEVIER
SAUNDERS

ELSEVIER
SAUNDERS

3251 Riverport Lane
St. Louis, Missouri 63043

SONOGRAPHY: PRINCIPLES AND INSTRUMENTS, Eighth Edition   ISBN: 978-1-4377-0980-3

Notices

Knowledge and best practice in this field are constantly changing. As new research and experience broaden our understanding, changes in research methods, professional practices, or medical treatment may become necessary.

Practitioners and researchers must always rely on their own experience and knowledge in evaluating and using any information, methods, compounds, or experiments described herein. In using such information or methods they should be mindful of their own safety and the safety of others, including parties for whom they have a professional responsibility.

With respect to any drug or pharmaceutical products identified, readers are advised to check the most current information provided (i) on procedures featured or (ii) by the manufacturer of each product to be administered, to verify the recommended dose or formula, the method and duration of administration, and contraindications. It is the responsibility of practitioners, relying on their own experience and knowledge of their patients, to make diagnoses, to determine dosages and the best treatment for each individual patient, and to take all appropriate safety precautions.

To the fullest extent of the law, neither the Publisher nor the authors, contributors, or editors, assume any liability for any injury and/or damage to persons or property as a matter of products liability, negligence or otherwise, or from any use or operation of any methods, products, instructions, or ideas contained in the material herein.

Library of Congress Cataloging-in-Publication Data

Kremkau, Frederick W.
  Sonography principles and instruments / Frederick W. Kremkau ; with contributions by Flemming Forsberg.—8th ed.
    p. ; cm.
  Ref. ed. of: Diagnostic ultrasound / Frederick W. Kremkau. 7th ed. c2006.
  Includes bibliographical references and index.
  ISBN 978-1-4377-0980-3 (hardcover : alk. paper) 1. Ultrasonic imaging. I. Forsberg, Flemming. II. Kremkau, Frederick W. Diagnostic ultrasound. III. Title.
  [DNLM: 1. Ultrasonography.   WN 208]
  RC78.7.U4K745 2011
  616.07′543—dc22

                                                        2010031016

Publisher: Jeanne Olson
Senior Developmental Editor: Linda Woodard
Publishing Services Manager: Catherine Jackson
Senior Project Manager: Karen M. Rehwinkel
Designer: Paula Catalano

Printed in China

Last digit is the print number: 9 8 7 6 5 4 3 2

*To students, instructors, program directors, and reviewers,
whose comments, questions, and suggestions lead to
improvements in the text with each new edition.*

Chastity Len Case, BS, RT(R), RDMS, RVT
Program Director
Asheville-Buncombe Technical Community College
Asheville, North Carolina

Jessica Chanaga, BA, RDCS, RVT
Clinical Coordinator
Florida Hospital College of Health Sciences
Orlando, Florida

Casey Clarke, BSRT, RT(R), RDMS, RDCS
Program Director, School of Diagnostic Medical Sonography
Northwestern Memorial Hospital
Chicago, Illinois

Karen M. Having, MSEd, RT, RDMS
Associate Professor
Southern Illinois University–Carbondale
Carbondale, Illinois

Ecaterina Mariana Hdeib, MA, RDMS
Clinical Assistant Professor, Diagnostic Medical Ultrasound Program
University of Missouri–Columbia
Columbia, Missouri

Mary K. Henne, MS, CNMT, RDMS, RVT
Clinical and Didactic Sonography Instructor
Columbia College of Nursing and Health Sciences
Milwaukee, Wisconsin

Frankie Lynn Martin, RT(R), DMS
Diagnostic Medical Sonography Program Director
Professor and Clinical Coordinator
Horry-Georgetown Technical College
Conway, South Carolina

Susanna Ovel, RDMS, RVT
Senior Sonographer/Trainer
Radiological Associates of Sacramento
Sacramento, California

Becky Stevens, RDMS, RT
Program Director
Bowling Green Technical College
Bowling Green, Kentucky

Anthony E. Swartz, BS, RT(R), RDMS
Maternal-Fetal Medicine Supervisor; Faculty, Physician
WakeMed Health and Hospitals
Raleigh, North Carolina

Matthew P. Varkey, BS, RDCS, RVT, RDMS
Adjunct Lecturer
School of Diagnostic Sonography
New York University;
Supervisor, Adult Echo Laboratory
New York University Medical Center
New York, New York

Ann Willis, MS, RDMS, RVT
Assistant Professor
Baptist College of Health Sciences
Memphis, Tennessee

Sonography: Principles and Instruments, eighth edition, is intended for sonography students, allied-health personnel, and physicians who seek understanding of the principles and instrumentation of diagnostic sonography. Applying these underlying principles in practice improves the quality of medical care involving sonography. The best sonographers and image interpreters understand these principles and apply them in their practice.

The purpose of this book is to explain how contemporary diagnostic sonography works. It serves as a principles textbook in sonography educational programs and helps readers handle artifacts properly, scan safely, and prepare for registry and board examinations. The content of the book is driven by the author's assessment of contemporary technology in the field and his experience in teaching this material in the medical-school classroom and at conferences and seminars. The book does not describe how to perform diagnostic examinations or how to interpret the results. Other Elsevier books cover these topics.

Although this latest edition includes newer developments in the field, the emphasis is on the fundamentals. For the sake of beginners, the text is simplified; yet at the same time it maintains its integrity and usefulness for more experienced users. Although the book is designed for *non*physicist and *non*engineering readers, digestion of the material will require some effort. Admittedly, for such readers, the material can be difficult. It cannot be made easy for everyone and still maintain the necessary understanding for appropriate application in practice. However, 35 years of lecturing and publication experience have convinced the author that the material *can* be understandable with reasonable preparation and effort on the part of the student. It is assumed that the student has completed courses in basic physics (including mechanics, waves, and electricity) and mathematics (including algebra, trigonometry, and statistics), which are normal prerequisites in sonography programs. The following topics are *not* covered in this textbook: the history of the development of sonography, therapy applications, and investigational techniques. They are covered in other books and journal articles.

DIFFERENCES BETWEEN EARLIER EDITIONS AND NATIONAL EXAMINATIONS

There are several differences between each new edition compared with earlier editions and compared with the content of registry and specialty-board examinations.

This is because this text is up to date with current technology, whereas examinations change more slowly because of the necessarily thorough and time-consuming process, which requires practice surveys, committee decisions, and item generation, review, and approval. Outmoded descriptions of technology and instrument features that are no longer largely present in the field are eliminated with each new edition. Thus the book tends to change more rapidly than the examinations. The philosophy of the book is to be, with each new edition, as consistent as possible with contemporary sonographic technology.

FEATURES

- Comprehensive coverage of the principles of diagnostic sonography
- Excellent preparation for the ARDMS SPI examination
- Latest developments in sonographic technology
- More than 1,000 color illustrations and images
- Hundreds of exercises with answers
- Comprehensive multiple-choice examination with annotated answers
- Consistent pedagogy, including learning objectives, chapter outlines, and key terms
- Key points lists set off by icons
- Descriptive subheadings
- Boxes and tables
- Math Review appendices
- Glossary

NEW TO THIS EDITION

- In the continuing attempt to simplify and condense the material in this text, the three chapters that covered Doppler principles in previous editions have been condensed into one chapter appropriate for all application areas of diagnostic ultrasound.
- Full color allows the display of over 120 color ultrasound scans in proximity to relevant discussions in the text, providing an accurate representation of what students will actually encounter in the clinical setting.
- Over 200 new illustrations and images demonstrate the latest and best images from the newest equipment.
- Expanded content on volume imaging, harmonics, and elastography keeps students up to date on the latest technology.

- Close alignment with the ARDMS physics examination specifications makes this the perfect text for studying for the SPI examination.

USING THIS TEXT

This eighth edition should be read in sequential chapter order, as each chapter builds on material previously presented. Key terms are listed at the beginning of each chapter and defined in the Glossary.

After studying this text, the student should be able to:

- Describe what ultrasound is
- Explain how ultrasound is sent into the body
- Explain how ultrasound detects and locates anatomic structures
- Discuss how echoes are received from the body and processed in the instrument
- Describe how anatomic information is presented on the display
- Explain how ultrasound detects and measures tissue motion and blood flow
- List the ways motion and flow information are presented
- Explain how flow detection is localized to a specific site in tissue
- List the common artifacts that can occur in diagnostic sonography
- Discuss how performance of sonographic instruments is tested
- Describe the risk and safety issues associated with diagnostic sonography

FOR THE INSTRUCTOR

The following resources are available at http://evolve.elsevier.com/Kremkau/ultrasound.

- *Instructor's Electronic Resource* containing an instructor's manual, PowerPoint slides, a test bank, and an image collection

- The instructor's manual includes outlines and summaries of textbook chapters, visual learning exercises, lab and learning assignments, and review questions
- The PPT presentation includes notes for instructors
- The test bank, available in Examview or Word, includes over 400 questions
- The image collection can be downloaded in PowerPoint or as jpeg files
- Extra study material for students, including a List of Symbols, a Compilation of Equations, a Physics Review, and Advanced Concepts
- Real-time videos of the following:
  - Use of a sonographic phantom as a patient surrogate
  - Effect of frequency on attenuation and penetration
  - Image formats of various transducer types
  - Impact of output and gain controls on the image
  - Color Doppler displays and control effects
  - Spectral Doppler displays and control effects
  - Aliasing artifact and ways to correct it

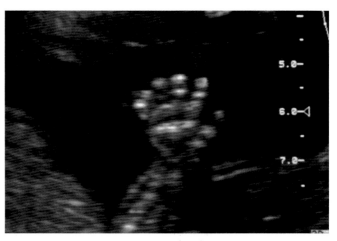

Any questions?

For assistance in illustration acquisition, the author thanks:

Jim Brown	Philips Ultrasound
Adelia Bullins	North Carolina Baptist Hospital
Kelli Bultman	GE Medical Systems
Pam Burgess	North Carolina Baptist Hospital
John D'Agostino	Tin Can Productions
Philippe Jeanty	Inner Vision Women's Ultrasound
Dana Meads	North Carolina Baptist Hospital
Cynthia Overturf	Philips Ultrasound
Cindy Owen	GE Medical Systems
Victoria Pyles	GE Medical Systems
Helen Routh	Philips Ultrasound
John Seksay	Toshiba America Medical Systems

For their cooperation and assistance he thanks:

American Institute of Ultrasound in Medicine (AIUM)
American Registry for Diagnostic Medical Sonography (ARDMS)
He acknowledges, with appreciation, Jeanne Olson for editorial advice and Linda Woodard for developmental assistance.

CONTENTS

1

Introduction

Bats, dolphins, and other animals have been using **ultrasound** long before human beings started applying it to their needs. These animals use ultrasound to detect, locate, determine the motion of, and capture prey; to avoid obstacles; to detect and avoid predators; and in the courtship of mates. One of the human applications of ultrasound techniques is **sonography** in diagnostic medicine. Diagnostic ultrasound encompasses sonography and Doppler ultrasound. Sonography is medical anatomic imaging employing ultrasound. Doppler ultrasound includes detection, quantization, and evaluation of tissue motion and blood flow using the **Doppler effect** with ultrasound.

SONOGRAPHY

The word *sonography* comes from the Latin *sonus* (sound) and the Greek *graphein* (to write). Diagnostic sonography is medical two-dimensional (2D) and three-dimensional (3D) anatomic and flow imaging using ultrasound. Ultrasound imaging is not a passive push-button activity but rather an interactive process involving sonographer (allied health professional who acquires the images), patient, ultrasound, transducer, instrument, and sonologist (physician who interprets the images). Understanding and application of the underlying physical and electronic principles presented in this book will strengthen the expertise of the sonographer and the sonologist and thus improve the quality of medical care involving diagnostic sonography.

 Medical imaging with ultrasound is called *sonography*.

An **image** (from the Latin term for "imitate") is a reproduction, representation, or imitation of the physical form of a person or object. An ultrasound image is the

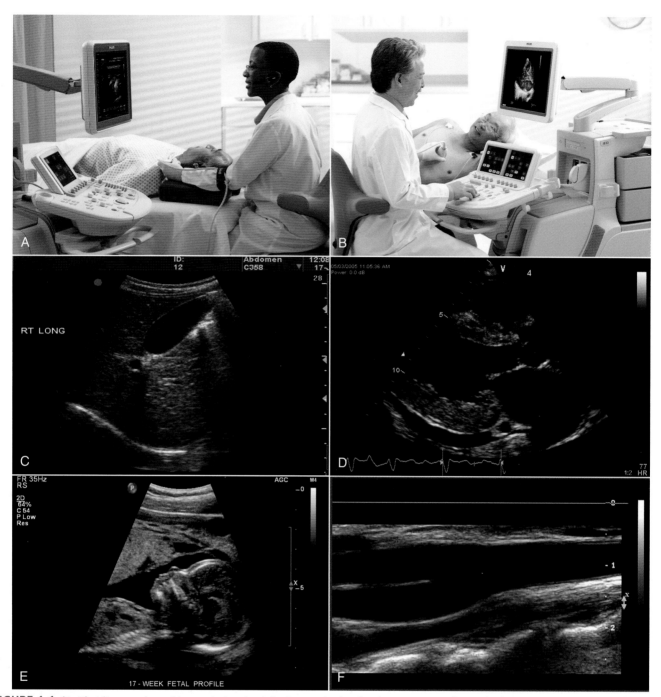

FIGURE 1-1 (A–B), Ultrasound provides a window into the human body, allowing us to see what we otherwise would not see: abdominal **(C),** cardiac **(D),** obstetric **(E),** and vascular **(F)** images.

visible counterpart of an invisible object, produced in an electronic instrument by the interaction of ultrasound with the object. Ultrasound provides a noninvasive way of looking inside the human body (Figure 1-1) to image otherwise unseen anatomy. Anatomic imaging with ultrasound is accomplished with a **pulse-echo technique.** Pulses of ultrasound are generated by a **transducer** and are sent into the patient (Figure 1-2), where they produce echoes at organ boundaries and within tissues. These echoes then return to the transducer, where they are detected and then presented on the display of a

sonographic instrument. The transducer (Figure 1-3) generates the ultrasound pulses and receives the returning echoes. Sonography requires knowledge of the location of origin and the strength of the echoes returning from the patient. The ultrasound instrument (Figure 1-4) processes the echoes and presents them as visible dots, which form the anatomic image on the display. The brightness of each dot corresponds to the echo strength, producing what then is known as a **gray-scale image.** The location of each dot corresponds to the anatomic location of the echo-generating structure. Positional information is determined by knowing the direction of the pulse when it enters the patient and by measuring the time it takes for each echo to return to the transducer. From a starting point on the display (usually at the top), the proper location for presenting the echo can then be

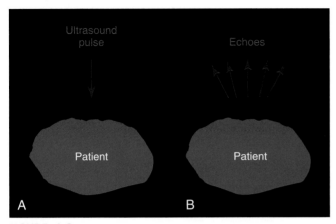

FIGURE 1-2 **Pulse-echo technique. A,** In diagnostic ultrasound, ultrasound pulses are sent into the tissues to interact with them and to obtain information about them. **B,** Echoes return from the tissues, providing information that enables anatomic imaging and observation of motion and flow, thus contributing to diagnosis.

determined. With knowledge of the sound speed, the echo arrival time is used to determine the depth of the structure that produced the echo.

 Sonography is accomplished with a pulse-echo technique.

 Echoes from anatomic structures represent these structures in a sonographic image.

If one pulse of ultrasound is sent into tissue, a series of dots (one line of echo information or one **scan line**) is displayed (Figure 1-5). Not all of the ultrasound pulse is reflected back from any interface. Rather, most of the original pulse continues on to be reflected back from deeper interfaces. The echoes from one pulse appear as one scan line (see Figure 1-5, *E-F*). If the process is repeated, but with different starting points for each subsequent pulse, a cross-sectional image of the anatomy is built up (Figure 1-6). Pulses travel in the same direction, even though they start from different points, and yield vertical parallel scan lines and a rectangular image as shown in Figure 1-7. These cross-sectional images are

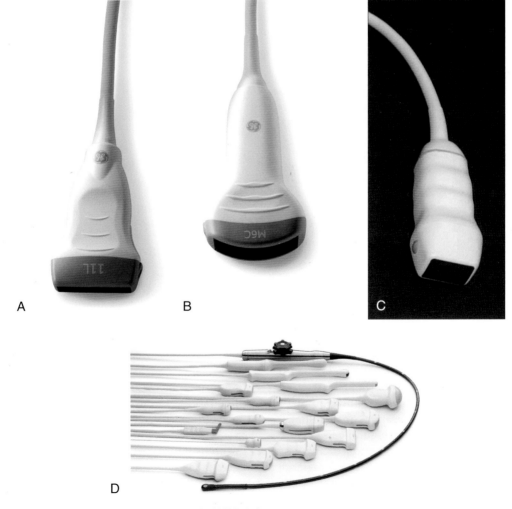

FIGURE 1-3 Transducers.

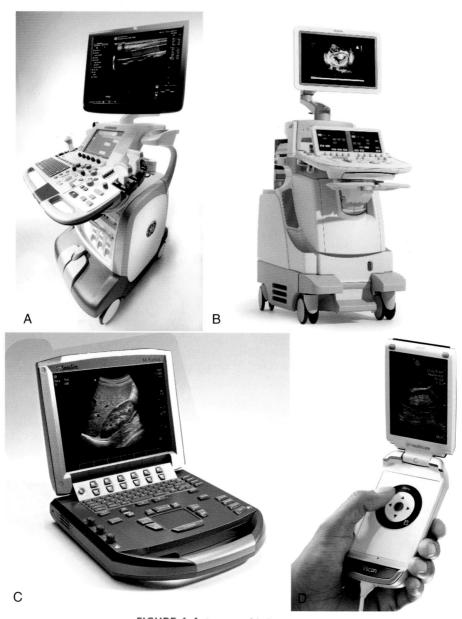

FIGURE 1-4 Sonographic instruments.

produced with vertical parallel scan lines that are so close together that they cannot be identified individually. The rectangular display resulting from this procedure often is called *a linear scan,* or **linear image,** referring to the linear-array transducer that is used to produce it. A second approach to sending ultrasound pulses through the anatomy to be imaged is shown in Figure 1-8. With this method, each pulse originates from the same starting point, but subsequent pulses go out in slightly different directions. This results in a sector scan, or **sector image,** which is shaped like a slice of pie (Figure 1-9). Figure 1-10 shows a format that is a combination of the two just described; that is, pulses (and scan lines) originate from different starting points (as in a linear image), but each pulse (and scan line) travels in a slightly different direction from that of the previous one (as in a sector

image). In this example, the starting points form a curved line across the top of the scan, rather than a straight line, as in the linear scans shown in Figure 1-7.

 Sonographic images are composed of many scan lines.

Sonographic scan formats commonly are limited to three types: (1) linear, (2) sector, and (3) their combination. Other formats may be used occasionally, but in any case, what is required is that ultrasound pulses be sent through all portions of the anatomy that are to be imaged. Each pulse generates a series of echoes, resulting in a series of dots (a scan line) on the display. The resulting cross-sectional image is composed of many (typically 96 to 256) of these scan lines. The scan format determines

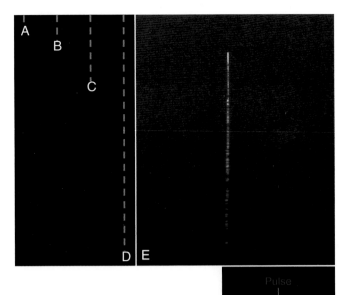

FIGURE 1-5 **One pulse of ultrasound generates a single scan line (series of echoes) as it travels through tissue.** Echoes are presented in sequence on a scan line as they return from tissue during pulse travel. **A,** The first echo is displayed. **B,** The second echo is added. **C,** Three more echoes are added. **D,** All the echoes from a single pulse have been received and displayed as a completed scan line. **E,** A complete scan line results from one emitted pulse. In practice, this is accomplished in less than one-thousandth of a second. **F,** According to the pulse-echo imaging principle, one pulse traveling through tissues produces a stream of echoes that become one scan line on the display.

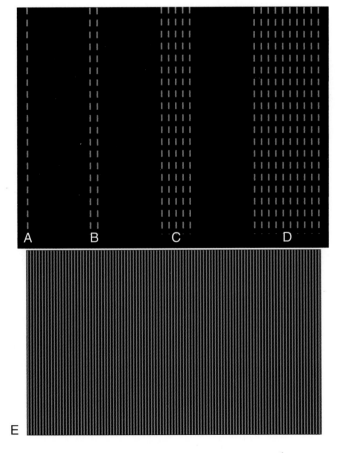

FIGURE 1-6 **A single rectangular image or scan (also called a *frame*) composed of many vertical parallel scan lines.** Each scan line represents a series of echoes returning from a pulse traveling through the tissues. **A,** One scan line from one pulse, as generated in Figure 1-5. **B,** A second scan line added. **C-D,** Five and ten scan lines, respectively. **E,** A complete frame consisting of (in this example) 100 scan lines.

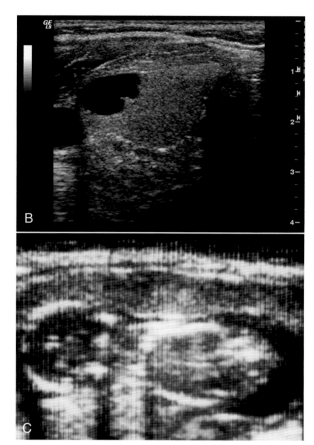

FIGURE 1-7 A, Ultrasound sent through a thin rectangular volume of tissue producing a rectangular image, commonly called a *linear image* or *linear scan*. **B,** Clinical linear (rectangular) scan. **C,** Poor-quality (by current standards) fetal image from the late 1970s, revealing the 120 vertical parallel scan lines that compose it.

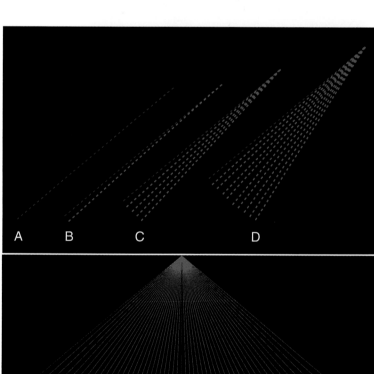

FIGURE 1-8 A single sector frame is progressively built up with 1 **(A),** 2 **(B),** 5 **(C),** 10 **(D),** and 100 **(E)** scan lines in sequence. All originate from a common origin and travel out in different directions.

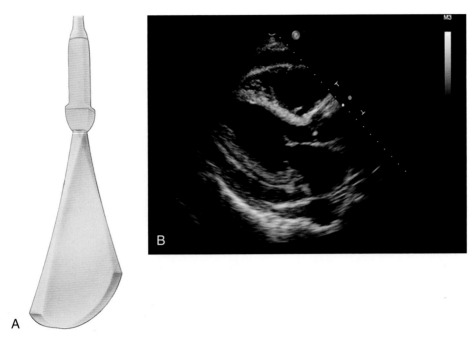

FIGURE 1-9 **A,** Ultrasound sent through a thin pie-slice–shaped volume of tissue, producing an image commonly called a *sector image* or *sector scan*. **B,** Sector scan of adult heart.

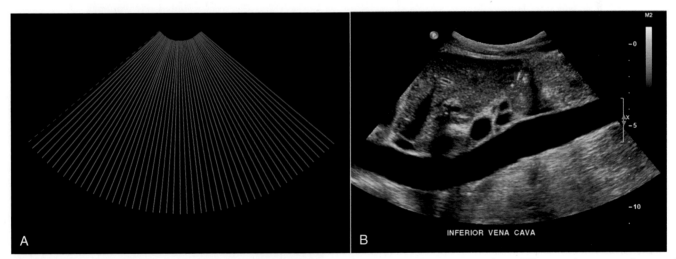

FIGURE 1-10 **A,** A modified form of a sector scan produced when pulses and scan lines originate from different points across the top of a sector display. **B,** Abdominal scan using the scan format shown in **A.**

the starting points and paths for individual scan lines, according to the starting point and path for each pulse used in generating each scan line. The clinical cross-sectional gray-scale sonographic images produced are sometimes called *B scans*, which implies that the images are produced by scanning the ultrasound through the imaged cross-section (i.e., sending pulses through all regions of the cross-section) and converting the echo strength into the brightness of each represented echo on the display (hence, B [brightness] scan). The terms *B scan* and *gray-scale scan* mean the same thing.

For decades, sonography was limited to 2D cross-sectional scans (or "slices") through the anatomy. Now 2D imaging has been enhanced to 3D scanning and imaging, also called *volume imaging*. This requires scanning the ultrasound through many adjacent 2D tissue cross-sections to build up a 3D volume of echo information like a loaf of sliced bread (Figure 1-11). This 3D volume of echoes can then be processed and interrogated to present 2D or 3D images of the anatomy.

 2D images are presented in linear (rectangular) and sector forms.

 Sonographic images are of 2D and 3D types.

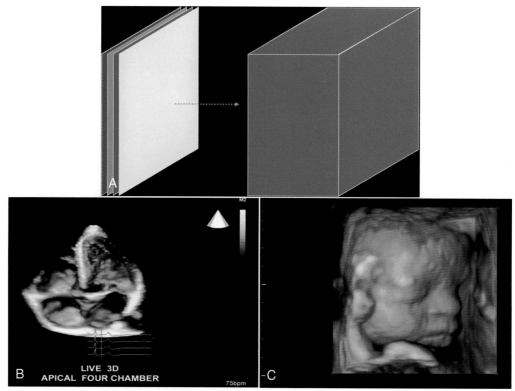

FIGURE 1-11 **Three-dimensional sonographic images. A,** Three-dimensional echo data acquired by obtaining many two-dimensional sections of echo information *(colored slices in illustration)* from the imaged anatomy, forming a three-dimensional volume of stored echo information *(blue box in illustration)*. **B,** Cardiac four-chamber view. **C,** Fetal head.

DOPPLER ULTRASOUND

Echoes produced by moving objects have frequencies that are different from the pulses sent into the body. This is called the *Doppler effect*, which is put to use in detecting and measuring tissue motion and blood flow. The use of Doppler radar in weather forecasting, aviation safety, and vehicle speed detection (police radar) has made this a household term. In addition to its use in everyday life (as demonstrated by the changing pitch of a siren or horn heard as the vehicle passes by), the Doppler effect has been applied to automatic door openers in public buildings (Figure 1-12) and to other motion-detecting devices. The Doppler effect is named after Christian Andreas Doppler, the Austrian physicist who conducted an extensive investigation into its nature.

 The Doppler effect is a change in frequency caused by moving objects.

Doppler ultrasound has been used in diagnostic medicine for decades. Long-standing applications include monitoring the fetal heart rate during labor and delivery and evaluating blood flow in the heart and in the arteries and veins of circulation. Rapid scanning and processing of Doppler data enable color-coded 2D and 3D presentations of Doppler information (**color-Doppler displays**) to be superimposed on gray-scale anatomic images (Figure 1-13). Doppler information is applied to loudspeakers for audible evaluation and to **spectral-Doppler**

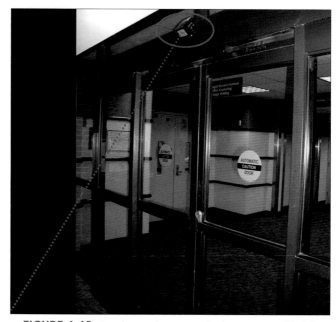

FIGURE 1-12 An ultrasonic automatic door opener *(circle)*.

displays for quantitative analysis (Figure 1-14). The spectral-Doppler operation includes anatomic imaging to determine the locations from which the spectral information is acquired (Figure 1-15).

 Doppler information is presented in audible, color-Doppler, and spectral-Doppler forms.

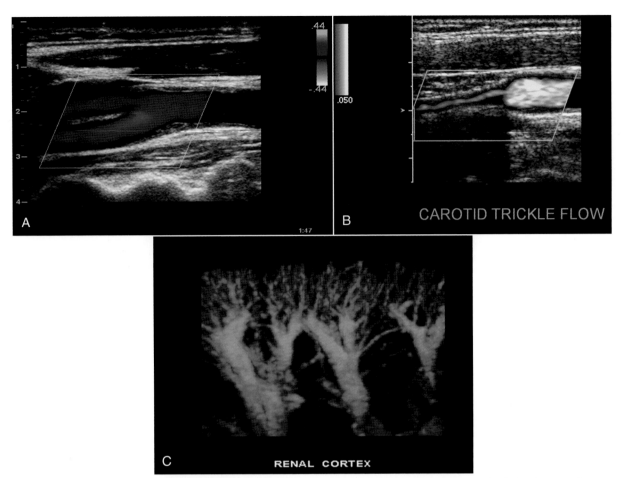

FIGURE 1-13 Color-Doppler displays of blood flow. Presented in forms called **(A)** *color-Doppler shift,* **(B)** *color-Doppler power,* and **(C)** *three-dimensional color-Doppler power displays.*

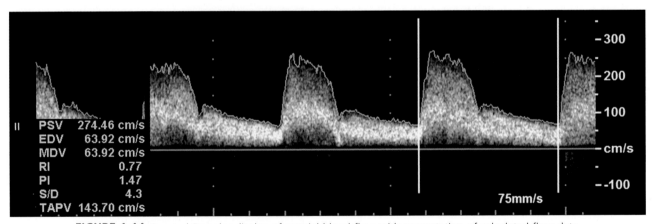

FIGURE 1-14 Spectral-Doppler display of arterial blood flow with presentation of calculated flow data.

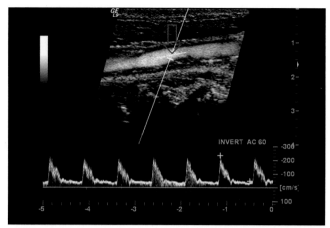

FIGURE 1-15 **Spectral-Doppler display of blood flow in the carotid artery.** The anatomic image shows the location *(arrow)* from which the spectral-Doppler information was acquired.

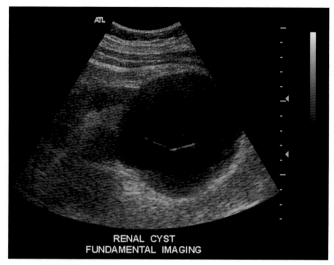

FIGURE 1-16 Illustration to accompany Exercise 9.

REVIEW

The key points presented in this chapter are the following:

- Medical imaging with ultrasound is called *sonography.*
- Sonography is accomplished with a pulse-echo technique.
- Echoes from anatomic structures represent these structures in a sonographic image.
- Sonographic images are composed of many scan lines.
- Sonographic images are of 2D and 3D types.
- 2D images are presented in linear (rectangular) and sector forms.
- The Doppler effect is a change in frequency caused by moving objects.
- Doppler information is presented in audible, color-Doppler and spectral-Doppler forms.

EXERCISES

Answers appear beginning on page 260.

1. The diagnostic ultrasound imaging (sonography) method has two parts:
   (1) Sending _____ of _____ into the body and (2) using _____ received from the anatomy to produce a(n) _____ of that anatomy.
   a. packs, sound, information, listing
   b. pulses, frequencies, echoes, description
   c. ultrasound, scans, power, image
   d. pulses, ultrasound, echoes, image

2. Ultrasound gray-scale scans are _____-_____ images of tissue cross-sections and volumes.
   a. pulse-echo
   b. virtual-anatomic
   c. pseudo-gray
   d. artificially presented

3. The brightness of an echo, as presented on the display, represents the _____ of the echo.
   a. strength   c. origin
   b. location   d. frequency

4. A linear scan is composed of many _____, _____ scan lines.
   a. horizontal, parallel
   b. horizontal, curved
   c. vertical, parallel
   d. vertical, curved

5. A sector scan is composed of many scan lines with a common _____.
   a. length   c. origin
   b. brightness   d. direction

6. A linear scan has a _____ shape.
   a. linear   c. square
   b. round   d. rectangular

7. A sector scan is shaped like a _____ of _____.
   a. slice, pie   c. scoop, pudding
   b. slice, bread   d. loaf, bread

8. A sector scan can have a(n) _____ or a _____ top.
   a. angled, straight   c. normal, inverted
   b. pointed, curved   d. curved, angled

9. Figure 1-16 is an example of an image in which the scan lines do not originate at a common _____.
   a. amplitude   c. origin
   b. disease   d. time

10. Sonography is accomplished by using a pulse-echo technique. The information of importance in doing this includes the _____ from which each echo originated and the _____ of each echo. From this information, the instrument can determine the echo _____ and _____ on the display.
   a. location, strength, location, brightness
   b. location, frequency, frequency, color
   c. anatomy, time, delay, color
   d. anatomy, strength, delay, brightness
11. The _____ is the interface between the patient and the instrument.
   a. sonographer   c. transducer
   b. Doppler   d. display
12. Transducers generate ultrasound _____ and receive returning _____.
   a. pulses, echoes
   b. waves, images
   c. echoes, pulses
   d. images, echoes
13. Three-dimensional echo information is presented on _____ displays.
   a. TV   c. 3D
   b. 2D   d. LED
14. Acquisition of a 3D echo data volume requires scanning the ultrasound through several tissue _____.
   a. angles   c. types
   b. orientations d. cross-sections
15. The Doppler effect is a change in echo _____.
   a. amplitude
   b. intensity
   c. impedance
   d. frequency
   e. arrival time
16. The change in Exercise 15 is a result of _____.
   a. pathology   c. pulses
   b. motion   d. echoes
17. The motion that produces the Doppler effect is that of the _____.
   a. transducer   c. display
   b. sound beam   d. reflector
18. In medical applications, the flow of _____ is commonly the source of the Doppler effect. Doppler information is applied to _____ for audible evaluation and to _____ for visual analysis.
   a. urine, loudspeakers, computers
   b. blood, earphones, computers
   c. lymph, earphones, displays
   d. blood, loudspeakers, displays
19. The visual display of Doppler information can be in the form of a _____-Doppler display or a _____-Doppler display.
   a. spectral, color
   b. gray-scale, color
   c. linear, sector
   d. static, temporal

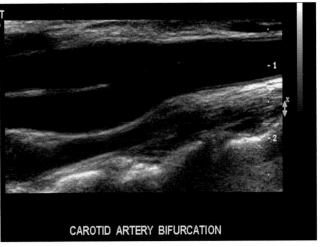

CAROTID ARTERY BIFURCATION

FIGURE 1-17 Illustration to accompany Exercise 21.

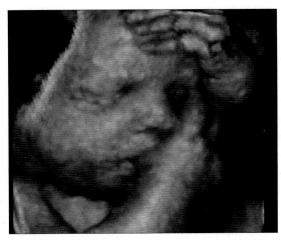

FIGURE 1-18 Illustration to accompany Exercise 22.

20. Color-Doppler displays can present Doppler-_____ and Doppler-_____ information in color.
   a. frequency, shift
   b. frequency, power
   c. shift, power
   d. bandwidth, shift
21. Figure 1-17 shows a _____.
   a. 2D linear image
   b. 2D sector image
   c. modified sector image
   d. 3D gray-scale image
   e. spectral display
22. Figure 1-18 shows a _____.
   a. 2D linear image
   b. 2D sector image
   c. modified sector image
   d. 3D gray-scale image
   e. spectral display

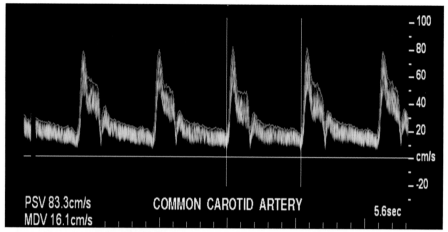

FIGURE 1-19 Illustration to accompany Exercise 23.

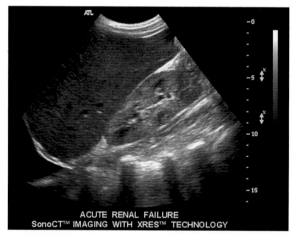

FIGURE 1-20 Illustration to accompany Exercise 24.

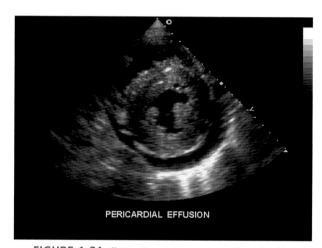

FIGURE 1-21 Illustration to accompany Exercise 25.

23. Figure 1-19 shows a _____.
    a. 2D linear image
    b. 2D sector image
    c. modified sector image
    d. 3D gray-scale image
    e. spectral display
24. Figure 1-20 shows a _____.
    a. 2D linear image
    b. 2D sector image
    c. modified sector image
    d. 3D gray-scale image
    e. spectral display

25. Figure 1-21 shows a _____.
    a. 2D linear image
    b. 2D sector image
    c. modified sector image
    d. 3D gray-scale image
    e. spectral display

Ultrasound

LEARNING OBJECTIVES

After reading this chapter, the student should be able to do the following:
- Explain what frequency is and why it is important in sonography
- Define ultrasound and describe how it behaves
- Discuss how harmonics are generated
- Compare continuous and pulsed ultrasound
- Describe the weakening of ultrasound as it travels through tissue
- Discuss the generation of echoes in tissue

OUTLINE

Sound
Waves
Frequency
Period
Wavelength
Propagation Speed
Harmonics
Pulsed Ultrasound
Pulse Repetition Frequency and Period
Pulse Duration

Duty Factor
Spatial Pulse Length
Frequency
Bandwidth
Attenuation
Amplitude
Intensity
Attenuation
Echoes
Perpendicular Incidence
Impedance

Oblique Incidence
Refraction
Scattering
Speckle
Contrast Agents
Range
Review
Exercises

KEY TERMS

Absorption
Acoustic
Acoustic variables
Amplitude
Attenuation
Attenuation coefficient
Backscatter
Bandwidth
Compression
Constructive interference
Continuous wave
Contrast agent
Coupling medium
Cycle
Decibel
Density
Destructive interference
Duty factor
Echo
Energy

Fractional bandwidth
Frequency
Fundamental frequency
Harmonics
Hertz
Impedance
Incidence angle
Intensity
Intensity reflection coefficient
Intensity transmission coefficient
Interference
Kilohertz
Longitudinal wave
Medium
Megahertz
Nonlinear propagation
Oblique incidence
Penetration
Period
Perpendicular

Perpendicular incidence
Power
Pressure
Propagation
Propagation speed
Pulse
Pulse duration
Pulse repetition frequency
Pulse repetition period
Pulsed ultrasound
Range equation
Rarefaction
Rayl
Reflection
Reflection angle
Reflector
Refraction
Scatterer
Scattering
Sound

Spatial pulse length
Speckle
Specular reflection
Stiffness

Strength
Transmission angle
Ultrasound
Wave

Wavelength
Work

Ultrasound is like the ordinary **sound** that we hear except that it has a **frequency** higher than what human beings can hear. As **ultrasound** travels through the human body, it interacts with the anatomy in ways that allow us to use it for diagnostic imaging. In this chapter, we consider what ultrasound is, how it is described, and how it travels through and interacts with the anatomy.

SOUND

Waves

Diagnostic sonography uses ultrasound to produce images of the anatomy and of flow. Ultrasound is a form of **sound**. Through our sense of hearing we experience sound daily. But what is sound? In spoken communication, sound is produced by a speaker and is heard by a listener. Sound travels from the speaker to the listener, so it is something that travels (i.e., propagates) through a **medium** such as air. But what is this sound that is traveling through air? Sound is a traveling variation in **pressure** (Figure 2-1, *A*). When the speaker speaks, variations in pressure are produced in the throat and mouth. These pressure variations travel through the air to the listener, where they stimulate the auditory response in the ear and brain.

In more general terms, we can say that sound is a **wave**. A **wave** is a traveling variation in one or more quantities, such as pressure. For example, a water wave is a traveling variation in water surface height. Dropping a pebble into a pond disturbs the surface of the water, causing it to move up and down. These up-and-down movements then travel across the surface of the pond so that motion, similar to what was generated where the pebble entered the water, eventually occurs at the far shore. Like water waves, sound involves mechanical motion in the medium through which it travels. The pressure variations in the sound wave cause the particles of the medium to vibrate back and forth.

 A wave is a traveling variation of some quantity or quantities.

Associated with pressure variations in a sound wave, **density** variations also exist. **Density** is the concentration of matter (mass per unit volume). Pressure, density, and particle vibration are called **acoustic variables** because they are quantities that vary in a sound wave (*acoustic* being derived from the Greek word for hearing). As sound travels through a medium, pressure and density go through **cycles** of increase and decrease, and particles

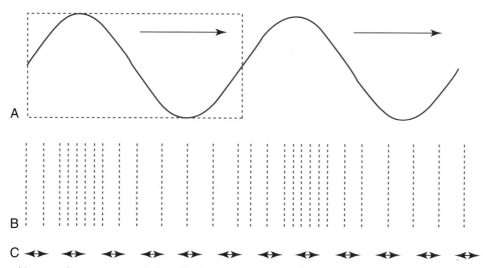

FIGURE 2-1 A, Sound is a traveling pressure variation. The box encloses one cycle of pressure variation. The pressure wave in this example is traveling to the right as indicated by the arrows. **B,** Sound is also a traveling density variation. Regions of compression (high density) and rarefaction (low density) travel along with the high- and low-pressure regions of the wave. **C,** Particles vibrate back and forth in a sound wave. This vibratory motion is parallel to the direction of travel of the wave. Such a wave is called a *longitudinal wave*. Thus, sound is a longitudinal, compressional pressure wave.

of the medium oscillate back and forth. At any point in the medium, pressure and density increase and decrease in repetitive cycles as the sound wave travels past that point. Regions of low pressure and density are called **rarefactions.** Regions of high pressure and density are called **compressions.** Compressions and rarefactions travel through a medium with a sound wave (Figure 2-1, *B*). Sound requires a medium to travel through; that is, it cannot pass through a vacuum. Sound is a mechanical compressional wave in which back-and-forth particle motion is parallel to the direction of wave travel (Figure 2-1, *C*). Such a wave is called a **longitudinal wave.**

 Sound is a traveling variation of acoustic variables.

 Acoustic variables include pressure, density, and particle motion.

Sound is described by terms that are used to describe all waves. These terms include *frequency, period, wavelength, propagation speed, amplitude,* and *intensity.* Amplitude and intensity are covered in the later section on **attenuation.**

Frequency

Frequency is a count of how many complete variations (cycles) that pressure (or any other acoustic variable) goes through in 1 second. In other words, frequency is the number of cycles that occur in a second. As shown in Figure 2-1, *A,* pressure starts at its normal (undisturbed) value. This would be the pressure in the medium if no sound were propagating through it. As a sound wave travels through a medium, the pressure at any point in the medium increases to a maximum value, returns to normal, decreases to a minimum value, and returns to normal. This describes a complete cycle of variation in pressure as an acoustic variable.

 A cycle is one complete variation in pressure or other acoustic variable.

The positive and negative halves of a pressure cycle correspond to compression and rarefaction, respectively. In other words, when the pressure is higher, the medium is more dense (more tightly packed), and when the pressure is lower, the medium is less dense. As a sound wave travels past some point in the medium, this cycle of increasing and decreasing pressure and density is repeated over and over. The number of times it is repeated in 1 second is called *frequency* (Figure 2-2). Thus frequency is the number of cycles that occur per second. Frequency units include **hertz** (Hz), **kilohertz** (kHz), and **megahertz** (MHz). One **hertz** is one cycle per second. One **kilohertz** is 1000 Hz. One **megahertz** is 1,000,000 Hz.

 Frequency is the number of cycles in a wave that occur in 1 second.

 One hertz is one cycle per second. The abbreviation for hertz is Hz.

 One kilohertz is 1000 cycles per second. The abbreviation for kilohertz is kHz.

 One megahertz is one million cycles per second. The abbreviation for megahertz is MHz.

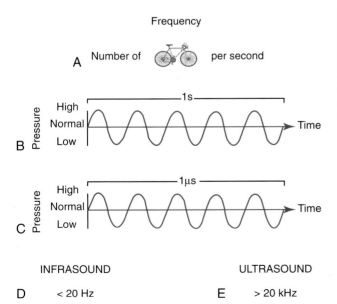

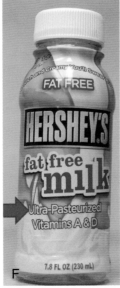

FIGURE 2-2 A, Frequency is the number of complete variations (cycles) that an acoustic variable (pressure, in this case) goes through in 1 second. **B,** Five cycles occur in 1 second; thus the frequency is five cycles per second, or 5 Hz. **C,** If five cycles occur within one millionth of a second, also known as a *microsecond* (1 μs) (i.e., five million cycles occurring in 1 second), the frequency is 5 MHz. **D,** Infrasound is sound that human beings cannot hear because the frequencies are too low (less than 20 Hz). **E,** Ultrasound is sound that human beings cannot hear because the frequencies are too high (greater than 20 kHz). **F,** Ultra *(arrow)* is a prefix meaning "beyond."

Human hearing operates in a frequency range of about 20 to 20,000 Hz, although there is great variation on the upper frequency limit in individuals. Sound having a frequency of less than 20 Hz is called *infrasound* because its frequency is too low for human hearing (infra is from the Latin word meaning "below"). Sound with a frequency of 20,000 Hz or higher is called *ultrasound* (ultra is from the Latin word meaning "beyond") because its frequency is too high for human hearing. Frequency is important in diagnostic ultrasound because of its impact on the resolution and **penetration** of sonographic images.

 Infrasound is sound of frequency too low for human hearing.

 Ultrasound is sound of frequency too high for human hearing.

Period

Period (T) is the time that it takes for one cycle to occur (Figure 2-3). In ultrasound, the common unit for period is the microsecond (μs). One microsecond is one millionth of a second (0.000001 second). For example, the period for 5 MHz ultrasound is 0.2 μs. This is because 5 MHz ultrasound contains five million cycles in a second so each cycle has only one fifth of a millionth of a second (0.2 μs) to occur. The importance of period will become apparent when **pulsed ultrasound** is considered in the next section. Table 2-1 lists common periods.

Period decreases as frequency increases because, as more cycles are packed into 1 second, there is less time for each one. Indeed, period equals 1 divided by frequency (f).

$$T(\mu s) = \frac{1}{f(MHz)}$$

 Period is the time that it takes for one cycle to occur.

 If frequency increases, period decreases.

Wavelength

Wavelength is the length of space that one cycle takes up (Figure 2-4). If we could stop a sound wave, visualize

TABLE 2-1	Common Ultrasound Periods and Wavelengths in Tissue	
Frequency (MHz)	**Period (μs)**	**Wavelength (mm)***
2.0	0.50	0.77
3.5	0.29	0.44
5.0	0.20	0.31
7.5	0.13	0.21
10.0	0.10	0.15
15.0	0.07	0.10

*Assuming a (soft tissue) propagation speed of 1.54 mm/μs (1540 m/s).

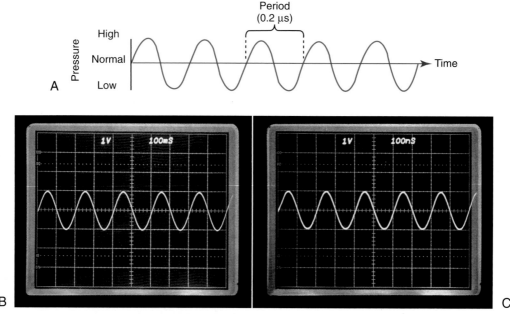

FIGURE 2-3 Period is the time it takes for one cycle to occur. A, Each cycle occurs in 0.2 μs, so the period is 0.2 μs. If one cycle takes 0.2 (or ⅕) millionths of a second to occur, it means that five million cycles occur in 1 second, so the frequency is 5 MHz. **B,** Photograph of a tracing of a 5-Hz wave. The total screen width represents 1 second. One can see that five cycles occur in 1 second and that each cycle takes one fifth (0.2) of a second to occur (period). If this were a pressure wave, it would be an example of infrasound (frequency is 5 Hz, i.e., less than 20 Hz). **C,** In this tracing, the total screen width is 1 μs. If five cycles occur in 1 μs, the period is 0.2 μs and the frequency is 5 MHz, as in **A.** If this were a pressure wave, it would be an example of ultrasound (frequency greater than 20 kHz).

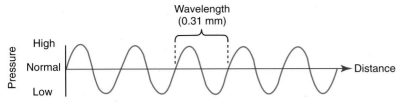

Wavelength
(0.31 mm)

High

Normal

Low

Pressure

Distance

FIGURE 2-4 Wavelength is the length of space over which one cycle occurs. In this figure, each cycle covers 0.31 mm. Thus the wavelength is 0.31 mm. This figure differs from Figures 2-2 and 2-3 in that the horizontal axis represents distance rather than time. For a propagation speed of 1.54 mm/μs and a frequency of 5 MHz, the wavelength is 0.31 mm.

it, and measure the distance from the beginning to the end of one cycle, the measured distance would be the wavelength of the sound wave. Wavelength is the length of a cycle from "front" to "back." More precisely, it could be called *cycle length*, but traditionally it has been called *wavelength*. For ultrasound, wavelength is commonly expressed in millimeters. One millimeter (1 mm) is one thousandth of a meter (0.001 m). The importance of wavelength will be evident when detail resolution of images is considered. Table 2-1 lists common wavelengths in sonography.

 Wavelength is the length of a cycle in space.

Propagation Speed

Propagation speed is the speed with which a wave moves through a medium. For sound, propagation speed is the speed at which a particular value of an acoustic variable moves (Figure 2-5), at which a cycle moves, and at which the entire wave moves. All of these are the same speed. Propagation speed units include meters per second (m/s) and millimeters per microsecond (mm/μs).

 Propagation speed is the speed at which a wave moves through a medium.

Wavelength (λ) depends on frequency and propagation speed. The relationship between the three is that wavelength is equal to propagation speed (c) divided by frequency.

$$\lambda \, (mm) = \frac{c \, (mm/\mu s)}{f \, (MHz)}$$

This equation predicts that wavelength decreases as frequency increases. This is confirmed in Table 2-1.

 If frequency increases, wavelength decreases.

An example of this relationship between frequency, wavelength, and propagation speed is seen by comparing Figures 2-3, *C*; 2-4; and 2-5. In these figures, frequency is 5 MHz, wavelength is 0.31 mm, and propagation speed is 1.54 mm/μs. These values apply to the same wave because they are a compatible set according to the following equation:

$$\lambda \, (mm) = \frac{c \, (mm/\mu s)}{f \, (MHz)} = \frac{1.54 \, mm/\mu s}{5 \, MHz} = 0.31 \, mm$$

Propagation speed is determined by the medium, primarily its **stiffness** (hardness). **Stiffness** is the resistance of a material to compression. Stiffness is the inverse of compressibility; that is, a compressible material such as a sponge has low stiffness, and a stiff (hard) material such as a rock has low compressibility. Stiffer media have higher sound speeds. Thus propagation speeds are lower in gases (which are highly compressible), higher in liquids, and highest in solids (which are nearly incompressible). The average propagation speed in soft tissues is 1540 m/s, or (in more relevant units for our purposes) 1.54 mm/μs. Values for soft tissues range from 1.44 to 1.64 mm/μs. Not surprisingly, because soft tissue is mostly water, these values are similar to those for liquids such as water.

 Propagation speeds are highest in solids and lowest in gases.

The average propagation speed of sound in tissues is 1.54 mm/μs.

In lung tissue, because it contains gas, the propagation speed of sound is much lower than in other soft tissues. However, this difference is not important because ultrasound does not penetrate air-filled lung well enough for imaging. In bone, because it is a solid, propagation speeds are higher (3 to 5 mm/μs) than in soft tissues. Soft tissue propagation speeds are within a few percent of the average, so the average can be assumed for all soft tissues with little error. Fat is furthest from the average, about 6% lower. Propagation speed is important because sonographic instruments use it to accurately locate echoes on the display.

Harmonics

The dependence of propagation speed on pressure causes strong sound (pressure) waves to change shape as they travel (Figure 2-6). The reason for this is that the higher-pressure portions of the wave travel faster than do the lower-pressure portions. This causes a wave that originally is shaped in a smooth curve form (called *sinusoidal*; illustrated in Figure 2-6, *A*) to progress toward a nonsinusoidal shape (Figure 2-6, *C*). **Propagation** in which

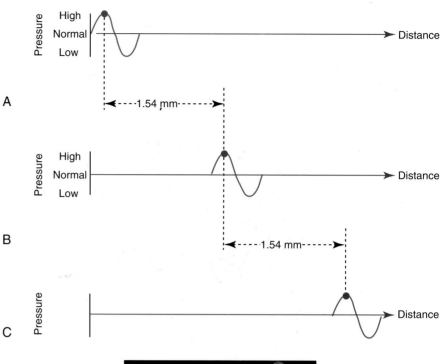

A

B

C

FIGURE 2-5 Propagation speed is the speed with which a particular value of an acoustic variable (also the rest of the cycle and, indeed, the entire wave) travels through a medium. **A,** The movement of a maximum *(identified by the dot)* is shown in this figure. **B,** 1 μs after **A.** **C,** 1 μs after **B** and 2 μs after **A.** The maximum *(dot)* moves 1.54 mm in 1 μs and 3.08 mm in 2 μs. The propagation speed is 1.54 mm/μs. The propagation speed in this figure (1.54 mm/μs), when divided by the frequency in Figure 2-3, *C* (5 MHz), equals the wavelength in Figure 2-4 (0.31 mm). **D,** Propagation speeds in soft tissue average 1540 m/s, or 1.54 mm/μs.

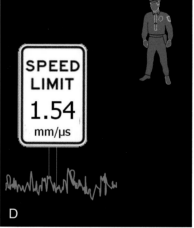

D

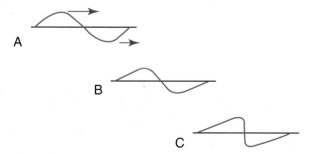

A

B

C

FIGURE 2-6 In nonlinear propagation, propagation speed depends on pressure. **A,** Higher-pressure portions of the wave travel faster than do the lower-pressure portions. **B-C,** Thus the wave changes shape as it travels. This change from the initial sinusoidal shape introduces harmonics that are even and odd multiples of the fundamental frequency.

speed depends on pressure and the shape of the wave changes is called **nonlinear propagation.** A continuous (not pulsed) sinusoidal waveform is characterized by a single frequency (equal to the number of cycles per second). Any other wave shape contains additional frequencies that are even and odd multiples of the original frequency. The original frequency is called **fundamental frequency.** The even and odd multiples are called *even* and *odd* **harmonics,** respectively. A frequency analysis of the wave in Figure 2-6, *A,* would yield a single (fundamental) frequency such as 2 MHz. Parts *B* and *C* would reveal, in addition to fundamental frequency, harmonics such as 4, 6, and 8 MHz. As the shape becomes less sinusoidal, the harmonics become stronger. Therefore they are stronger in part *C* than in part *B.* Using harmonic frequency echoes (harmonic imaging is discussed later) improves the quality of sonographic images.

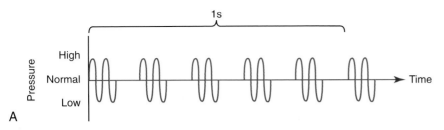

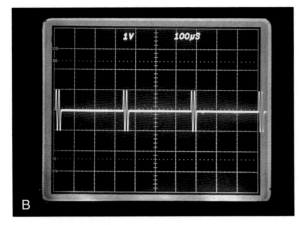

FIGURE 2-7 Pulse repetition frequency is the number of pulses occurring in 1 second. A, Five pulses (containing two cycles each) occur in 1 second; thus the pulse repetition frequency is 5 Hz. **B,** In this photograph, three pulses occur in 1 millisecond (or one thousandth of a second); thus the pulse repetition frequency is 3 kHz. The total screen width is 1 ms.

 Harmonics are even and odd multiples of fundamental frequency.

PULSED ULTRASOUND

Thus far we have discussed terms (*frequency*, *period*, *wavelength*, and *propagation speed*) that are sufficient to describe **continuous wave** (or CW) ultrasound where cycles repeat indefinitely. For sonography and most of Doppler ultrasound, **pulsed ultrasound** is used rather than *continuous wave*. An ultrasound **pulse** is a few cycles of ultrasound. Pulses are separated in time with gaps of no ultrasound. Ultrasound pulses are described by some additional parameters that we will discuss now.

 With continuous wave ultrasound, cycles repeat indefinitely. Pulsed ultrasound consists of pulses separated by gaps in time. A pulse is a few cycles of ultrasound.

Pulse Repetition Frequency and Period

Pulse repetition frequency (PRF) is the number of pulses occurring in 1 second (Figure 2-7). Diagnostic ultrasound involves a few thousand pulses per second, so pulse repetition frequency is commonly expressed in kilohertz (kHz). One kilohertz is 1000 Hz. **Pulse repetition period** (PRP) is the time from the beginning of one pulse to the beginning of the next (Figure 2-8). Its common units are milliseconds (ms, one thousandth

of a second). Pulse repetition period is the reciprocal of pulse repetition frequency. Pulse repetition period decreases as pulse repetition frequency increases because, as more pulses occur in a second, there is less time from one to the next.

$$PRP\,(ms) = \frac{1}{PRF\,(kHz)}$$

The pulse repetition frequency is controlled automatically by sonographic instruments to satisfy requirements that are discussed later. With Doppler techniques, the operator controls pulse repetition frequency, also described in later chapters. Pulse repetition frequency is important because it determines how fast images are generated. For example, for a pulse repetition frequency of 5 kHz, 5000 pulses are produced each second, generating 5000 scan lines per second. If, for example, there are 100 scan lines in each image, 50 images will be produced per second. Later this will be called *frame rate*. It will determine how well rapidly moving structures can be followed.

 Pulse repetition frequency is the number of pulses occurring in a second.

 Pulse repetition period is the time from the beginning of one pulse to the beginning of the next one.

 If pulse repetition frequency increases, pulse repetition period decreases.

Pulse Duration

Pulse duration (PD) is the time that it takes for one pulse to occur (Figure 2-8). Pulse duration is equal to the

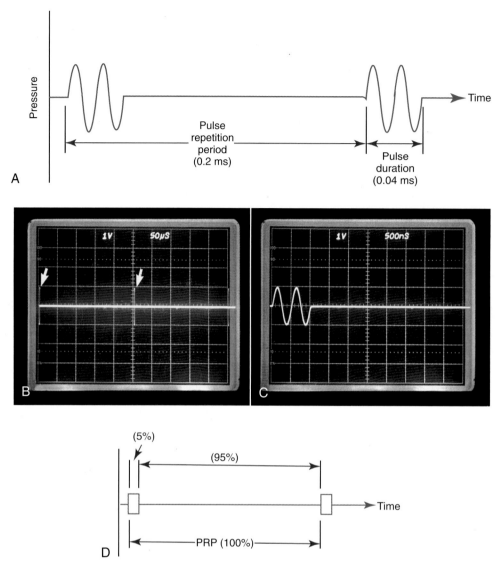

FIGURE 2-8 Pulse repetition period is the time from the beginning of one pulse to the beginning of the next. A, The pulse repetition period is 0.2 ms (200 μs). Therefore the pulse repetition frequency is 5 kHz. Pulse duration is the time that it takes for one pulse to occur. Pulse duration is equal to the period multiplied by the number of cycles in the pulse. The pulse duration is 40 μs. Duty factor is the fraction of time that the sound is on. The duty factor is 40/200, which equals 0.2, or 20%. **B,** This photograph shows that the pulse repetition period is 0.25 ms. (The pulse repetition frequency is 4 kHz.) The period is 0.5 μs, as shown expanded in **C,** and the pulse duration is 1 μs. From one pulse to the next (pulse repetition period of 0.25 ms, or 250 μs), the sound is on (pulse duration) for 1 μs. The duty factor in this example is 0.004, or 0.4%. The screen width is 0.5 ms in **B** and 5 μs in **C. D,** Duty factor is the fraction of time that pulsed ultrasound is actually on. In this example, the pulse repetition period (PRP) represents 100% of the time from the start of one pulse to the start of the next one. Of this time, the sound is on 5% of the time (pulse duration divided by pulse repetition period) and off 95% of the time.

period (the time for one cycle) times the number of cycles in the pulse (n) and is expressed in microseconds. Sonographic pulses are typically two or three cycles long. Shorter pulses, compared with longer ones, improve the quality of sonographic images. Doppler ultrasound pulses are typically 5 to 30 cycles long.

$$PD\,(\mu s) = n \times T\,(\mu s)$$

 Sonographic pulses are typically two or three cycles long. Doppler pulses are typically 5 to 30 cycles long.

Pulse duration decreases if the number of cycles in a pulse is decreased or if the frequency is increased (reducing the period). The instrument operator chooses the frequency.

 Pulse duration is the time for a pulse to occur.

 If frequency is increased, period is decreased, reducing pulse duration. If the number of cycles in a pulse is reduced, pulse duration is decreased. Shorter pulses improve the quality of sonographic images.

Duty Factor

Duty factor (DF) is the fraction of time that pulsed ultrasound is on (Figure 2-8, D). Continuous wave ultrasound is on 100% of the time. Pulsed ultrasound, by definition, is not on all of the time. The duty factor indicates how much of the time the ultrasound is on. Longer pulses increase the duty factor because the sound is on more of the time.

 Duty factor is the fraction of time that pulsed ultrasound is on.

Higher pulse repetition frequencies increase duty factor because there is less "dead" time between pulses. Thus the duty factor increases with increasing pulse duration or pulse repetition frequency. Duty factor has no units because it is a fraction with time in both the numerator and denominator. Thus duty factor is simply expressed as a decimal, such as 0.10 or 0.25, or as a percentage, such as 10% or 25%. The importance of duty factor will become evident when intensities and safety issues are discussed later. The duty factor is equal to pulse duration divided by pulse repetition period. The reason for this is that pulse duration represents the amount of time that the sound is on, and pulse repetition period is the time from one pulse to the next. Thus the ratio of the two represents the fraction of time that pulsed ultrasound is on.

$$DF = \frac{PD\,(\mu s)}{PRP\,(\mu s)} = \frac{PD\,(\mu s) \times PRF\,(kHz)}{1000\,(kHz/MHz)}$$

The factor of 1000 converts kilohertz to megahertz to be consistent with microseconds of pulse duration. Multiplying the duty factor by 100 expresses it as a percentage. For example, if the pulse duration is 2 μs and the pulse repetition period is 250 μs, then

$$DF = \frac{2}{250} = 0.008 = or\ 0.8\%$$

A range of duty factors is encountered in diagnostic ultrasound because of the various conditions chosen by the instrument and the operator. Typical duty factors for sonography are in the range of 0.1% to 1.0%. For Doppler ultrasound, because of longer pulse durations, the range of typical duty factors is 0.5% to 5.0%.

 If pulse duration increases, duty factor increases.

 If pulse repetition frequency increases, pulse repetition period decreases and duty factor increases.

Spatial Pulse Length

If we could stop a pulse, visualize it, and measure the distance from its beginning to its end, the measured distance would be **spatial pulse length** (SPL). Spatial pulse length is the length of a pulse from front to back (Figure 2-9, A). Spatial pulse length is equal to the length of each cycle times the number of cycles in the pulse. The length of each cycle is wavelength. Thus spatial pulse length increases with wavelength and increases with the number of cycles in the pulse.

$$SPL\,(mm) = n \times \lambda\,(mm)$$

 Spatial pulse length is the length of space that a pulse takes up.

Because wavelength decreases with increasing frequency, spatial pulse length decreases with increasing frequency (Figure 2-9, B-C). Units for spatial pulse length are millimeters. Spatial pulse length is an important quantity when considering image resolution. Shorter pulse lengths improve resolution.

 If the number of cycles in a pulse increases, spatial pulse length increases. If frequency increases, wavelength and spatial pulse length decrease.

 Shorter pulses improve sonographic image resolution.

Frequency

Recall that frequency expresses the number of cycles in a wave that occurs in a second. This is fine for continuous wave ultrasound; however, in pulsed ultrasound, gaps exist between pulses, so some of the cycles are missing. For example, 5-MHz frequency continuous wave ultrasound has five million cycles occurring in a second. But what about 5-MHz pulsed ultrasound? The frequency, 5 MHz, gives the number of cycles per second, as if the wave were a continuous wave, even though it is not. The actual number of cycles occurring in a second for pulsed ultrasound depends on duty factor. For example, if the duty factor is 0.01, or 1%, the ultrasound is on only one hundredth of the time, and the actual number of cycles per second is 50,000, or 50 kHz. The quiet time between pulses eliminates 99% of the cycles in this example, even though the frequency implies that there are five million cycles per second. However, the frequency for pulsed ultrasound is still given as 5 MHz because the behavior of the pulses (regarding period, wavelength, propagation speed, and other characteristics such as attenuation) is like that of 5-MHz continuous wave ultrasound.

Bandwidth

In contrast to continuous wave ultrasound, which can be described by a single frequency, ultrasound pulses

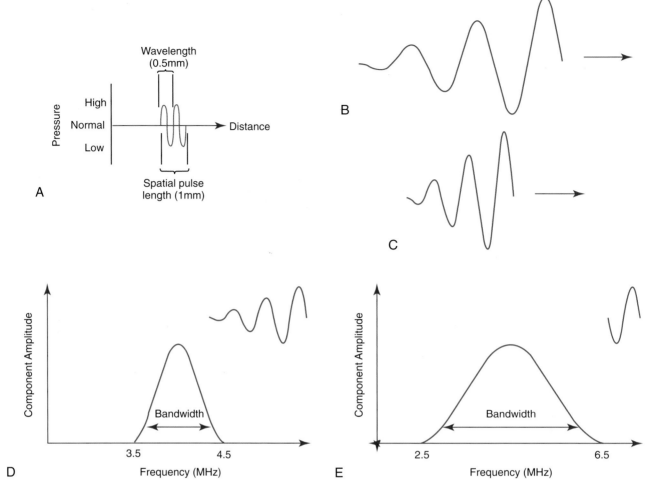

FIGURE 2-9 A, Spatial pulse length is the length of space over which a pulse occurs. Spatial pulse length is equal to wavelength multiplied by the number of cycles in the pulse. In this figure, the wavelength is 0.5 mm, there are two cycles in each pulse, and the spatial pulse length is 0.5 × 2, or 1 mm. This figure differs from Figures 2-7, *A*, and 2-8, *A*, in that the horizontal axis represents distance rather than time. **B-C,** Three-cycle damped (decreasing in amplitude) pulses of ultrasound traveling to the right. **B** shows lower-frequency pulse with longer wavelength and spatial pulse length. **C** shows higher-frequency pulse with shorter wavelength and spatial pulse length. **D-E,** Plots of the frequencies present in two ultrasound pulses. Component amplitude is the amplitude of each frequency component present. Bandwidth is the range of frequencies present. Compare the bandwidth for a narrowband, longer pulse **(D)** with the bandwidth for a broadband, shorter pulse **(E).**

contain a range of frequencies called **bandwidth** (Figure 2-9, *D-E*). The shorter the pulse (the fewer the number of cycles), the higher are the number of frequencies present in it (broader bandwidth). **Fractional bandwidth** is bandwidth divided by operating frequency. **Fractional bandwidth** is unitless. It describes how large the bandwidth is compared with operating frequency. The reciprocal of fractional bandwidth (operating frequency divided by bandwidth) is called *quality factor* (Q).

 Bandwidth is the range of frequencies contained in a pulse.

ATTENUATION

We now consider the magnitude of the cyclic variations in a continuous or pulsed ultrasound wave. Amplitude

and intensity are indicators of the **strength** of the sound. They are related to how loud the sound would be if it could be heard. Ultrasound, however, cannot be heard, so loudness is irrelevant. Nevertheless, amplitude and intensity are important indicators of how strong or "intense" the ultrasound is.

Amplitude

Amplitude is the maximum variation that occurs in an acoustic variable. **Amplitude** is a measure of how far a variable gets away from its normal, undisturbed value (its value if there were no sound present). Amplitude is the maximum value minus the normal (undisturbed or no-sound) value (Figure 2-10, *A*). Amplitude is expressed in units that are appropriate for the acoustic variable considered. For example, megapascals (MPa) are the units for pressure amplitude.

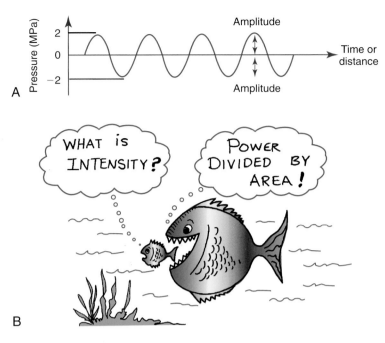

A

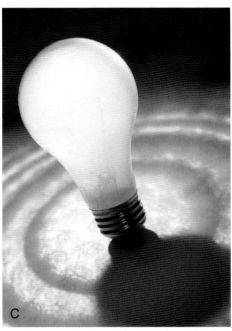

B

C

FIGURE 2-10 A, Amplitude is the maximum amount of variation that occurs in an acoustic variable (pressure, in this case). In this figure, the amplitude is 2 MPa. **B,** Intensity is the power in a sound wave divided by the area over which the power is spread (the beam area). **C,** A watt is the unit of power for a light bulb.

Intensity

Intensity (I) is the rate at which **energy** (the ability to do work) passes through a unit area. It is equal to **power** (P, the rate at which energy travels along a beam) in a wave divided by the area (A) over which the power is spread (Figure 2-10, B). Ultrasound is generated by transducers in the form of beams, somewhat like laser beams, but as sound instead of light. The average intensity of a sound beam is the total power in the beam divided by the cross-sectional area of the beam.

$$I\,(mW/cm^2) = \frac{P\,(mW)}{A\,(cm^2)}$$

Increasing power increases intensity. Increasing area decreases intensity because power is less concentrated. Decreasing area (focusing) increases intensity because power is more concentrated.

> If beam power increases, intensity increases. If beam area decreases (focusing), intensity increases.

Energy is the capability to do **work**. Sound, heat, light, and mechanical motion are forms of energy. Power is the rate at which energy is transferred from one part of a system to another (e.g., a lamp plugged into a wall outlet) or from one location to another (e.g., traveling

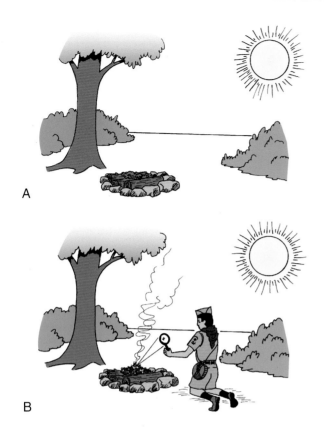

A

B

FIGURE 2-11 A, Sunlight does not normally ignite a fire. **B,** However, when the sunlight is focused, intensity increases, and ignition can occur.

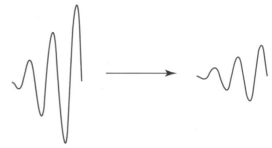

FIGURE 2-12 An ultrasound pulse is weakened (reduction of amplitude) as it travels through a medium (in this case from left to right). This weakening is called *attenuation*.

down a laser or ultrasound beam). Power is energy transferred divided by time required to transfer energy, that is, the transfer rate. Power units include watts (W) (Figure 2-10, C) and milliwatts (mW). One milliwatt is one thousandth of a watt. Beam area is expressed in centimeters squared (cm^2). Intensity units include milliwatts per centimeter squared (mW/cm^2) and watts per centimeter squared (W/cm^2). Intensity is an important quantity in describing the sound that is sent into the body by a transducer and in discussing bioeffects and safety. An analogy may be made to the effect of sunlight on dry kindling (Figure 2-11). Sunlight normally will not ignite the kindling, but if the same light power from the sun is concentrated into a small area (increased intensity) by focusing it with a magnifying glass, the kindling can be ignited. In this example, increasing intensity produces an effect, even though power remains the same. The beam area is determined by the transducer, in particular, how it focuses the beam. Intensity is proportional to amplitude squared. Thus, if amplitude is doubled, intensity is quadrupled. If amplitude is halved, intensity is quartered.

Attenuation

Attenuation (a) is the weakening of sound as it propagates (Figure 2-12). It is important to understand attenu-

ation because (1) it limits imaging depth and (2) its weakening effect on the image must be compensated by the diagnostic instrument. With an unfocused beam in any medium, such as tissue, amplitude and intensity will decrease as the sound travels through the medium. This reduction in amplitude and intensity as sound travels is called *attenuation* (Figure 2-13). Attenuation encompasses the **absorption** (conversion of sound to heat) of sound as it travels and the **reflection** and **scattering** of the sound (**echoes**) as it encounters tissue interfaces and heterogeneous tissues. Absorption is the dominant factor contributing to attenuation of ultrasound in soft tissues. The generation of echoes by the reflection and scattering of sound is crucial to sonographic imaging but contributes little to attenuation in most cases. **Decibels** are the units used to quantify attenuation. The **attenuation coefficient** (a_c) is the attenuation that occurs with each centimeter the sound wave travels. Its units are decibels per centimeter (dB/cm). The farther the sound travels, the greater is the attenuation.

Decibels are useful units for making comparisons. For example, they describe the relationships between various measured sound levels (Figure 2-14) and the threshold of human hearing (the weakest sound we can hear). Table 2-2 gives examples of various values. Decibels involve the logarithm of the ratio of two powers or intensities. In the case of attenuation, they are the intensities before and after attenuation has occurred. Two decibel values have particular usefulness: 3 dB corresponds to an intensity ratio of one half, that is, an intensity reduction of 50%; and 10 dB corresponds to an intensity ratio of one tenth, that is, an intensity reduction of 90% (Figures 2-13 and 2-15).

Example 2-1
Compare the following two intensities in decibels:

$$I_1 = 20\,mW/cm^2, I_2 = 10\,mW/cm^2.$$

I_2 is one half of I_1. Therefore, I_2 is 3 dB less than I_1.

Example 2-2
Compare (in decibels) I_2 with I_1, where $I_1 = 10\,mW/cm^2$ and $I_2 = 0.01\,mW/cm^2$.

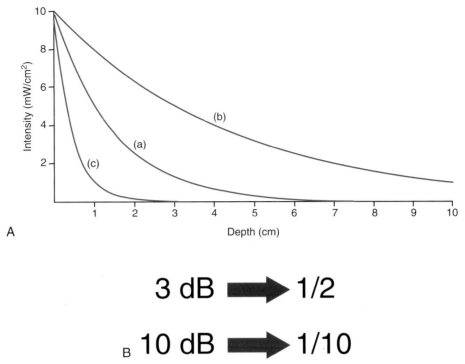

A

B

$3\,dB \Longrightarrow 1/2$

$10\,dB \Longrightarrow 1/10$

FIGURE 2-13 Attenuation of sound as it travels through a medium. A, In example *(a)*, the intensity decreases by 50% for each 1 cm of travel. This corresponds to an attenuation coefficient of 3 dB/cm. In example *(b)*, the attenuation coefficient is 1 dB/cm, whereas in *(c)*, the attenuation coefficient is 10 dB/cm. **B,** Two easy-to-remember values for decibels and their corresponding intensity reductions are (1) a 3-dB attenuation corresponds to an intensity reduction (50%) to one half the original value, and (2) a 10-dB attenuation corresponds to an intensity reduction (90%) to one tenth the original value.

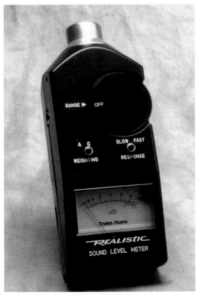

FIGURE 2-14 A sound level meter based on decibels.

TABLE 2-2	Sound Levels
Sound	**Level (dB)**
Pain threshold	130
Rock concert	115
Chain saw	100
Lawn mower	90
Vacuum cleaner	75
Normal conversation	60
Whisper	30
Hearing threshold	0

Each factor of 10 is equivalent to 10 dB. I_1 is 1000 times I_2, so I_2 is 30 dB less than I_1.

Example 2-3

As sound passes through tissue, its intensity at one point is 1 mW/cm²; at a point 10 cm farther along, it is 0.1 mW/cm². What are the attenuation and attenuation coefficient values?

Because intensity is reduced to one tenth from the first point to the second, attenuation is 10 dB. The attenuation coefficient is attenuation divided by the separation between the two points. In this case,

$$a_c = \frac{10\,dB}{10\,cm} = 1\,dB/cm$$

Table 2-3 lists various values of intensity ratio and percent values with corresponding decibel values of attenuation. To determine attenuation in decibels, multiply the attenuation coefficient by sound path length (L) (how far the sound has traveled) in centimeters.

$$a\,(dB) = a_c\,(dB/cm) \times L\,(cm)$$

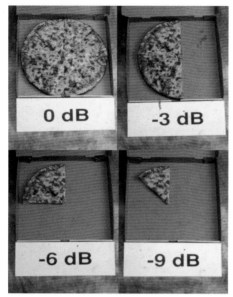

FIGURE 2-15 Each reduction of 3 dB corresponds to removing half the pizza.

TABLE 2-3	Attenuation for Various Intensity Ratios*	
Attenuation (dB)	Intensity Ratio	Percent Intensity Ratio
0	1.00	100
1	0.79	79
2	0.63	63
3	0.50	50
4	0.40	40
5	0.32	32
6	0.25	25
7	0.20	20
8	0.16	16
9	0.13	13
10	0.10	10
15	0.032	3.2
20	0.010	1.0
25	0.003	0.3
30	0.001	0.1
35	0.0003	0.03
40	0.0001	0.01
45	0.00003	0.003
50	0.00001	0.001
60	0.000001	0.0001
70	0.0000001	0.00001
80	0.00000001	0.000001
90	0.000000001	0.0000001
100	0.0000000001	0.00000001

*The intensity ratio is the fraction of the original intensity remaining after attenuation.

 If the attenuation coefficient increases, attenuation increases.

TABLE 2-4	Average Attenuation Coefficients in Tissue		
Frequency (MHz)	Average Attenuation Coefficient for Soft Tissue (dB/cm)	Intensity Reduction in 1-cm Path (%)	Intensity Reduction in 10-cm Path (%)
2.0	1.0	21	90
3.5	1.8	34	98
5.0	2.5	44	99.7
7.5	3.8	58	99.98
10.0	5.0	68	99.999

 If path length increases, attenuation increases.

Attenuation increases with increasing frequency. Persons who live in apartments or dormitories experience this fact when they hear mostly the bass notes through the wall from a neighbor's sound system. For soft tissues, there is approximately (values of 0.3 to 0.7 are used by authors for various purposes) 0.5 dB of attenuation per centimeter for each megahertz of frequency (Table 2-4). In other words, the average attenuation coefficient in decibels per centimeter for soft tissues is approximately equal to one half the frequency in megahertz. To calculate the attenuation in decibels, multiply one half the frequency in megahertz by path length in centimeters.

$$a\,(dB) = \frac{1}{2}\,(dB/cm\text{-}MHz) \times f\,(MHz) \times L\,(cm)$$

 As frequency increases, attenuation increases.

The intensity ratio corresponding to that number of decibels may be obtained from Table 2-3. This ratio is equal to the fraction of the intensity (at the beginning of the path) that remains at the end of the path. If the intensity at the beginning is known, the intensity at the end may be found by multiplying the beginning intensity by the intensity ratio. A summary of this four-step process follows:

1. Multiplying the frequency by one half yields the approximate attenuation coefficient.
2. Multiplying the attenuation coefficient by path length yields attenuation.
3. The intensity ratio is then determined for the decibel value calculated in step 2 (using Table 2-3). This is the fraction of the original intensity remaining at the end of the path.
4. Multiplying the intensity ratio by the intensity at the start of the path yields the intensity at the end of the path.

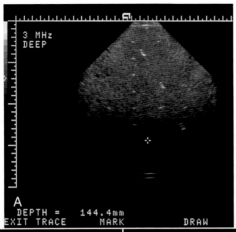

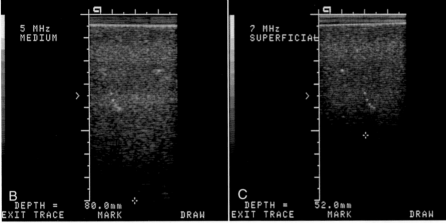

FIGURE 2-16 Examples of penetration in a tissue-equivalent phantom at 3 MHz **(A)**, 5 MHz **(B)**, and 7 MHz **(C)**. Penetration decreases as frequency increases.

Example 2-4

If 4-MHz ultrasound with 10 mW/cm² intensity is applied to a soft tissue surface, what is the intensity 1.5 cm into the tissue?

Step 1: Multiply frequency by one half to yield an attenuation coefficient of 2 dB/cm.

Step 2: Multiply the attenuation coefficient (2 dB/cm) by path length (1.5 cm) to yield an attenuation of 3 dB.

Step 3: From Table 2-3, an attenuation of 3 dB corresponds to an intensity ratio of 0.5. Thus 50% of intensity remains after the sound travels through this path.

Step 4: Multiply the intensity ratio (0.5) by the intensity at the beginning of the path (10 mW/cm²) to yield the intensity at the end of the path. The result is 5 mW/cm².

TABLE 2-5	Common Values for Attenuation Coefficient and Penetration	
Frequency (MHz)	**Attenuation Coefficient (dB/cm)**	**Penetration (cm)**
2.0	1.0	30
3.5	1.8	17
5.0	2.5	12
7.5	3.8	8
10.0	5.0	6
15.0	7.5	4

Attenuation is higher in the lung than in other soft tissues because of the air present in the organ. Attenuation is higher in bones than in soft tissues.

A practical consequence of attenuation is that it limits the depths of images (**penetration**) obtained. Penetration decreases as frequency increases (Figure 2-16). Table 2-5 lists attenuation coefficients and typical imaging depths for various frequencies in soft tissue.

If frequency increases, penetration decreases.

The depths needed to reach various parts of human anatomy determine the frequencies used in diagnostic ultrasound, which range from 2 to 15 MHz for most applications. Within this range, lower frequencies are used for deeper penetration and higher frequencies for superficial applications and invasive transducers (rectal, vaginal, and esophageal). Even higher frequencies (up to 50 MHz) are used for some specialized applications, including skin and ophthalmologic imaging and intravascular imaging with catheter-mounted transducers. Frequencies less than 2 MHz are used in large-animal applications.

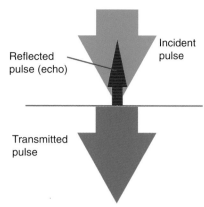

FIGURE 2-17 Reflection and transmission at a boundary with perpendicular incidence. The incident pulse is partially reflected (echo) with the remainder (transmitted pulse) continuing into the second medium. The strengths of the reflected and transmitted pulses are determined by the impedances of the two media at the boundary.

ECHOES

Ultrasound is useful as an imaging tool because of the reflection and scattering of sound waves at organ and tissue interfaces and scattering within heterogeneous tissues. The reflected and scattered sound waves produce the pattern of echoes that is necessary for diagnostic pulse-echo imaging with ultrasound. These phenomena are considered in this section.

Perpendicular Incidence

Perpendicular incidence denotes a direction of travel of the ultrasound wave **perpendicular** to the boundary between two media (Figure 2-17). The incident sound may be reflected back into the first medium or transmitted into the second medium; most often, both occur. When there is perpendicular incidence, reflected sound travels back through the first medium in a direction opposite to the incident sound (i.e., the reflected sound returns to the sound source). In the case of perpendicular incidence, the transmitted sound does not change direction; it moves through the second medium in the same direction as the incident sound did in the first. The intensities of the reflected sound (the **echo**) and the transmitted sound depend on the incident intensity at the boundary and the impedances of the media on either side of the boundary.

Impedance

Impedance (z) determines how much of an incident sound wave is reflected back into the first medium and how much is transmitted into the second medium. Impedance is equal to the density (ρ) of a medium multiplied by its propagation speed. Impedance units are **rayls**. Impedance increases if density is increased or if propagation speed is increased. Average soft tissue impedance is 1,630,000 rayls.

$$z \, (\text{rayls}) = \rho \, (\text{kg/m}^3) \times c \, (\text{m/s})$$

 If density increases, impedance increases. If propagation speed increases, impedance increases.

Dividing reflected (echo) intensity by the incident intensity yields the fraction of the incident intensity that is reflected. This fraction is called the **intensity reflection coefficient** (IRC). For example, if the incident intensity (I_i) is 10 mW/cm^2 and echo, or reflected, intensity (I_r) is 1 mW/cm^2, the intensity reflection coefficient is one tenth, or 0.1. In this case, one tenth (10%) of the incident sound is reflected. Dividing the transmitted intensity (I_t) by incident intensity yields the fraction of the incident intensity that is transmitted into the second medium. This fraction is called the **intensity transmission coefficient** (ITC). For example, if incident intensity is 10 mW/cm^2 and the transmitted intensity is 9 mW/cm^2, the intensity transmission coefficient is nine tenths, or 0.9. In this case, nine tenths (90%) of the incident sound is transmitted into the second medium. The reflection and transmission coefficients must add up to 1 (i.e., 100%) to account for all the incident sound intensity (what is not reflected at the boundary must be transmitted into the second medium). The two foregoing examples are really the same example, because if 10% of the sound is reflected back into the first medium, then 90% is transmitted into the second medium; that is, all (100%) of the incident sound arriving at the boundary is accounted for.

For perpendicular incidence, the reflection coefficient depends on the impedances as follows:

$$IRC = \frac{I_r \left(W/cm^2 \right)}{I_i \left(W/cm^2 \right)} = \left[\frac{(z_2 - z_1)}{(z_2 + z_1)} \right]^2$$

From this relationship between the reflection coefficient and the impedances, we see that the coefficient depends on the difference between the impedances. The more different the impedances are, the stronger is the echo. The more alike the impedances are, the weaker is the echo. If the media impedances are the same, the difference between them is zero, and there is no echo.

 If the difference between the impedances increases, the intensity reflection coefficient (and echo intensity) increases.

The transmission coefficient depends on the reflection coefficient as follows:

$$ITC = \frac{I_t \left(W/cm^2 \right)}{I_i \left(W/cm^2 \right)} = 1 - IRC$$

Because the coefficients must add up to 1 (100%), larger reflection coefficients mean smaller transmission coefficients, and vice versa. As you would expect, if more of the incident sound is reflected (stronger echo), less remains to travel into the second medium.

 If intensity reflection coefficient increases, the intensity transmission coefficient decreases.

If the impedances are equal, there is no echo, and the transmitted intensity is equal to incident intensity. This is what we expect: if no sound is reflected at a boundary, then all of it travels into the second medium as if there were no boundary. Conversely, we can conclude that if there is no reflection, the media impedances must be equal. If the impedances are equal, then there is no echo, and the transmitted intensity equals the incident intensity.

For perpendicular incidence and equal impedances, there is no reflection, and transmitted intensity equals the incident intensity. If there is a large difference between the impedances, there will be nearly total reflection (an intensity reflection coefficient close to 1, and an intensity transmission coefficient close to 0). An example of this is an air–soft tissue boundary. For this reason, a gel **coupling medium** is used to provide a good sound path from the transducer to the skin (eliminating the thin layer of air that would reflect the sound, preventing entrance of the sound into the body).

Example 2-5
For impedances of 40 and 60 rayls, determine the intensity reflection and transmission coefficients.

$$IRC = \left[\frac{(60-40)}{(60+40)} \right]^2 = \left(\frac{20}{100} \right)^2 = 0.2^2 = 0.2 \times 0.2 = 0.04$$

$$ITC = 1 - 0.04 = 0.96$$

In Example 2-5, the intensity reflection coefficient can be expressed as 4%, and the intensity transmission coefficient as 96%. The sum of the two coefficients is 100%, underscoring the fact that all of the incident intensity must be reflected or transmitted.

If the incident intensity is known, the reflected and transmitted intensities can be calculated by multiplying the incident intensity by the intensity reflection coefficient and the intensity transmission coefficient, respectively.

Example 2-6
For Example 2-5, if the incident intensity is 10 mW/cm², calculate the reflected and transmitted intensities.

From Example 2-5, the intensity reflection and transmission coefficients are 0.04 and 0.96, respectively, so

$$I_r = 10 \times 0.04 = 0.4 \, mW/cm^2$$

$$I_t = 10 \times 0.96 = 9.6 \, mW/cm^2$$

The coefficients give the fractions of the incident intensity that are reflected and transmitted. By multiplying the coefficients by 100, these fractions are expressed in percentages. They must always add up to 1 (or 100%). In Example 2-5, all of the incident intensity is accounted for (0.4 mW/cm² reflected, 9.6 mW/cm² transmitted, for a total of 10 mW/cm², or 100% of the incident intensity).

Oblique Incidence

Oblique incidence denotes a direction of travel of the incident ultrasound that is not perpendicular to the

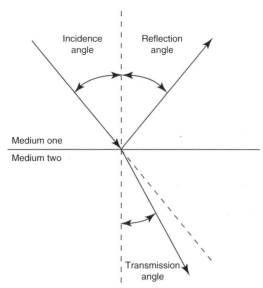

FIGURE 2-18 Reflection and transmission at a boundary with oblique incidence. Incidence and reflection angles are equal. The transmission angle depends on the incidence angle and the media propagation speeds.

boundary between two media (Figure 2-18). This is a common situation in diagnostic ultrasound. The direction of travel with respect to the boundary is given by the **incidence angle** (θ_i) as shown in Figure 2-18. In geometry, angles are measured from a line perpendicular to the surface. For perpendicular incidence, the incidence angle is zero. The reflected and transmitted directions are given by the **reflection angle** (θ_r) and **transmission angle** (θ_t), respectively. The incidence angle always equals the reflection angle.

$$\theta_i \, (degrees) = \theta_r \, (degrees)$$

This phenomenon is observed in optics also (e.g., a laser beam reflecting off a mirror). The transmission angle depends on the propagation speeds in the media. Note that for oblique incidence, the reflected sound does not return to the transducer but travels off in some other direction.

Refraction

If the direction of sound changes as it crosses a boundary, it means that the transmission angle is different from the incidence angle. A change in the direction of sound when it crosses a boundary is called **refraction** (from the Latin term meaning "*to turn aside*"). If the propagation speed through the second medium is greater than through the first medium, then the transmission angle is greater than the incidence angle (Figure 2-19).

$$\text{If } c_1 < c_2, \text{ then } \theta_i < \theta_t. \text{ If } c_1 > c_2, \text{ then } \theta_i > \theta_t$$

The changes are approximately proportional. For example, if the speed increases by 1% as the sound enters the second medium, the transmission angle will be about 1% greater than the incidence angle. Similarly, if the

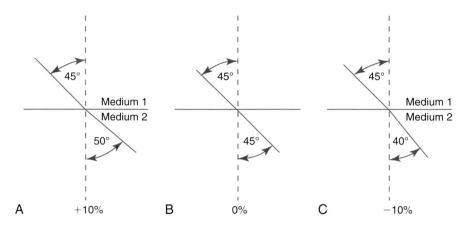

FIGURE 2-19 Transmission angles for an incidence angle of 45 degrees and propagation speeds through medium 2 that are 10% greater than **(A)**, equal to **(B)**, and 10% less than **(C)** propagation speed through medium 1.

speed in the second medium is less than in the first, the transmission angle is less than the incidence angle. No refraction occurs if the propagation speeds are equal. Also, if the incidence angle is zero (perpendicular incidence), there is no refraction, even though there may be different propagation speeds in the media. Thus the two requirements for refraction to occur are as follows:

1. Oblique incidence
2. Different propagation speed on either side of the boundary

Refraction is important because when it occurs, lateral position errors (refraction artifacts) occur on an image.

Example 2-7

If the incidence angle is 20 degrees, the propagation speed in the first medium is 1.7 mm/μs, and the propagation speed in the second medium is 1.6 mm/μs, what are the reflection and transmission angles? The incidence and reflection angles are always equal, so the reflection angle is 20 degrees.

The ratio of the media speeds is 1.6/1.7, which is equal to 0.94. This means that there is a 6% reduction in speed when the sound crosses the boundary. Because the speed decreases by 6%, the transmission angle is 6% less than the incidence angle, that is, 94% of the incidence angle ($0.94 \times 20 = 19$ degrees).

Refraction occurs with light, sound, and any other type of wave. It is the principle on which lenses operate. Refraction is also the cause of the distorted view of objects seen in a fish bowl or swimming pool. As with sound, when light crosses a boundary obliquely and a change in the speed of the light occurs, the direction of the light changes.

Scattering

The discussion thus far has assumed that a boundary is flat and smooth. The resulting reflections are called **specular** (from the Latin term meaning *"mirror-like"*)

reflections. If, however, the size of the reflecting object is comparable with that of the wavelength or smaller, or if a larger object does not have a smooth surface, the incident sound will be scattered. Scattering is the redirection of sound in many directions by rough surfaces or by heterogeneous media (Figure 2-20), such as (cellular) tissues, or particle suspensions, such as blood. These cases are analogous to light in which **specular reflections** occur at mirrors. But with rougher surfaces such as a white wall, light is scattered at the surface and mixed up as it travels back to the viewer's eyes. Therefore an observer does not see his or her reflected image when facing a wall. When light passes through fog, which is a suspension of water droplets in air, it is scattered as well. This limits the viewer's ability to see through fog. Although scattering inhibits vision (we cannot see ourselves reflected in a wall, and we cannot see well through fog), it is of great benefit in sonographic imaging. The reason is that with ultrasound, the goal is to see the "wall" (tissue interface) itself, not the reflection of "oneself" (the transducer in this case). The sonographer also desires to see the "fog" (tissue parenchyma) itself, not just the objects beyond it.

Backscatter (sound scattered back in the direction from which it originally came) intensities from rough surfaces and heterogeneous media vary with frequency and **scatterer** size. Normally, scatter intensities are less than boundary specular-reflection intensities, and they increase with increasing frequency. The intensity received by the sound source from specular reflections is highly angle dependent. Scattering from boundaries helps make echo reception less dependent on incidence angle. Unlike the reflection from specular boundaries, scattering permits ultrasound imaging of tissue boundaries that are not necessarily perpendicular to the direction of the incident sound (Figure 2-21, *A-B*). Scattering also allows imaging of tissue parenchyma (Figure 2-21, *C*) in addition to organ boundaries. Scattering is relatively independent of the direction of the incident sound and therefore is more characteristic of the scatterers. Most surfaces in the body are rough for imaging purposes. Reflections from smooth boundaries (e.g., vessel intima)

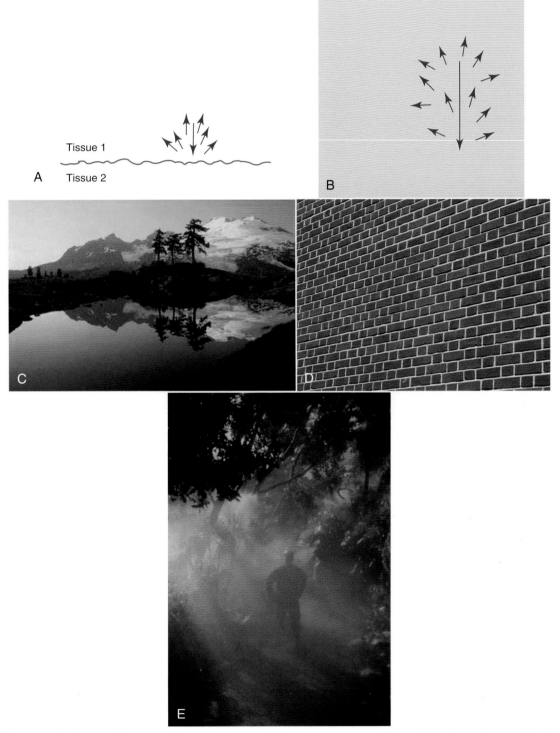

FIGURE 2-20 A sound pulse may be scattered by a rough boundary between tissues **(A)** or within tissues due to their heterogeneous character **(B).** The differences between a specular surface (smooth lake) **(C),** a scattering surface (brick wall) **(D),** and a scattering medium (fog) **(E)** are illustrated.

depend not only on the acoustic properties at the boundaries but also on the angles involved.

Speckle

An ultrasound pulse, with its finite length and width, simultaneously encounters many scatterers at any instant

in its travel. Thus several echoes are generated simultaneously within the pulse as it interacts with these scatterers. The echoes may arrive at the transducer in such a way that they reinforce (**constructive interference**) or partially or totally cancel (**destructive interference**) each other (Figure 2-22, *A-B*). As the ultrasound beam is scanned through the tissues, with scatterers moving into and out

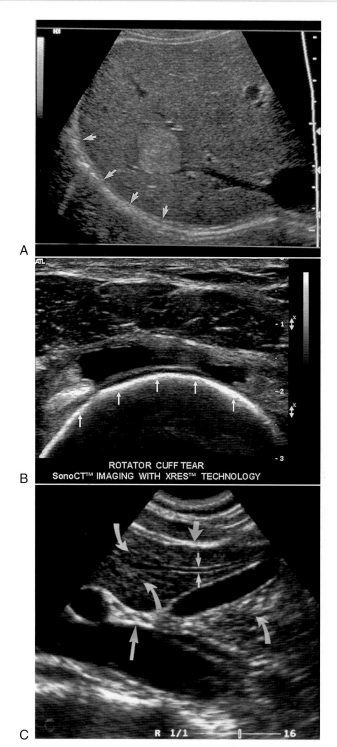

A

B   ROTATOR CUFF TEAR
SonoCT™ IMAGING WITH XRES™ TECHNOLOGY

C   R 1/1   16

FIGURE 2-21 **A,** Longitudinal abdominal scan in which the diaphragm is imaged, even where it is not *(arrows)* perpendicular to the beam and scan lines. **B,** Strong echoes *(arrows)* from a tissue boundary. **C,** Abdominal scan showing echoes from tissue boundaries *(straight arrows)* and regions of scattering from within tissues *(curved arrows),* allowing parenchymal imaging.

of the beam, the **interference** alternates between being constructive and being destructive, resulting in a displayed dot pattern—a grainy appearance—that does not directly represent scatterers but rather represents the interference pattern of the scatterer distribution scanned.

This phenomenon is called acoustic **speckle** and is similar to the speckle observed with lasers. Speckle is a form of acoustic noise in sonographic imaging (Figure 2-22, C).

Contrast Agents

Liquid suspensions that can be injected into the circulation intravenously to increase echogenicity have been developed. These materials are called ultrasound **contrast agents**.[1,2] Contrast agents must be capable of easy administration, nontoxic and stable for a sufficient examination time, small enough to pass through capillaries, and large enough and echogenic enough to improve sonography through an alteration in ultrasound–tissue interaction. Almost all agents contain microbubbles of gas that are stabilized by a protein, lipid, or polymer shell (although free gas microbubbles and solid particle suspensions have been used). These agents enhance echogenicity from vessels and perfused tissues in gray-scale sonography and Doppler ultrasound and "opacify" (fill normally anechoic regions with echoes) cardiac chambers (Figure 2-23). Contrast agents produce echoes because of the impedance mismatch between the suspended particles and the suspending medium (i.e., blood). Microbubbles in suspension are especially strong echo producers because the impedance of the gas is so much less than that of the suspending liquid. Bubbles also expand and contract unequally— that is, nonlinearly—under the influence of an ultrasound pulse. This means that echoes that contain harmonics of the incident pulse frequency are produced. Because bubbles generate stronger harmonics than does tissue, detecting harmonic frequency echoes increases the contrast between the contrast agent and the surrounding tissue. This is called *contrast harmonic imaging* or *harmonic contrast imaging*. Encapsulation of the gas slows its diffusion back into the solution, lengthening the duration of the contrast effect. To further slow diffusion out of an encapsulated bubble, low-solubility gases such as perfluorocarbons are used. Three agents are currently approved for clinical cardiac use (left ventricular opacification and endocardial border detection) in the United States: (1) Definity (octafluoropropane-containing liposomes), (2) Imagent (dimyristoyl lecithin), and (3) Optison (perfluoropropane-filled albumin). In addition to these, other agents—such as Sonazoid, Levovist, and SonoVue—are approved for use in Canada, Europe, and Japan. Contrast agents improve (1) lesion detection when lesion echogenicity is similar to that of the surrounding tissue, (2) lesion characterization by showing both the arterial and portal phases of the agent in real time, and (3) Doppler ultrasound detection when Doppler signals are weak (deep, slow, and small-vessel flows), often rescuing an otherwise failed examination. Ultrasound pulses of sufficiently high pressure-amplitude can fragment the bubbles, allowing the gas to dissolve and eliminating the contrast effect. Subsequent

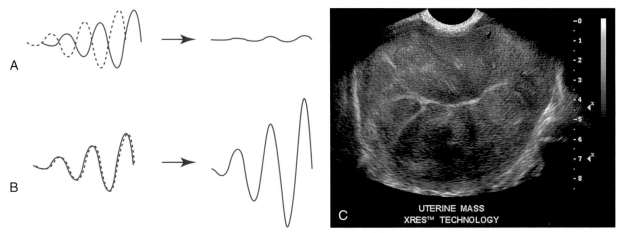

FIGURE 2-22 A, Two similar echoes with slightly different arrival times sum to a nearly zero amplitude (destructive interference). **B,** Two similar echoes arriving nearly simultaneously sum to nearly double amplitude (constructive interference). **C,** Speckle, the grainy appearance of the tissues, is seen in this image.

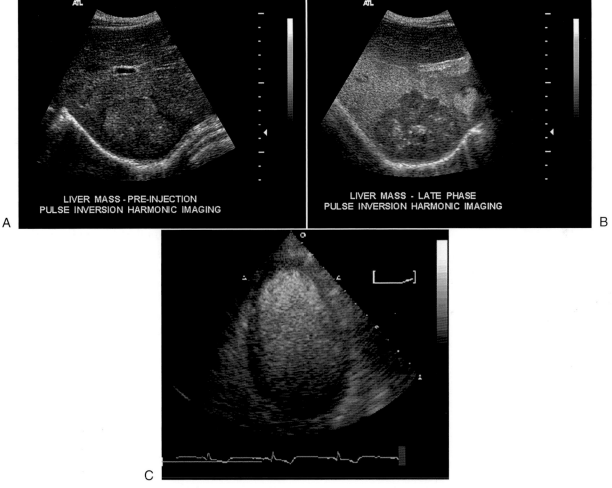

FIGURE 2-23 Contrast agents enhance echogenicity from perfused tissues. Liver mass before **(A)** and after **(B)** injection of contrast agent. The agent has perfused the normal tissue better than the mass, yielding an improved contrast difference between them. **C,** Left ventricular opacification with a contrast agent.

lower-amplitude imaging then can show the return of the contrast effect, thus giving an indication of tissue or organ perfusion rate.

Range

Now that sound propagation, reflection, and scattering have been considered, we can discuss an important aspect of sonography: the determination of the distance (range) from the transducer to an echo-generating structure and thus the appropriate location for each echo's placement on its scan line. To position the echoes properly on the display, two items of information are required:

1. The direction from which the echo came (which is assumed to be the direction in which the emitted pulse is launched)
2. The distance to the **reflector** or scatterer where the echo was produced

With regard to point 2 above, the instrument cannot measure distance directly; rather, it measures travel time and determines the distance from it. Similarly, directly measuring the distance between two cities would be inconvenient (a long measuring tape would be required), but we could determine the distance by asking someone to drive from one city to the other and observe the time required. Of course, we would not know when the person arrived at the other city if we were not riding along, so we would instruct the driver to return immediately after arriving at the destination (Figure 2-24) to give us that information. Let us say that the round trip took exactly 4 hours. What was the distance traveled? We, of course, cannot determine the answer unless we

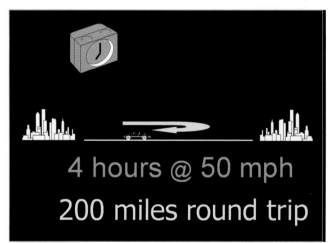

FIGURE 2-24 The distance between two cities can be determined by driving from one city to the other and returning. Multiplying the speed of travel by one half the round-trip travel time yields the distance between the cities. If the speed is 50 mph and the round-trip travel time is 4 hours, the distance between the cities is 100 miles. In this example, the round-trip distance traveled is 200 miles, obtained by multiplying the speed (50 mph) by the elapsed travel time (4 hours).

know the speed traveled. If the driver was traveling at a speed of exactly 50 mph for the entire round trip (a difficult achievement), then we can determine that the distance traveled was 200 miles (50 mph × 4 hours). Therefore the distance to the city is 100 miles. Note that the total distance was halved because round-trip travel time was used to determine the one-way distance.

Thus the distance (d) to a reflector is calculated from the propagation speed and pulse round-trip travel time (t) according to the **range equation**:

$$d\,(mm) = \frac{1}{2}[c\,(mm/\mu s) \times t\,(\mu s)]$$

 As round-trip time increases, calculated reflector distance increases.

To determine the distance from the source to the reflector, the propagation speed in the intervening medium must be known or assumed, and the pulse round-trip time must be measured. The reason that the factor ½ appears is that the round-trip time is the time for the pulse to travel to and return from the reflector. However, only the distance to the reflector is the desired information. The average propagation speed in soft tissue (1.54 mm/μs) is assumed in using the range equation. As multiplying 1.54 by ½ yields 0.77, the distance (millimeters) to the reflector can be calculated by multiplying 0.77 by the round-trip time (microseconds).

In the problem involving determining the distance between cities, 50 mph is equivalent to 0.83 mile/min or 1.20 min/mile. Thus, at this speed, 2.4 minutes of round-trip travel are required for each mile of distance separating the cities. Similarly, sound speed in tissue is 1.54 mm/μs, so 0.65 μs is required for each millimeter of travel; thus 6.5 μs are required for 1 cm of travel. Therefore 13 μs of round-trip travel time are required for each centimeter of distance from the transducer to the reflector. To confirm this, substitution of 13 μs for t in the foregoing range equation yields a reflector distance of 10 mm (1 cm):

$$d = \frac{1}{2}(c \times t) = \frac{1}{2}(1.54 \times 13) = \frac{1}{2}(20) = 10\,mm = 1\,cm$$

All this leads to the important 13 μs/cm rule: the pulse round-trip travel time is 13 μs for each centimeter of distance from source to reflector (Table 2-6; Figure 2-25). Figure 2-26 illustrates the correspondence between echo arrival time and reflector depth.

Example 2-8

If an echo returns 104 μs after a pulse was emitted by a transducer, at what depth is the echo-producing structure located?

1. Using the range equation:

$$d\,(mm) = 0.77\,mm/\mu s \times 104\,\mu s = 80\,mm = 8.0\,cm$$

2. Using the 13 µs/cm rule:

$$d(mm) = \frac{104\,\mu s}{13\,\mu s/cm} = 8\,cm$$

Table 2-7 gives common values for several parameters of sonography. Table 2-8 summarizes how various parameters change with frequency.

TABLE 2-6	Pulse Round-Trip Travel Time for Various Reflector Depths
Depth (cm)	**Travel Time (µs)**
0.5	6.5
1	13
2	26
3	39
4	52
5	65
10	130
15	195
20	260

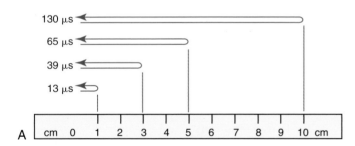

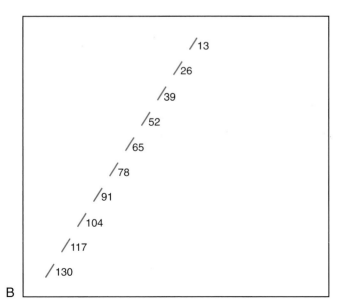

FIGURE 2-25 A, Echo arrival times for 1-, 3-, 5-, and 10-cm reflector distances. **B,** Echoes from 1-, 2-, 3-, 4-, 5-, 6-, 7-, 8-, 9-, and 10-cm depths arrive at the times (microseconds) indicated.

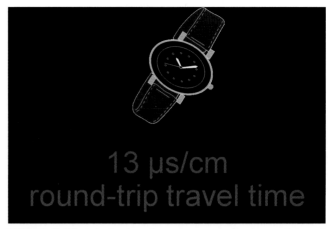

FIGURE 2-26 Substituting the average speed of sound in soft tissues into the range equation yields the 13 µs/cm round-trip travel time rule.

TABLE 2-7	Sonographic Parameters in Tissue	
Symbol or Range of Parameter	**Abbreviation**	**Common Values**
Frequency	f	2–15 MHz
Period	T	0.07–0.5 µs
Wavelength	λ	0.1–0.8 mm
Propagation speed	c	1.44–1.64 mm/µs
Impedance	z	1,300,000–1,700,000 rayls
Pulse repetition frequency	PRF	4–15 kHz
Pulse repetition period	PRP	0.07–0.25 ms
Cycles per pulse	n	1–3
Pulse duration	PD	0.1–1.5 µs
Spatial pulse length	SPL	0.1–2.5 mm
Duty factor	DF	0.1%–1%
Pressure amplitude	p	0.1–4 MPa
Intensity*	I_{SPTA}	0.01–100 mW/cm²
Attenuation coefficient	a_c	1–8 dB/cm

*Spatial-peak, temporal average.

TABLE 2-8	Dependence of Various Factors on Increasing (↑) Frequency	
Symbol or Dependence Parameter	**Abbreviation**	**(↑ Increase; ↓Decrease)**
Period	T	↓
Wavelength	λ	↓
Pulse duration	PD	↓
Spatial pulse length	SPL	↓
Attenuation	a	↑
Penetration	pen	↓

REVIEW

The key points presented in this chapter are the following:

- Sound is a wave of pressure and density variations and particle vibration.
- Ultrasound is sound having a frequency greater than 20 kHz.
- Frequency denotes the number of cycles occurring in a second.
- Harmonic frequencies are generated as sound travels through tissue.
- Wavelength is the length of a cycle in space.
- Propagation speed is the speed of sound through a medium.
- The medium determines propagation speed.
- The average propagation speed of sound through soft tissue is 1.54 mm/μs.
- Pulsed ultrasound is described by pulse repetition frequency (PRF), pulse repetition period, pulse duration, duty factor, and spatial pulse length.
- Amplitude and intensity describe the strength of sound.
- Attenuation is the weakening of sound caused by absorption, reflection, and scattering.
- Attenuation increases with frequency and path length.
- The average attenuation coefficient for soft tissues is 0.5 dB/cm for each megahertz of frequency.
- Imaging depth decreases with increasing frequency.
- Impedance is the density of a medium times propagation speed.
- When sound encounters boundaries between media with different impedances, part of the sound is reflected and part transmitted.
- With perpendicular incidence, and if the two media have the same impedance, there is no reflection.
- The greater the difference in the impedances of the media at a boundary, the greater is the intensity of the echo that is generated at the boundary.
- With oblique incidence, the sound is refracted at a boundary between media for which propagation speeds are different.
- Incidence and reflection angles at a boundary are always equal.
- Scattering occurs at rough media boundaries and within heterogeneous media.
- Contrast agents are used to enhance echogenicity in sonography and Doppler ultrasound.
- Pulse-echo round-trip travel time (13 μs/cm) is used to determine the distance to a reflector.

EXERCISES

1. A wave is a traveling variation in quantities called *wave* _____
   a. *lengths*   c. *cycles*
   b. *variables*   d. *periods*
2. Sound is a traveling variation in quantities called _____ *variables*.
   a. *wave*   c. *density*
   b. *pressure*   d. *acoustic*
3. Ultrasound is sound with a frequency greater than _____ Hz.
   a. 2
   b. 15
   c. 20,000
   d. 1540
4. Acoustic variables include _____, _____, and particle motion.
   a. stiffness, density
   b. hardness, impedance
   c. amplitude, intensity
   d. pressure, density
5. Which of the following frequencies is in the ultrasound range?
   a. 15 Hz
   b. 15,000 Hz
   c. 15 kHz
   d. 30,000 Hz
   e. 0.004 MHz
6. Which of the following is *not* an acoustic variable?
   a. Pressure
   b. Propagation speed
   c. Density
   d. Particle motion
7. Frequency is the number of _____ an acoustic variable goes through in a second.
   a. cycles
   b. amplitudes
   c. pulse lengths
   d. duty factors
8. The unit of frequency is _____, which is abbreviated _____.
   a. hertz, Hz
   b. megahertz, mHz
   c. kilohurts, khts
   d. cycles, cps
9. Period is the _____ that it takes for one cycle to occur.
   a. length
   b. amplitude
   c. time
   d. height
10. Period decreases as _____ increases.
   a. wavelength
   b. pulse length
   c. frequency
   d. bandwidth

11. Wavelength is the length of _____ over which one cycle occurs.
    a. time
    b. space
    c. propagation
    d. power
12. Propagation speed is the speed with which a(n) _____ moves through a medium.
    a. wave
    b. particle
    c. frequency
    d. attenuation
13. Wavelength is equal to _____ _____ divided by _____.
    a. propagation speed, frequency
    b. media density, stiffness
    c. pulse length, frequency
    d. wave amplitude, period
14. The _____ and _____ of a medium determine propagation speed.
    a. amplitude, intensity
    b. wavelength, period
    c. impedance, attenuation
    d. density, stiffness
15. Propagation speed increases if _____ is increased.
    a. amplitude
    b. frequency
    c. density
    d. stiffness
16. The average propagation speed in soft tissues is _____ m/s or _____ mm/μs.
    a. 10, 3
    b. 1540, 1.54
    c. 3, 10
    d. 1.54, 1540
17. Propagation speed is determined by the _____.
    a. frequency
    b. amplitude
    c. wavelength
    d. medium
18. Place the following in order of increasing sound propagation speed:
    a. gas, solid, liquid
    b. solid, liquid, gas
    c. gas, liquid, solid
    d. liquid, solid, gas
19. The wavelength of 7-MHz ultrasound in soft tissues is _____ mm.
    a. 1.54
    b. 0.54
    c. 0.22
    d. 3.33
20. Wavelength in soft tissues _____ as frequency increases.
    a. is constant   c. increases
    b. decreases   d. weakens
21. It takes _____ μs for ultrasound to travel 1.54 cm in soft tissue.
    a. 10
    b. 0.77
    c. 154
    d. 100
22. Propagation speed in bone is _____ that in soft tissues.
    a. lower than
    b. equal to
    c. higher than
    d. 10 m/s greater than
23. Sound travels fastest in _____.
    a. air
    b. helium
    c. water
    d. steel
24. Solids have higher propagation speeds than liquids because they have greater _____.
    a. density
    b. stiffness
    c. attenuation
    d. propagation
25. Sound travels slowest in _____.
    a. gases
    b. liquids
    c. tissue
    d. bone
26. Sound is a _____ _____ wave.
27. If propagation speed is doubled (a different medium) and frequency is held constant, the wavelength is _____.
28. If frequency in soft tissue is doubled, propagation speed is _____.
29. If wavelength is 2 mm and frequency is doubled, the wavelength becomes _____ mm.
30. Waves can carry _____ from one place to another.
31. From given values for propagation speed and frequency, which of the following can be calculated?
    a. Amplitude
    b. Impedance
    c. Wavelength
    d. a and b
    e. b and c
32. If two media have different stiffnesses, the one with the higher stiffness will have the higher propagation speed. True or false?
33. The second harmonic of 3 MHz is _____ MHz.
34. The odd harmonics of 2 MHz are _____ MHz.
    a. 1, 3, 5
    b. 2, 4, 6
    c. 6, 9, 12
    d. 6, 10, 14
    e. 10, 12, 14

35. The even harmonics of 2 MHz are _____ MHz.
    a. 1, 3, 5
    b. 2, 4, 6
    c. 4, 8, 12
    d. 6, 10, 14
    e. 10, 12, 14
36. Nonlinear propagation means that _____.
    a. the sound beam does not travel in a straight line
    b. propagation speed depends on frequency
    c. propagation speed depends on pressure
    d. the waveform changes shape as it travels
    e. more than one of the above
37. As a wave changes from sinusoidal form to saw-tooth form, additional _____ appear that are _____ and _____ multiples of the _____. They are called _____.
38. If the density of a medium is 1000 kg/m^3 and the propagation speed is 1540 m/s, the impedance is _____ rayls.
39. If two media have the same propagation speed but different densities, the one with the higher density will have the higher impedance. True or false?
40. If two media have the same density but different propagation speeds, the one with the higher propagation speed will have the higher impedance. True or false?
41. Impedance is _____ multiplied by _____ _____.
42. The abbreviation CW stands for _____.
43. Pulse repetition frequency is the number of _____ occurring in 1 second.
44. Pulse repetition _____ is the time from the beginning of one pulse to the beginning of the next.
45. Pulse repetition period _____ as pulse repetition frequency increases.
46. Pulse duration is the _____ it takes for a pulse to occur.
47. Spatial pulse length is the _____ of _____ that a pulse occupies as it travels.
48. _____ _____ is the fraction of time that pulsed ultrasound is actually on.
49. Pulse duration equals the number of cycles in the pulse multiplied by _____.
50. Spatial pulse length equals the number of cycles in the pulse multiplied by _____.
51. The duty factor of continuous wave sound is _____.
52. If the wavelength is 2 mm, the spatial pulse length for a three-cycle pulse is _____ mm.
53. The spatial pulse length in soft tissue for a two-cycle pulse of frequency 5 MHz is _____ mm.
54. The pulse duration in soft tissue for a two-cycle pulse of frequency 5 MHz is _____ μs.

55. For a 1-kHz pulse repetition frequency, the pulse repetition period is _____ ms.
56. For Exercises 54 and 55 together, the duty factor is _____.
57. How many cycles are there in 1 second of continuous wave 5-MHz ultrasound?
    a. 5
    b. 500
    c. 5000
    d. 5,000,000
    e. None of the above
58. How many cycles are there in 1 second of pulsed 5-MHz ultrasound with a duty factor of 0.01 (1%)?
    a. 5
    b. 500
    c. 5000
    d. 5,000,000
    e. None of the above
59. In Exercise 58, how many cycles did pulsing eliminate?
    a. 100%
    b. 99.9%
    c. 99%
    d. 50%
    e. 1%
60. For pulsed ultrasound, the duty factor is always _____ _____ one.
61. _____ is a typical duty factor for sonography.
    a. 0.1
    b. 0.5
    c. 0.7
    d. 0.9
62. Amplitude is the maximum _____ that occurs in an acoustic variable.
63. Intensity is the _____ in a wave divided by _____.
64. The unit for intensity is _____.
65. Intensity is proportional to _____ squared.
66. If power is doubled and area remains unchanged, intensity is _____.
67. If area is doubled and power remains unchanged, intensity is _____.
68. If both power and area are doubled, intensity is _____.
69. If amplitude is doubled, intensity is _____.
70. If a sound beam has a power of 10 mW and a beam area of 2 cm^2, the spatial average intensity is _____ mW/cm^2.
71. Attenuation is the reduction in _____ and _____ as a wave travels through a medium.
72. Attenuation consists of _____, _____, and _____.
73. The attenuation coefficient is attenuation per _____ of sound travel.

74. Attenuation and the attenuation coefficient are given in units of _____ and _____, respectively.

75. For soft tissues, there is approximately _____ dB of attenuation per centimeter for each megahertz of frequency.

76. For soft tissues, the attenuation coefficient at 3 MHz is approximately _____.

77. The attenuation coefficient in soft tissue _____ as frequency increases.

78. For soft tissue, if frequency is doubled, attenuation is _____. If path length is doubled, attenuation is _____. If both frequency and path length are doubled, attenuation is _____.

79. If frequency is doubled and path length is halved, attenuation is _____.

80. Absorption is the conversion of _____ to _____.

81. Can absorption be greater than attenuation in a given medium at a given frequency?

82. Is attenuation in bone higher or lower than in soft tissue?

83. The imaging depth (penetration) _____ as frequency increases.

84. If the intensity of 4-MHz ultrasound entering soft tissue is 2 W/cm^2, the intensity at a depth of 4 cm is _____ W/cm^2.

85. If the intensity of 40-MHz ultrasound entering soft tissue is 2 W/cm^2, the intensity at a depth of 4 cm is _____ W/cm^2.

86. The depth at which half-intensity occurs in soft tissues at 7.5 MHz is _____.
    a. 0.6 cm
    b. 0.7 cm
    c. 0.8 cm
    d. 0.9 cm
    e. 1.0 cm

87. When ultrasound encounters a boundary with perpendicular incidence, the _____ of the tissues must be different to produce a reflection (echo).

88. With perpendicular incidence, two media _____ and the incident _____ must be known to calculate the reflected intensity.

89. With perpendicular incidence, two media _____ must be known to calculate the intensity reflection coefficient.

90. For an incident intensity of 2 mW/cm^2 and impedances of 49 and 51 rayls, the reflected intensity is _____ mW/cm^2, and the transmitted intensity is _____ mW/cm^2.

91. If the impedances of the media are equal, there is no reflection. True or false?

92. With perpendicular incidence, the reflected intensity depends on the _____.
    a. density difference
    b. impedance difference
    c. impedance sum
    d. b and c
    e. a and b

93. Refraction is a change in _____ of sound when it crosses a boundary. Refraction is caused by a change in _____ _____ at the boundary.

94. Under what two conditions does refraction *not* occur?
    a. _____
    b. _____

95. The low speed of sound in fat is a source of image degradation because of refraction. If the incidence angle at a boundary between fat (1.45 mm/μs) and kidney (1.56 mm/μs) is 30 degrees, the transmission angle is _____ degrees.

96. Redirection of sound in many directions as it encounters rough media junctions or particle suspensions (heterogeneous media) is called _____.

97. Backscatter helps make echo reception less dependent on incident angle. True or false?

98. What must be known to calculate the distance to a reflector?
    a. Attenuation, speed, and density
    b. Attenuation and impedance
    c. Attenuation and absorption
    d. Travel time and speed
    e. Density and speed

99. No reflection will occur with perpendicular incidence if the media _____ are equal.

100. Scattering occurs at smooth boundaries and within homogeneous media. True or false?

3

Transducers

LEARNING OBJECTIVES

After reading this chapter, the student should be able to do the following:
- Describe the construction of a transducer and the function of each part
- Explain how a transducer generates ultrasound pulses
- Explain how a transducer receives echoes
- Describe a sound beam and list the factors that affect it
- Discuss how sound beams are focused and automatically scanned through anatomy
- Compare linear, convex, phased, and vector arrays
- Define detail resolution
- Differentiate between three aspects of detail resolution
- List the factors that determine detail resolution

OUTLINE

Construction and Operation
  Piezoelectric Element
  Damping Material
  Matching Layer
  Coupling Medium
  Invasive Transducers
Beams and Focusing
  Near and Far Zones
  Focusing

Automatic Scanning
  Linear Array
  Convex Array
  Phased Array
  Electronic Focus
  Variable Aperture
  Section Thickness Focus
  Grating Lobes
  Vector Array

Reception Steering, Focus, and
  Aperture
Detail Resolution
  Axial Resolution
  Lateral Resolution
  Useful Frequency Range
Review
Exercises

KEY TERMS

Aperture
Apodization
Array
Axial
Axial resolution
Beam
Composite
Convex array
Crystal
Curie point
Damping
Detail resolution
Disk
Dynamic aperture
Dynamic focusing
Element
Elevational resolution

Far zone
Focal length
Focal region
Focal zone
Focus
Grating lobes
Lateral
Lateral resolution
Lead zirconate titanate
Lens
Linear
Linear array
Linear phased array
Linear sequenced array
Matching layer
Natural focus
Near zone

Operating frequency
Phased array
Phased linear array
Piezoelectricity
Probe
Resolution
Resonance frequency
Scanhead
Sector
Sensitivity
Side lobes
Sound beam
Source
Transducer
Transducer assembly
Ultrasound transducer
Vector array

This chapter describes transducers, the devices that generate and receive ultrasound. Transducers form the connecting link between the ultrasound–tissue interactions described in Chapter 2 and the instruments described in Chapters 4 and 5. The sound produced by these transducers is confined in beams rather than traveling in all directions away from the **source**. These beams are focused and are automatically scanned through tissue by the transducers.

CONSTRUCTION AND OPERATION

A **transducer** converts one form of energy to another. **Ultrasound transducers** (Figure 3-1) convert electric energy into ultrasound energy, and vice versa. The electric voltages applied to transducers are converted to ultrasound. Ultrasound echoes incident on the transducers produce electric voltages. Loudspeakers (Figure 3-2, A), microphones (Figure 3-2, B), and intercoms accomplish similar functions with audible sound.

Some transducers include internally some parts of the electronics that are otherwise located in the instrument.

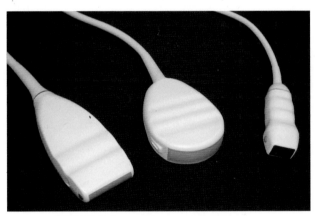

FIGURE 3-1 Transducers of various types.

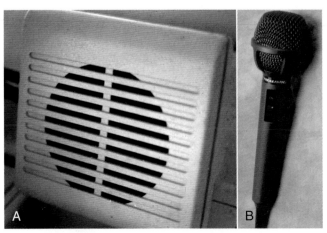

FIGURE 3-2 A, Loudspeaker. **B,** Microphone.

Piezoelectric Element

Ultrasound transducers operate according to the principle of **piezoelectricity**. The word *piezoelectricity* is derived from the Greek *piezo*, meaning "to press," and *elektron*, meaning "amber," the organic plant resin that was used in early studies of electricity. This principle states that some materials, when deformed by an applied pressure, produce a voltage. Conversely, piezoelectricity also results in the production of a pressure when an applied voltage deforms these materials. Various formulations of **lead zirconate titanate** are used commonly as materials in the production of modern ultrasound transducer elements. Ceramics such as these are not naturally piezoelectric. They are made piezoelectric during their manufacture by being placed in a strong electric field while they are at a high temperature. If a critical temperature (the **Curie point**) subsequently is exceeded, the **element** will lose its piezoelectric properties. These ceramics often are combined with a nonpiezoelectric polymer to create materials that are called piezocomposites. These **composites** have lower impedance and improved bandwidth, **sensitivity**, and **resolution**.

 Piezoelectric elements convert electric voltages into ultrasound pulses and convert returning echoes back into voltages.

Single-element transducers take the form of **disks** (Figure 3-3, A). **Linear array** transducers contain numerous elements that have a rectangular shape (Figure 3-3, B). When an electric voltage is applied to the faces of either type, the thickness of the element increases or decreases, depending on the polarity of the voltage (Figure 3-3, C). The term *transducer element* (also called *piezoelectric element*, *active element*, or **crystal**) refers to the piece of piezoelectric material (Figure 3-3, D) that converts electricity to ultrasound, and vice versa. Elements, with their associated case and **damping** and matching materials (Figure 3-3, E), are called **transducer assembly**, **probe**, **scanhead** or, simply, *transducer*.

Transducers typically are driven by one cycle of alternating voltage for sonographic imaging. This single-cycle–driving voltage produces a two- or three-cycle ultrasound pulse. Longer-driving voltages, typically 5 to 30 cycles, are used for Doppler techniques. This operation produces an alternating pressure that propagates from the transducer as a sound pulse (Figure 3-4, A). The frequency of the sound produced is equal to the frequency of the driving voltage, which must be reasonably near the **operating frequency** (f_o) of the transducer for operation with acceptable efficiency. The operating frequency (sometimes called **resonance frequency**) is the preferred, or natural, frequency of operation for the element. Operating frequency is determined by the following:

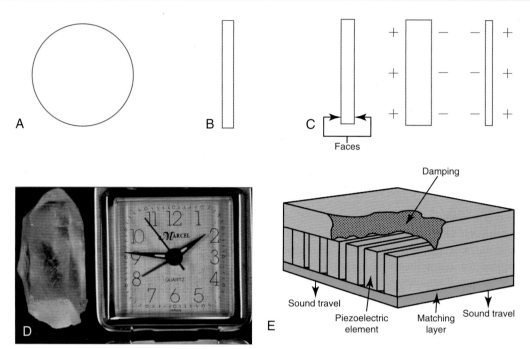

FIGURE 3-3 A, Front view of a disk transducer element. **B,** Front view of a rectangular element. **C,** Side view of either element with no voltage applied to faces (normal thickness), with voltage applied (increased thickness), and with opposite voltage applied (decreased thickness). **D,** Thin slices of quartz crystals *(on left)* are used in electric clocks, watches, and other devices. **E,** The internal parts of a transducer assembly (scanhead or probe). The damping (backing) material reduces pulse duration, thus improving axial resolution. The matching layer improves sound transmission into the tissues. Not included in this illustration are a lens and a protective/insulating layer that commonly are attached to the front of the assembly.

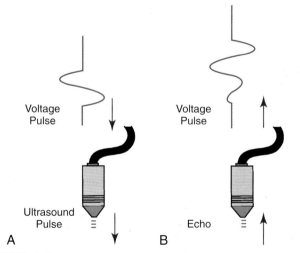

FIGURE 3-4 A transducer converts electric voltage pulses into ultrasound pulses **(A)** and converts received echoes into electric voltage pulses **(B).**

TABLE 3-1	Transducer Element Thickness* for Various Operating Frequencies
Frequency (MHz)	**Thickness (mm)**
2.0	1.0
3.5	0.6
5.0	0.4
7.5	0.3
10.0	0.2

*Assuming an element propagation speed of 4 mm/µs.

producing higher-pitched sounds (Figure 3-5, *C*). The transducer converts the returning echo into an alternating voltage pulse (Figure 3-4, *B*).

$$f_0 (MHz) = \frac{c_t \, (mm/\mu s)}{2 \times th \, (mm)}$$

 Thinner elements operate at higher frequencies.

- The propagation speed of the element material (c_t)
- The thickness (th) of the transducer element

Operating frequency is such that the thickness of the element corresponds to half a wavelength in the element material. Typical diagnostic ultrasound elements are 0.2 to 1 mm thick (Table 3-1) and have propagation speeds of 4 to 6 mm/µs. Because wavelength decreases as frequency increases, thinner elements yield higher frequencies (Figure 3-5). This is analogous to smaller bells

With wide-bandwidth transducers (e.g., those having a fractional bandwidth of at least 70%), voltage excitation can be used selectively to operate the same transducer at more than one frequency (Figure 3-6). The transducer is driven at one of two or three selectable frequencies by voltage pulses with the selected frequency. The two or three frequencies must fall within

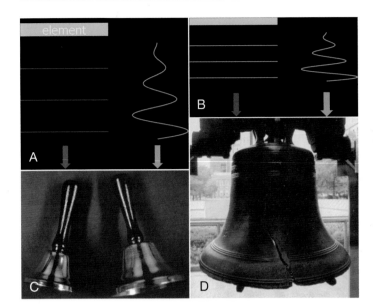

FIGURE 3-5 A, Thicker elements operate at lower frequencies. **B,** Thinner elements operate at higher frequencies. **C-D,** Smaller and larger bells ring with higher and lower pitches, respectively.

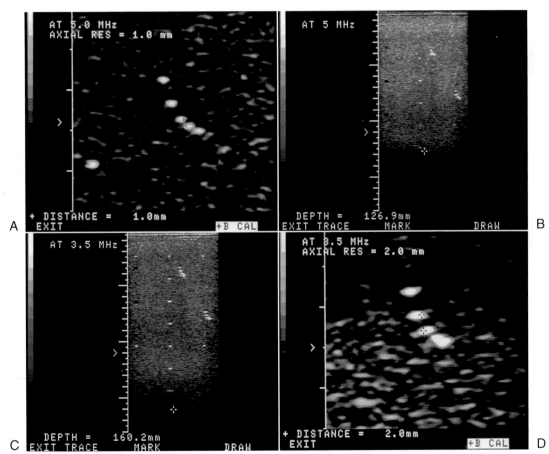

FIGURE 3-6 Multihertz operation allows the transducer to provide (at a higher frequency) selectively better detail resolution **(A)** with reduced penetration **(B)** or (at a lower frequency) deeper penetration **(C)** with some degradation of resolution **(D).**

the transducer bandwidth. Choosing the higher frequency yields better **detail resolution**. If the resulting penetration is not sufficient for the study at hand, however, a lower frequency can be selected (resulting in some degradation in resolution). Push-button frequency switching is quicker, more convenient, and more cost effective than changing of transducers. Wide bandwidth also allows harmonic imaging, where echoes of twice the frequency sent into the body are received to improve the image.

Damping Material

Pulse repetition frequency is equal to the voltage pulse repetition frequency. This is the number of voltage pulses sent to the transducer each second, which is determined by the instrument driving the transducer. Pulse duration is equal to period multiplied by number of cycles in the pulse. Damping (also called *backing*) material, a mixture of metal powder and a plastic or epoxy resin, is attached

to the rear face of the transducer elements to reduce the number of cycles in each pulse (Figures 3-3, *E*, and 3-7). Damping reduces pulse duration and spatial pulse length and improves resolution. This method of damping is analogous to packing foam rubber around a bell that is rung by a tap with a hammer. The rubber reduces the time that the bell rings following the tap. The rubber also reduces the loudness of the ringing. In the case of ultrasound transducers, the damping material additionally reduces the ultrasound amplitude and thus decreases the efficiency and sensitivity (ability to detect weak echoes) of the system (an undesired effect). This is the price paid for reduced spatial pulse length (a desired effect resulting in improved resolution) with damping. Typically, pulses of two to three cycles are generated with (damped) diagnostic ultrasound transducers. Shortening the pulses broadens their bandwidth. Typical bandwidths for modern transducers range from 50% to 100%. An example of a 100% bandwidth is a 5-MHz operating frequency with a bandwidth of 5 MHz, that is, from 2.5 to 7.5 MHz.

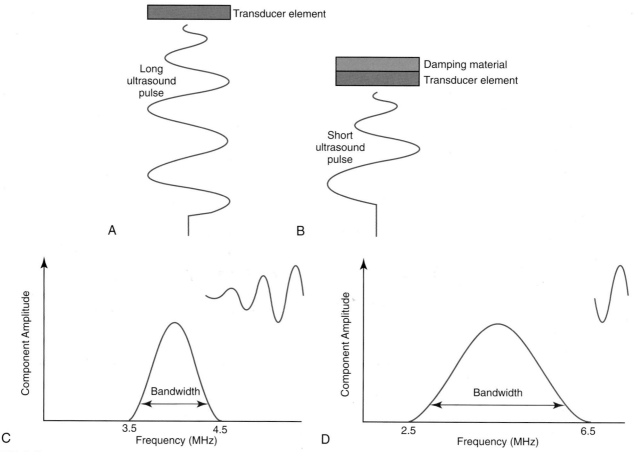

FIGURE 3-7 A, Without damping, a transducer element produces a long ultrasound pulse of many cycles. **B,** With damping material on the rear face of the transducer element, a short ultrasound pulse of a few cycles is produced. This figure shows each pulse traveling (down) away from the transducer in space so that the bottom end is the beginning or leading edge of the pulse as it travels down. **C-D,** Plots of the frequencies present in the ultrasound pulses (from **A** and **B,** respectively). Component amplitude is the amplitude of each frequency component present. Bandwidth is the frequency range within which the amplitudes exceed some reference value. Compare the frequency spectrum for a narrowband, undamped pulse **(C)** with the frequency spectrum for a broadband, damped pulse **(D).**

Composites and damping material shorten pulses and improve resolution.

 Transducers intended for continuous wave Doppler ultrasound use are not damped because pulses are not used in this application. These transducers have higher efficiencies because energy is not lost to damping material.

Matching Layers

Because the transducer element is a solid (having high density and sound speed), it has an impedance that is about 20 times that of tissues. Without compensation, this factor would cause about 80% of the emitted intensity to be reflected at the skin boundary. Thus most of the sound energy would not enter the body. A returning echo also would have about 80% of its intensity reflected, so only a small portion would enter the transducer. Therefore, the received echo intensity for a perfect (100%) reflector would be only 4% ($0.2 \times 1.00 \times 0.2$) because only about 20% of the intensity enters and only about 20% of the echo intensity exits the body. To solve this problem, a **matching layer** is usually placed on the transducer face (Figure 3-3, *E*). This material has an impedance of some intermediate value between those of the transducer element and the tissue. The material reduces the reflection of ultrasound at the transducer element surface, thereby improving sound transmission across it. This is analogous to the coating on eyeglasses or camera lenses that reduces light reflection at the air–glass boundary. Many frequencies (the bandwidth) and wavelengths are present in short ultrasound pulses. Thus multiple matching layers improve sound transmission across the element–tissue boundary better than does a single layer. Typically, two layers are used, although in some cases, one or three layers are used. The lower impedance of piezocomposite elements assists in the impedance-matching process, allowing more of the ultrasound energy to exit the front of the element into the patient rather than being lost as heat in the damping material.

Coupling Medium

Because of its very low impedance, even a very thin layer of air between the transducer and the skin surface reflects virtually all the sound, preventing any penetration into the tissue. For this reason, a coupling medium, usually an aqueous gel (Figure 3-8), is applied to the skin before transducer contact. This eliminates the air layer and facilitates the passage of sound into and out of the tissue. Thus the combination of matching layers with the coupling medium enables the efficient passage of ultrasound into the body and the return of echoes from the body into the transducer.

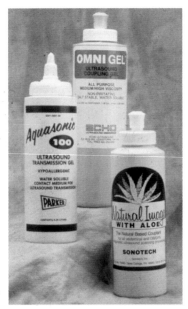

FIGURE 3-8 Coupling gel improves sound transmission into and out of the patient by eliminating air reflection.

 Matching layers and coupling media facilitate the passage of ultrasound across the transducer–skin boundary.

Invasive Transducers

Some transducers are designed to enter the body (Figure 3-9) via the vagina, rectum, esophagus, or a blood vessel (catheter-mounted type). These approaches allow the transducer to be placed closer to the anatomy of interest, thus avoiding intervening tissues (e.g., lung or gassy bowel) and reducing the sound transmission path length. This reduction in path length, which yields lower attenuation, allows higher frequencies to be used and improves resolution.

BEAMS AND FOCUSING

A continuous wave ultrasound **beam** is filled with ultrasound similarly to a flashlight beam being filled with light. A pulsed beam is not. What is meant by "the beam," then, in the case of pulsed ultrasound? The term *beam* refers to the width of a pulse as it travels away from the transducer. Generally, the width in the scan plane is not the same as the width perpendicular to the scan plane. The width in the scan plane determines the **lateral resolution**, whereas the width perpendicular to the scan plane determines the extent of the section thickness artifact.

A single-element disk transducer operating in continuous wave mode provides a simple approximation to beams produced by sonographic transducers. The transducer produces a **sound beam** with a width that varies according to the distance from the transducer face, as

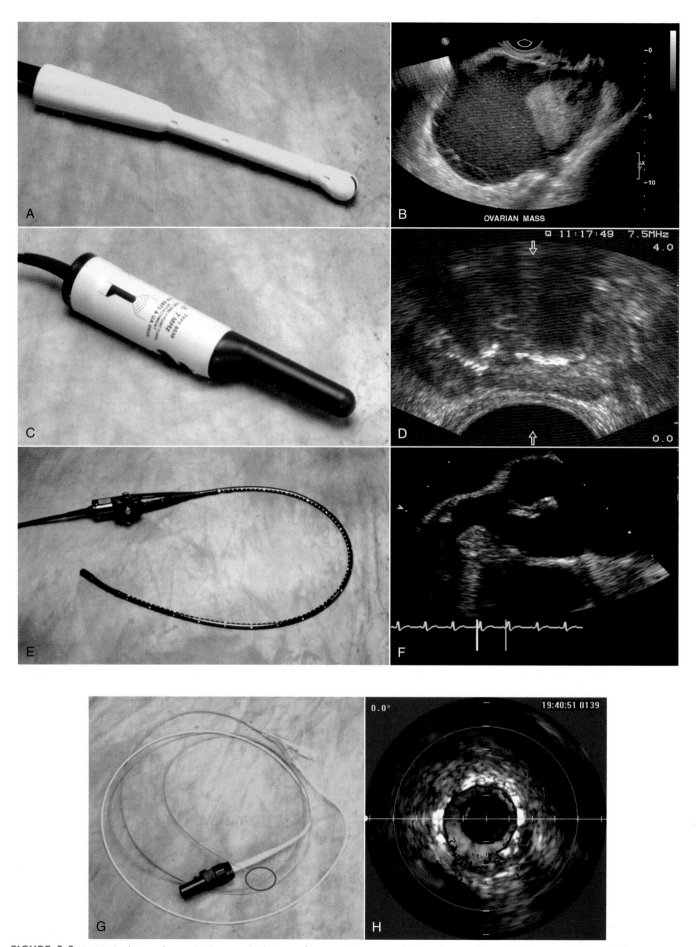

FIGURE 3-9 A, Vaginal transducer. **B,** Transvaginal view of an ovarian mass. **C,** Rectal transducer. **D,** Transrectal view of the prostate. **E,** Transesophageal probe for echocardiography. **F,** Transesophageal view of the adult heart. **G,** Catheter-mounted transducer *(circle)* for viewing the interior of a blood vessel. **H,** Interior view of a blood vessel.

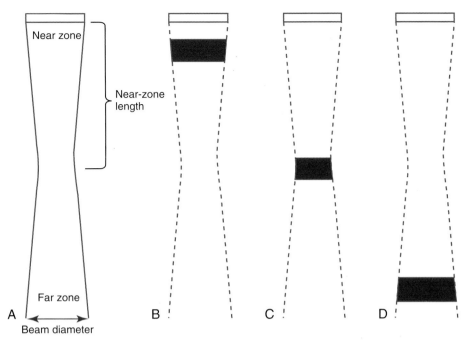

FIGURE 3-10 A, Beam width for a single-element unfocused disk transducer operating in continuous wave mode. The near zone is the region between the disk and the minimum beam width. The far zone is the region beyond the minimum beam width. Intensity varies within the beam, with variations being greatest in the near zone. This beam approximates the changing pulse diameter as an ultrasound pulse travels away from a transducer. **B,** An ultrasound pulse shortly after leaving the transducer. **C,** Later, the ultrasound pulse is located at the end of the near-zone length, where its width is at a minimum. **D,** Still later, the pulse is in the far zone, where its width is increasing as it travels.

shown in Figure 3-10. The intensity is not uniform throughout the beam, but the beam shown includes nearly all the power in the beam. Sometimes, significant intensity travels out in some directions not included in this beam. These additional beams are called side lobes. They are a source of artifacts.

Near and Far Zones

The region extending from the element to a distance of one near-zone length is called the near zone, *near field,* or Fresnel zone. The beam width decreases with increasing distance from the transducer in the near zone. Near-zone length (NZL; also called *near-field length*) is determined by the size and operating frequency of the element. Near-zone length increases with increasing frequency or element size, which is also called *aperture* (ap).

 An ultrasound beam consists of near and far zones.

 If aperture increases, near-zone length increases.

 If frequency increases, near-zone length increases.

TABLE 3-2	Near-Zone Length (NZL) for Unfocused Elements	
Frequency (MHz)	**Width (mm)**	**NZL (cm)**
2.0	19	12
3.5	13	10
3.5	19	20
5.0	6	3
5.0	10	8
5.0	13	14
7.5	6	4
10.0	6	6

Table 3-2 lists near-zone lengths for various disk element frequencies and diameters. The region that lies beyond a distance of one near-zone length is called the far zone, *far field,* or Fraunhofer zone. The beam width increases with increasing distance from the transducer in the far zone.

 Aperture is the size of a source of ultrasound (single element or group of elements).

What is somewhat surprising but true is that even in the case of this flat, unfocused transducer element, there is some beam narrowing. This narrowing is sometimes called *natural focus*. Modern diagnostic transducer **arrays** contain rectangular elements. Beams

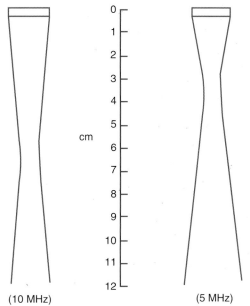

FIGURE 3-11 Beams for disk transducers having a diameter of 6 mm at two frequencies. Higher frequencies produce smaller beam diameters (at a distance greater than 4 cm in this case) and longer near-zone lengths.

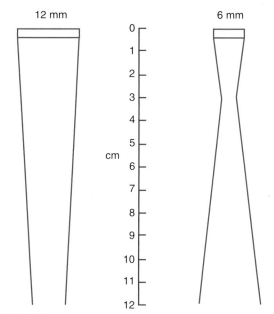

FIGURE 3-12 Beams for 5-MHz disk transducers of two diameters. The larger transducer *(left)* produces the longer near-zone length. A smaller transducer *(right)* can produce a larger-diameter beam in the far zone. In this example, the beam diameters are equal at a distance of 8 cm.

from rectangular elements are similar but not identical to those from disk elements.

Example 3-1

For a 10-mm, 5-MHz flat (unfocused) disk transducer, what are the beam widths at the near-zone length and at two times the near-zone length?

At the end of the near zone, the beam width is approximately equal to one half the width of the transducer element, or 5 mm. At double the near-zone length, the beam diameter is approximately equal to the diameter of the transducer element, or 10 mm.

The effects of frequency and aperture on near-zone length are shown in Figures 3-11 and 3-12, respectively. An increase in frequency or in aperture increases near-zone length. At a sufficient distance from the transducer, an increase in frequency or transducer size can decrease the beam diameter, as shown in the figures.

The beam in Figure 3-10, *A,* is for continuous wave mode, but it can be used to describe pulses in the rest of the figure. The beam for pulses is similar to, but not exactly the same as, that for continuous sound.

Focusing

To improve resolution, diagnostic transducers are focused. Focusing sound in the same manner as focusing light reduces beam width. Sound may be focused (Figure 3-13) by using curved (rather than flat) transducer elements, by using a **lens,** or by phasing (discussed later). Focusing moves the end of the near zone toward the transducer and narrows the beam. Beam width is

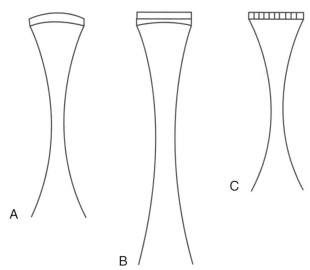

FIGURE 3-13 Sound focusing by a curved transducer element, lens, or phased array. Lenses focus because the propagation speed through them is higher than that through tissues. Refraction at the surface of the lens forms the beam in such a way that a focal region occurs. The operation of phased arrays is described later in this chapter. **A,** Curved transducer element. **B,** Lens. **C,** Phased array.

decreased in the **focal region** and in the area between it and the transducer, but it is widened in the region beyond (Figure 3-14). **Focal length** (fl) is the distance from the transducer to the center of the focal region. Focusing can be accomplished only in the near zone of a transducer. **Focal zone** length (called *depth of field* in photography) is the distance between equal beam widths that are some multiple (e.g., ×2) of the minimum value (at the **focus**).

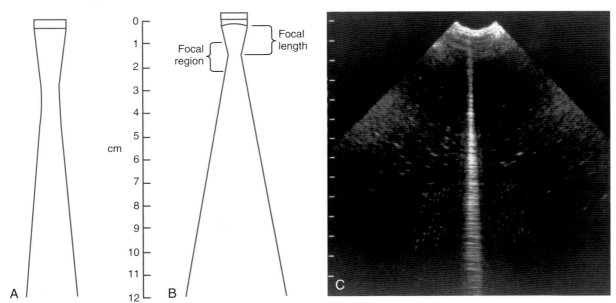

FIGURE 3-14 Beam diameter for a 6-mm, 5-MHz transducer without **(A)** and with **(B)** focusing. Focusing reduces the minimum beam width compared with that produced without focusing. However, well beyond the focal region, the width of the focused beam is greater than that of the unfocused beam. **C,** A focused beam. This is an ultrasound image of a beam profile test object containing a thin vertical scattering layer down the center. Scanning this object generates a picture of the beam (the pulse width at all depths). In this case, the focus occurs at a depth of about 4 cm (this image has a total depth of 15 cm). Depth markers (in 1-cm increments) are indicated on the left edge of the figure.

 Focusing can be achieved only in the near zone of a beam.

As the element or lens is increasingly curved (or phase-delay curvature in a **phased array** is increased), the focus moves closer to the transducer and becomes "tighter" (i.e., the beam width at the focus decreases). The limit to which a beam can be narrowed depends on wavelength, aperture, and focal length.

AUTOMATIC SCANNING

Not only must the transducer emit ultrasound pulses and receive echoes, but it must also send the pulses through the many anatomic paths required to generate an image. This sometimes is called *scanning, sweeping,* or *steering* the beam through the tissue cross-sections to be imaged. Scanning is done rapidly and automatically so that many images, called *frames,* can be acquired and presented in rapid sequence within a second. Presenting images in a rapid sequential format, like a movie, is called *real-time sonography.*

Automatic scanning of a sound beam is performed electronically, providing a means for sweeping the sound beam through the tissues rapidly and repeatedly.

Electronic scanning is performed with arrays. Transducer arrays are transducer assemblies with several transducer elements. The elements are rectangular and are arranged in a straight line (**linear array;** Figures 3-3, *E,* and 3-15, *A*) or curved line (**convex array;** Figure 3-15, *B*). **Linear** is the adjectival form of the word "line." Convex means "bowed outward."

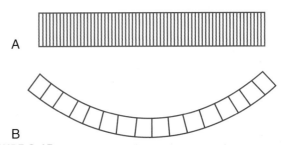

FIGURE 3-15 A, Front view of a linear array with 64 rectangular elements. **B,** Side view of a convex array with 16 elements.

Linear Array

Arrays are operated in two ways, called *sequencing* and *phasing.* A more complete name for what is commonly called a *linear array* is **linear sequenced array.** This array contains a straight line of rectangular elements, each about a wavelength wide, and is operated by applying voltage pulses to groups of elements in succession (Figure 3-16). Each group of elements acts like a larger transducer element, providing a large enough aperture to confine the ultrasound to a fine enough beam for satisfactory resolution. As different groups are energized, the origin of the sound beam moves across the face of the transducer assembly from one end to the other, thus producing the same effect as would manual linear scanning with a single element the size (aperture) of the energized groups. Such electronic scanning, however, can be done rapidly and consistently without involving moving parts or a coupling liquid. If this electronic scanning is repeated rapidly enough, real-time presentation (many images per second) of visual information can

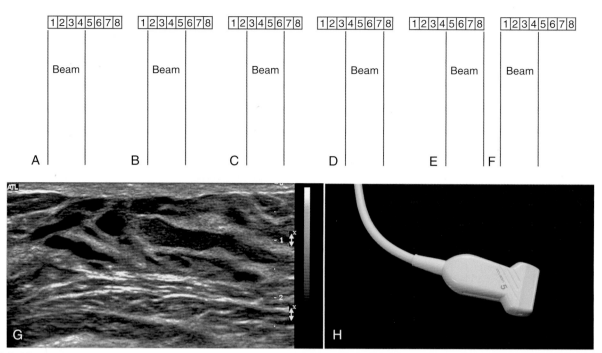

FIGURE 3-16 **A linear sequenced array** *(side view).* A voltage pulse is applied simultaneously to all elements in a small group: first to elements 1 to 4 (for example) as a group **(A),** then to elements 2 to 5 **(B),** and so on across the transducer assembly **(C-E).** The process is then repeated **(F). G,** An image generated from a linear array. **H,** A linear array transducer.

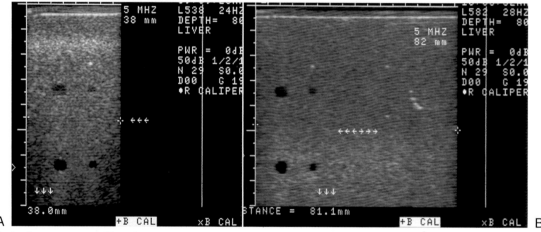

FIGURE 3-17 **The linear image width is determined by the length of the linear array used. A,** In this example, a 5-MHz, 38-mm linear array (L538) produces an image that is 38 mm wide. **B,** A 5-MHz, 82-mm linear array (L582) produces an image that is 81 mm wide.

result. Real-time presentation requires scanning the beam across the transducer assembly several times per second. The aperture is the size of the group of elements energized to produce each pulse. The width of the entire image is approximately equal to the length of the array (Figure 3-17). The linear image consists of parallel scan lines produced by pulses originating at different points across the surface of the array (and across the top of the image) but all traveling in the same vertical direction (parallel) (Figure 1-6). This produces a rectangular image, as shown in Figures 3-16, *G,* and 3-17.

> A linear array produces rectangular images composed of many parallel, vertical scan lines.

The pulsing sequence described in Figure 3-16 (eight elements, pulsed in groups of four) yields only five scan lines to make up the image. This would certainly be a poor-quality image. A 128-element array pulsed in groups of four would yield a 125-line display. Pulsing these elements individually (rather than in groups of four) would yield a 128-line display, but the small aperture (a single element less than 1 mm in size) would cause excessive beam spreading and poor resolution. If the pulsing sequence alternated groups of three and four elements (e.g., elements 1 to 3, then 1 to 4, 2 to 4, 2 to 5, 3 to 5, 3 to 6, 4 to 6, 4 to 7, and on through the array), the number of scan lines would be doubled, to 250, thereby increasing scan-line density and improving the quality of the image.

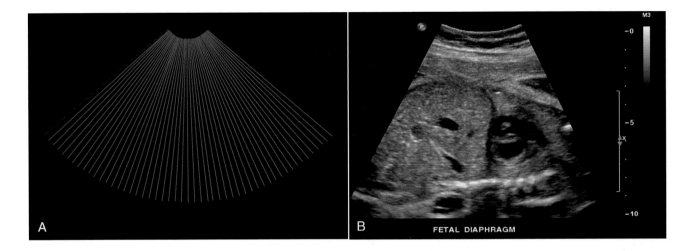

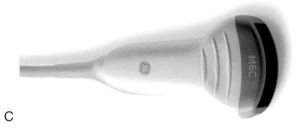

FIGURE 3-18 **A,** Convex arrays send pulses out in different directions from different points across the curved array surface. **B,** A sector-type image with a curved top is produced by a convex array. **C,** A convex array transducer.

Convex Array

A convex array, also called a *curved array*, is constructed as a curved line of elements rather than a straight one. The operation of a convex array is identical to that of the linear sequenced array (sequencing groups of elements from one end of the array to the other), but because of the curved construction, the pulses travel out in different directions, producing a sector-type image (Figure 3-18). The complete name for this transducer is *convex sequenced array*.

 The convex array operates similarly to the linear array but produces a sector image.

Phased Array

A **linear phased array** (commonly called *phased array*) contains a compact straight line of elements, each about one quarter of a wavelength wide. The phased array is operated by applying voltage pulses to most or all elements (not a small group) in the assembly, but with small (less than 1 μs) time differences (called *phasing*) between them, so that the resulting sound pulse is sent out in a specific path direction, as shown in Figure 3-19. If the same time delays were used each time the process was repeated, the subsequent pulses would travel out in the same direction repeatedly. However,

the time delays automatically are changed slightly with each successive repetition so that subsequent pulses travel out in slightly different directions, and the beam direction continually changes (Figure 3-20). This process results in the sweeping of the beam, with beam direction changing with each pulse, to produce a sector image (Figure 3-20, *F*), the same effect as with manual rotation of a single element. Such electronic sector scanning, however, can be done rapidly and consistently without involving moving parts or a coupling liquid. The phased array is sometimes called an *electronic sector transducer*.

 A phased array scans the beam in sector format with short time delays.

Phasing is applied to some linear and convex arrays to steer the beam from each element group in several directions by sending out several pulses from each group with different phasing. Thus echoes can be generated from a specific anatomic location with several viewing angles. The echo information from these multiple views is processed to present an image of improved quality. This is a form of electronic "compounding" of an image. This is discussed in more detail in the next chapter.

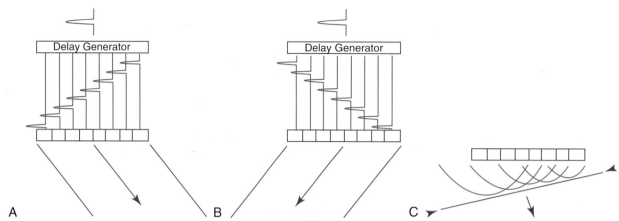

FIGURE 3-19 A linear phased array (*side view*). A, When voltage pulses are applied in rapid progression from left to right, one ultrasound pulse is produced that is directed to the right. **B,** Similarly, when voltage pulses are applied in rapid progression from right to left, one ultrasound pulse is produced that is directed to the left. **C,** The delays in **A** produce a pulse the combined pressure wavefront of which *(arrowheads)* is angled from lower left to upper right. A wave always travels perpendicular to its wavefront, as indicated by the arrow.

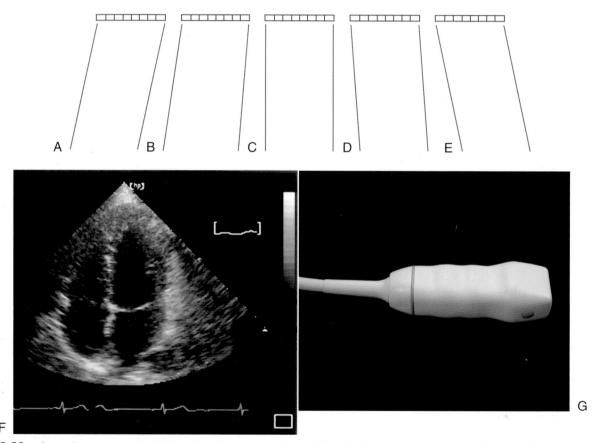

FIGURE 3-20 A five-pulse sequence in which each pulse travels out in a different direction. A, The rapid voltage-application progression is from right to left across the array. **B,** A right-to-left progression with slightly shorter time delays. **C,** No delays (all elements energize simultaneously). **D,** A left-to-right progression. **E,** A left-to-right progression with slightly longer delays. **F,** A cardiac sector image produced by a phased array. The image comes to a point at the top. **G,** A phased array transducer.

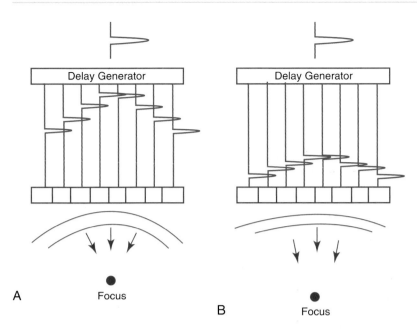

FIGURE 3-21 By putting curvature in the phase delay pattern, a pulse is focused. A, Greater curvature places the focus closer to the transducer. **B,** Less curvature moves the focus deeper.

Electronic Focus

In addition to steering the beam, the phased array can focus the beam as well (Figure 3-21). An increase in the curved delay pattern (greater time delays between elements) moves the focus closer to the transducer, whereas a decrease (shorter delays) in curvature moves it deeper. Thus phasing provides electronic control of the location of the focus (Figure 3-22). Multiple foci can be used to achieve, in effect, a long focus (Figure 3-23). One pulse can be focused at only one depth. Therefore multiple foci require multiple pulses (per scan line), each focused at a different depth. Echoes from the focal region of each pulse are displayed, and the rest are discarded. The resulting image is a montage of the focal regions of the different pulses, which improves detail resolution. However, using multiple pulses per scan line takes more time, and the frame rate is reduced, which degrades temporal resolution (discussed later). Thus temporal resolution is sacrificed for an improvement in detail resolution.

 Electronic focusing is accomplished with a curved pattern of phased delays. An increase or decrease in the curvature of the delay pattern moves the focus shallower or deeper, respectively.

Phasing is also applied to linear arrays to provide electronic focal control (Figure 3-24). The term **phased linear array** indicates that phased focus control is applied to a linear sequenced array. Rather than each group of elements being pulsed simultaneously, as in Figure 3-16, the outer elements are pulsed slightly ahead of the inner ones (Figure 3-24, C). This produces a curved pulse that is focused at a depth determined by the delay between the firing of the outer and inner elements. These pulses are focused, but not steered, by phasing. They still travel straight down to produce parallel vertical scan lines and a rectangular display. In a similar way, phased focusing is applied to convex arrays as well.

Variable Aperture

Recall that aperture, focal length, and wavelength determine the beam width at the focus. To maintain the same beam width at the focus for increasing focal lengths, the aperture must also be increased. This means that, in fact, not all elements of a phased array are used to generate all pulses. Smaller groups are used for short focal lengths, whereas larger groups are used for foci of increasing depth (Figure 3-25).

Section Thickness Focus

A single line of elements can electronically focus or steer only in the scan plane. Focus (fixed at one depth) can be achieved in the third dimension with a lens or with curved elements. With at least three rows of elements—that is, a two-dimensional array—phasing can be applied to focus the third dimension electronically. Electronic focusing in the third dimension eliminates the need for a lens or curved elements. Two-dimensional arrays as large as 3000 elements are commercially available. This dimension, perpendicular to the scan plane, is called *slice thickness dimension* or *section thickness dimension*. Beam width in this dimension is important with regard to section thickness artifacts, also called *partial-volume artifacts*. This third dimension and its associated section thickness are shown in Figures 1-7, *A*, and 1-9, *A*.

Grating Lobes

In addition to side lobes, which single-element transducers have, arrays have **grating lobes**, which are additional beams resulting from their multi-element

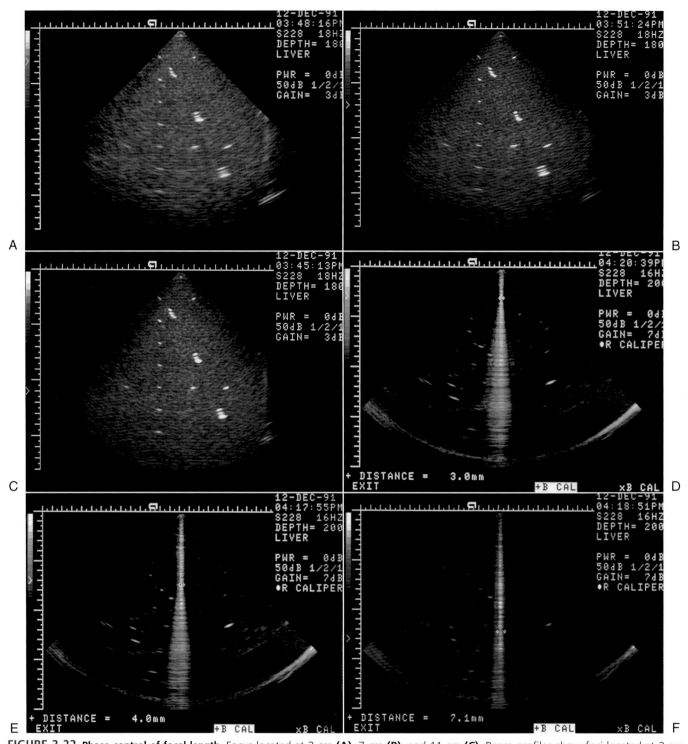

FIGURE 3-22 Phase control of focal length. Focus located at 3 cm **(A)**, 7 cm **(B)**, and 11 cm **(C)**. Beam profiles show foci located at 3 cm **(D)**, 7 cm **(E)**, and 13 cm **(F)**.

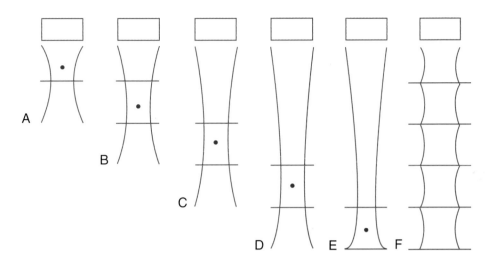

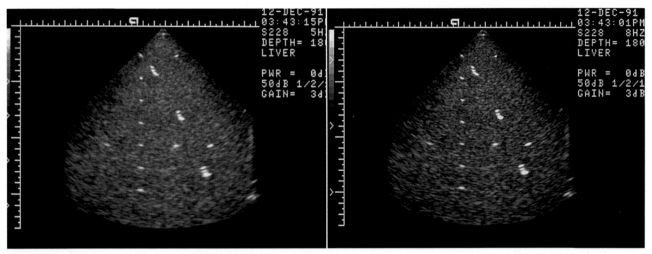

FIGURE 3-23 Multiple-transmit focus uses a pulse for each focus. In this example, five pulses focused at different depths **(A-E)** are needed to produce a montage image **(F)** with an effectively long focus (narrow beam). Only the echoes from the focal region of each pulse are used to produce the image. The rest are discarded. **G,** Five foci at 2, 5, 8, 12, and 16 cm. **H,** Triple foci at 3, 9, and 15 cm. Note the reduced frame rates (5 and 8 Hz, compared with 18 and 16 Hz in Figure 3-22).

structure. **Grating lobes** can be reduced by driving the elements in a group nonuniformly (i.e., with different voltage amplitudes). Outer elements are driven at lower amplitudes than are inner elements. Echo reception sensitivity is also less for outer elements. This is called *apodization*. Because optimal apodization changes continually with focusing and steering, it is called *dynamic apodization*. The downside of **apodization** is that there is some broadening of the main beam with degradation of resolution. Subdicing of each element into a group of smaller crystals is also done to weaken grating lobes and to reduce interelement interaction for improved electronic focusing. The subelements are tied together electrically so that they function as one element.

Vector Array

Phasing can be applied to each element group in a linear sequenced array to steer pulses in various directions, in addition to initiating them at various starting points across the array. **Vector array** is the name applied to this type of transducer (Figure 3-26). This transducer converts the image format of a linear array from rectangular to **sector**. Scan lines originate from different points across the top of the display and travel out in different directions. The image format is similar to that of a convex array except that the contact surface (footprint) is smaller and the top of the display is flat. More elements can be used at a time, allowing for larger apertures than can be achieved with convex arrays. Phasing can be applied to linear sequenced arrays as well in such a way that each pulse travels in the same direction (but not straight down). This converts a rectangular display to a parallelogram-shaped display useful in color Doppler imaging (Figure 3-26, *D*).

 The vector array is a combination of linear and phased array operations. It presents a sector display with a nonzero width at the top.

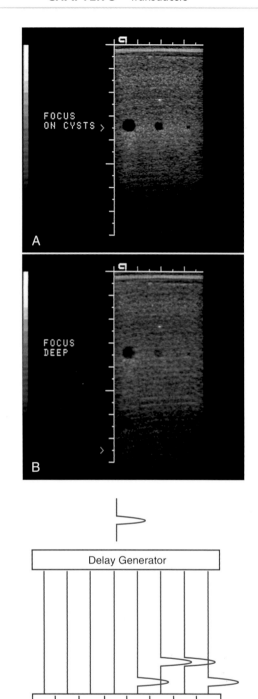

FIGURE 3-24 **A,** A phased linear array with the focus located at 3.5 cm produces a clear image of the small cystic object. **B,** When the focus is located at 7.5 cm (less phase delay curvature), a loss of image quality results for cystic objects. **C,** Phased delays are applied to each element group to focus the pulse.

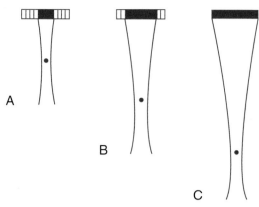

FIGURE 3-25 **Variable aperture.** To maintain comparable focal beam width at different depths, more array elements are used (increasing the aperture) as the focus is moved deeper. **A,** Four elements. **B,** Eight elements. **C,** Twelve elements.

Reception Steering, Focus, and Aperture

When an array is receiving echoes, the electric outputs of the elements can be timed so that the array is sensitive in a particular direction, with a listening focus at a particular depth (Figure 3-27). This reception focus depth may be increased continually as the transmitted pulse travels through tissues and the echoes arrive from deeper and deeper locations. This continually changing reception focus is called **dynamic focusing.** Dynamic focusing is similar to the continual change in focusing that occurs with a video camera, for example, when filming a child riding away on a bicycle. The combination of transmission focus (particularly multizone focusing) and dynamic reception focus improves detail resolution over large depth ranges in images. As the focus continually changes during echo reception, the aperture increases to maintain a constant focal width. This is called **dynamic aperture.** The terms used to describe arrays describe their construction and function as shown in Table 3-3. Boxes 3-1 and 3-2 and Tables 3-4 and 3-5 summarize transducer types, terminology, characteristics, and display formats.

 With phasing, the reception "beam" is steered and dynamically focused.

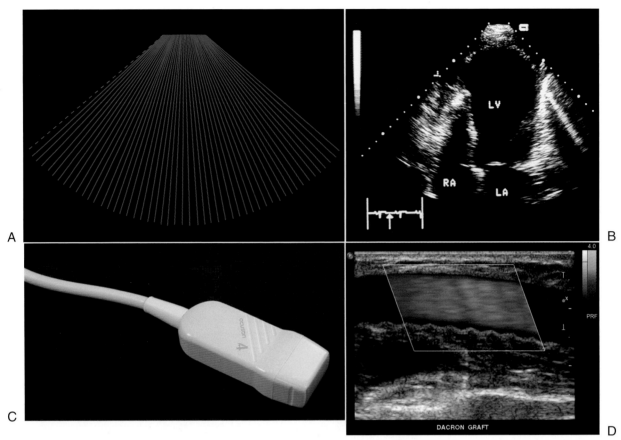

FIGURE 3-26 A, A vector array sends pulses out in different directions from different starting points across the flat surface of the array. **B,** A cardiac scan produced by a vector array. **C,** A vector array transducer. **D,** A phased linear array producing a parallelogram-shaped color Doppler display.

BOX 3-1	Common Transducer Types

- Linear array
- Convex array
- Phased array
- Vector array

TABLE 3-3	Terms Used to Describe Arrays		
Term	**Construction**	**Scanning**	**Focusing**
Array	√		
Linear	√		
Sequenced		√	
Convex	√		
Phased		√	√

BOX 3-2	Array Terminology

- (Phased) linear (sequenced) array
- (Phased) convex (sequenced) array
- (Linear) phased array
- (Phased and sequenced) (linear) vector array

  The words in parentheses are implied in the abbreviated common terminology.

TABLE 3-4	Transducer Characteristics		
Type	**Beam Scanned by Sequencing**	**Beam Scanned by Phasing**	**Beam Focused by Phasing**
Linear array	√		√
Convex array	√		√
Phased array		√	√
Vector array	√	√	√

TABLE 3-5	Display Formats				
Type	**Rectangle or Parallelogram**	**Sector**	**Flat Top**	**Curved Top**	**Pointed Top**
Linear array	√		√		
Convex array		√		√	
Phased array		√			√
Vector array		√	√		

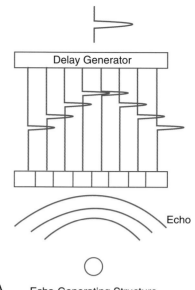

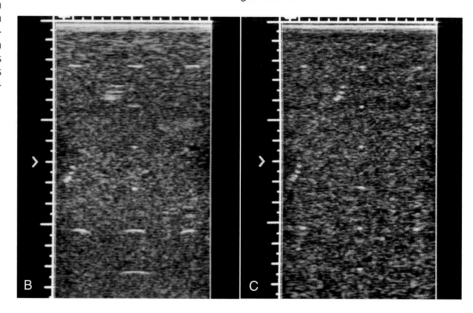

FIGURE 3-27 **A,** A spherically shaped echo arrives at array elements at different times, producing noncoincident voltages in the various channels. If simply combined, a weak, long voltage (with poor resolution and sensitivity) would result. However, with proper delays, the voltages are made to coincide, producing a strong, short (good resolution and sensitivity) voltage. As echoes return from deeper and deeper locations, their curvature is reduced. Thus the delay correction must be reduced as echoes return. This is called dynamic focusing. **B,** Dynamic focus is off. **C,** When the dynamic focus is on, resolution improves.

DETAIL RESOLUTION

Imaging resolution has three aspects:

1. Detail
2. Contrast
3. Temporal

Contrast and temporal resolutions relate more directly to instruments. Detail resolution (Figure 3-28) relates more directly to transducers and is therefore discussed in this section. If two reflectors are not separated sufficiently, they produce overlapping (not distinct) echoes that are not separated on the instrument display. Rather, the echoes merge together and appear as one. Thus the echoes are not resolved. If distinct (separated by a gap) echoes are not generated initially in the anatomy, the reflectors will not be separated on the display. In ultrasound imaging, the two aspects to detail resolution are **axial** and **lateral,** which depend on the different characteristics of ultrasound pulses as they travel through tissues.

Axial Resolution

Axial resolution (AR) is the minimum reflector separation required along the direction of sound travel (along the scan line) to produce separate echoes (Figure 3-29). The important factor in determining axial resolution is spatial pulse length. Axial resolution is equal to one half the spatial pulse length.

$$AR\,(mm) = \frac{SPL\,(mm)}{2}$$

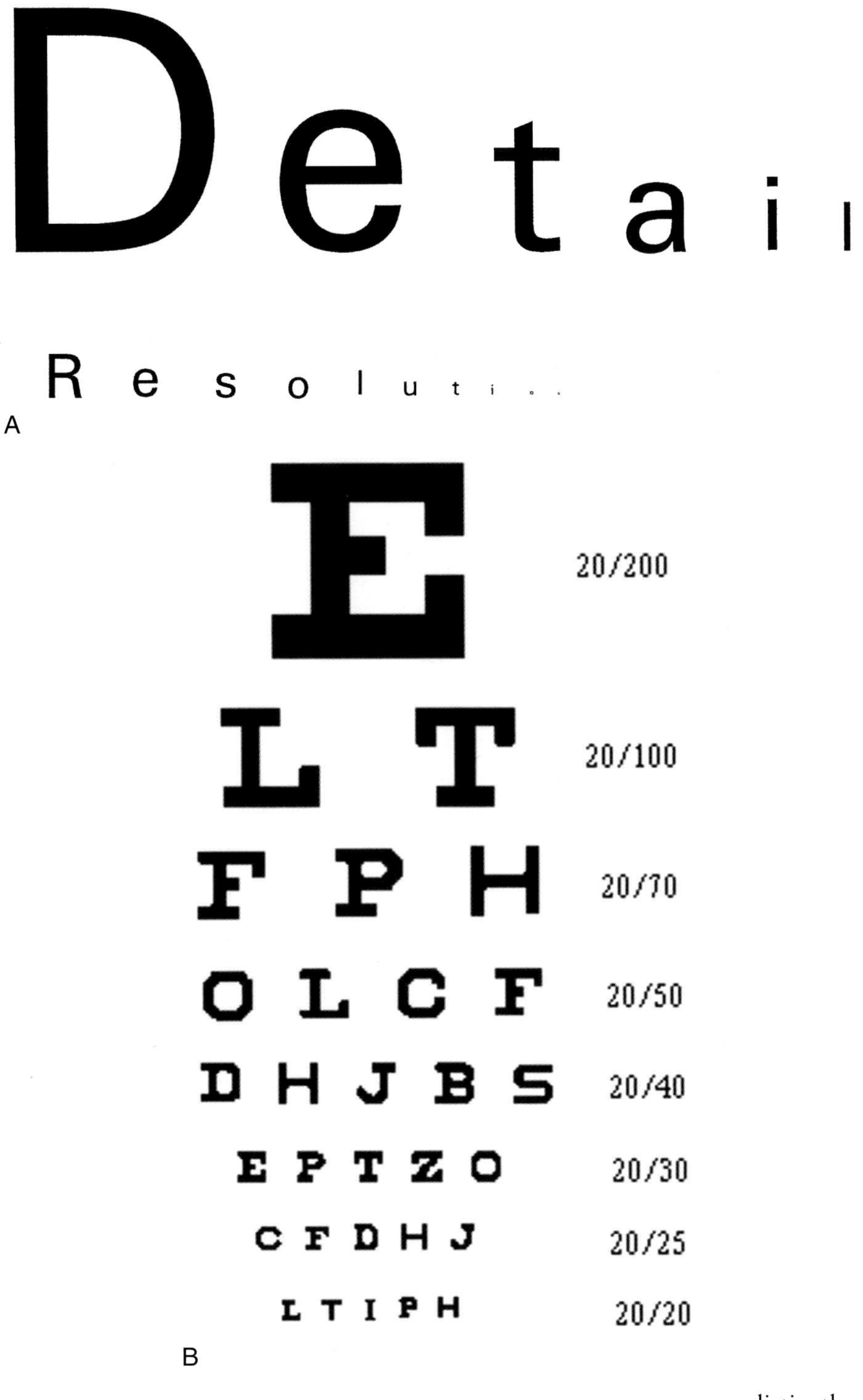

Detail

Resolution

A

E	20/200
L T	20/100
F P H	20/70
O L C F	20/50
D H J B S	20/40
E P T Z O	20/30
C F D H J	20/25
L T I P H	20/20

B

FIGURE 3-28 A, Excellent detail resolution is the ability to image fine detail. Smaller is better, that is, tinier details can be discerned. **B,** Snellen vision testing chart.

Axial resolution is the minimum reflector separation necessary to resolve reflectors along scan lines. Axial resolution (millimeters) equals spatial pulse length (millimeters) divided by 2.

Note that the numeric value of detail resolution decreases as frequency increases. Axial resolution is like a shopping-mall sale, a weight-loss program, or a golf score: smaller is better. The smaller the axial resolution, the finer is the detail that can be displayed; thus the two reflectors can be closer along the sound path and still be seen distinctly, thereby allowing tinier objects to be displayed. To improve axial resolution, spatial pulse length must be reduced. Because spatial pulse length is wavelength multiplied by number of cycles in the pulse, one or both of these factors must be reduced. Wavelength is reduced by increasing frequency. The number of cycles in each pulse is reduced by transducer damping. Because the number of cycles per pulse has been reduced to a minimum (one to three) by transducer design, the only way the instrument operator can improve axial resolution further is to increase frequency. With an increase in frequency, however, comes a reduction in penetration

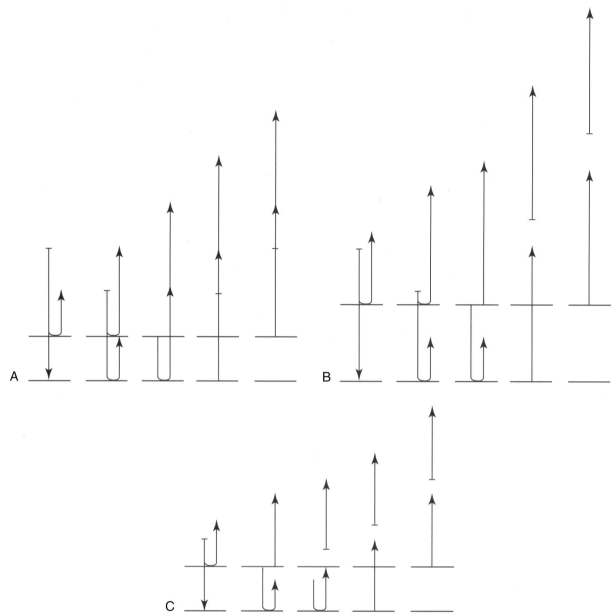

FIGURE 3-29 Axial resolution. Action proceeds in time from left to right in each part of the figure. **A,** The separation of the reflectors is less than half the spatial pulse length, so echo overlap occurs. Separate echoes are not produced. The reflectors are not resolved on the display. **B,** The reflector separation is increased so that it is greater than half the spatial pulse length. Echo overlap does not occur. Separate echoes are produced, and the reflectors are resolved on the display. **C,** The reflector separation is the same as in *A*, but resolution is achieved by shortening the pulse so that separate echoes are produced.

(imaging depth) because attenuation increases as frequency increases. Thus, in sonographic imaging, there is a trade-off between resolution and penetration with changing frequency. This is, in fact, an image quality–quantity trade-off.

Lateral Resolution

Lateral resolution (LR) is the minimum reflector separation in the direction perpendicular to the beam direction (that is, across scan lines) that can produce two separate echoes when the beam is scanned across the reflectors

(Figure 3-30). Lateral resolution is equal to the beam width (w_b) in the scan plane.

$$LR \, (mm) = w_b \, (mm)$$

 Lateral resolution is the minimum reflector separation necessary to resolve reflectors across scan lines. Lateral resolution (millimeters) equals beam width (millimeters).

As with axial resolution, smaller lateral resolution is better. A smaller value indicates an improvement (finer detail and the ability to image tinier objects). Just as

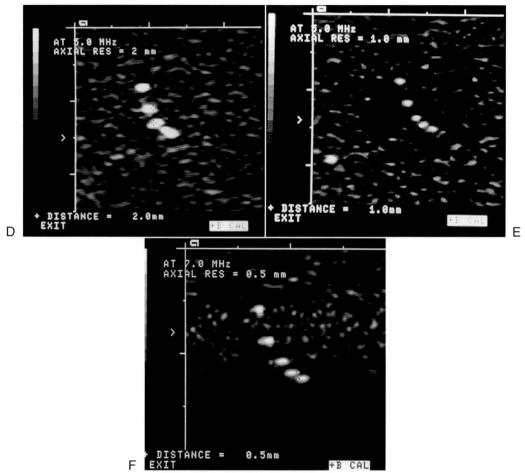

FIGURE 3-29, cont'd **D-F,** Axial resolution improves as frequency increases: **D,** 3.5 MHz, with a resolution of 2.0 mm; **E,** 5.0 MHz, with a resolution of 1.0 mm; **F,** 7.0 MHz, with a resolution of 0.5 mm.

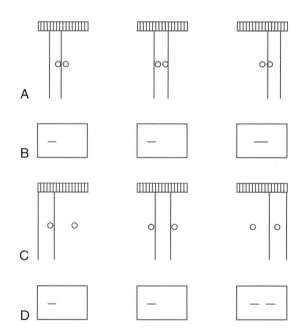

FIGURE 3-30 **Lateral resolution.** Reflector separation (perpendicular to beam direction) is less than beam diameter in **A** and **B,** whereas in **C** and **D,** reflector separation is greater than beam diameter. Action proceeds in time from left to right in each part of the figure. **A,** The beam first encounters the left reflector, then is reflected by both reflectors, and finally is reflected by the right reflector. **B,** This scanning sequence results in continual reflection from one or both reflectors. Separate echoes are not produced, and the reflectors are not resolved. **C,** The beam encounters the left reflector, then fits between both reflectors (yielding no echo), and finally is reflected by the right reflector. **D,** Separate echoes are produced, and the reflectors are resolved on the display.

beam width varies with distance from the transducer, so, too, does lateral resolution. If the lateral separation between two reflectors is greater than the beam diameter, two separate echoes are produced when the beam is scanned across them. Thus the echoes are resolved, or detected, as separate reflectors.

 For detail resolution, smaller is better.

 If frequency increases, detail resolution improves, but penetration decreases.

Lateral resolution is improved by reducing the beam diameter, that is, by focusing (Figure 3-31). Figure 3-32 shows a focused beam. The lateral smearing of a thin layer of scatterers indicates the beam width and lateral resolution at various depths. The best resolution is obtained at the focus (Figure 3-33; see also Figure 3-24). Diagnostic ultrasound transducers often have better axial resolution than lateral resolution, although the two may be comparable in the focal region of strongly focused beams. Figure 3-34 shows examples of typical detail resolution.

Section thickness can be considered a third aspect of detail resolution and therefore is sometimes called **elevational resolution**. Elevational resolution contributes to section thickness artifact, also called *partial-volume artifact*. This artifact is a filling in of what should be anechoic structures such as cysts. This filling in occurs when the section thickness is larger than the size of the structure. Thus echoes from outside the structure are included in the image, and the structure appears to be echoic. The thinner the section thickness, the less is its negative impact on sonographic images. Focusing in the section-thickness plane reduces section thickness artifacts.

Useful Frequency Range

To meet resolution and penetration requirements reasonably, the useful frequency range for most diagnostic applications is 2 to 15 MHz. The lower portion of the range is useful when increased depth (e.g., in an obese subject) or high attenuation (e.g., in transcranial studies) is encountered. The higher portion of the frequency range is useful when little penetration is required (e.g., in imaging breast, thyroid, or superficial vessels or in pediatric imaging). In most large patients, 3 to 5 MHz is a satisfactory frequency; however, in thin patients and in children, 7.5 and 10 MHz often can be used. If frequencies less than 2 MHz are used, detail resolution is insufficient. If frequencies higher than 15 MHz (less than 15 MHz in deeper applications) are used, the depth is not sufficient in many applications. In the case of ophthalmologic, dermatologic, and intravascular imaging (the latter involving use of catheter-mounted transduc-

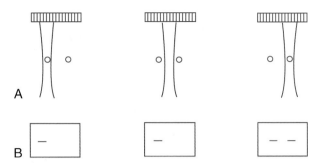

FIGURE 3-31 A, Two separate echoes are generated because the beam is focused and is narrower than the reflector separation. **B,** The two reflectors are resolved on the display. Without focusing, in this case, they would not have been resolved.

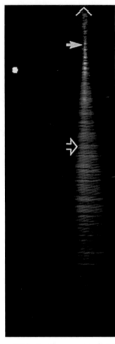

FIGURE 3-32 Beam width is shown as lateral smearing of a thin vertical scattering layer in a test object. The beam indicates the lateral resolution at each depth. In this example, beam width is about 2 mm at the focus **(closed arrow)** and about 10 mm at a depth of 6 cm *(open arrow)*, well beyond the focus.

TABLE 3-6	Typical Imaging Depth and Axial Resolution (Two-Cycle Pulse) in Tissue	
Frequency (MHz)	**Imaging Depth (cm)**	**Axial Resolution (mm)**
2.0	30	0.77
3.5	17	0.44
5.0	12	0.31
7.5	8	0.20
10.0	6	0.15
15.0	4	0.10

ers), frequencies up to 50 MHz are used because penetration of only a few millimeters is sufficient. Table 3-6 lists values for typical imaging depths and axial resolutions for various frequencies.

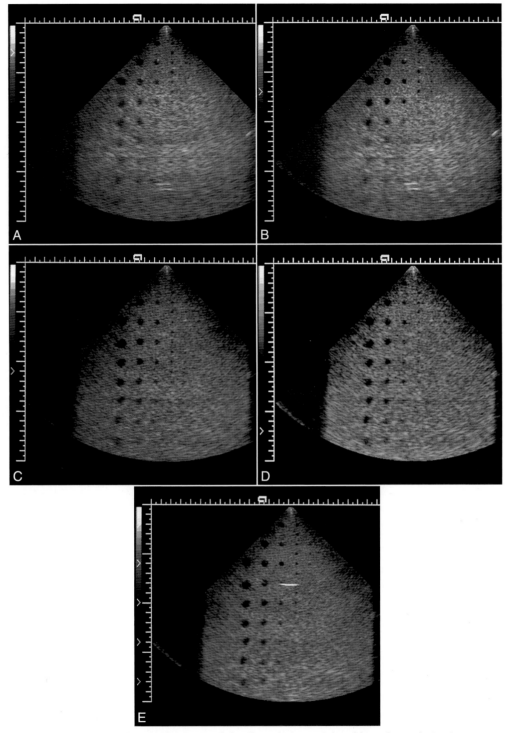

FIGURE 3-33 Imaging of small cysts involves both aspects of detail resolution: axial and lateral. Resolution improves at various depths as the focus is located there. Focus at 3 cm **(A)**, 7 cm **(B)**, 11 cm **(C)**, and 17 cm **(D)**. With multiple foci **(E)**, resolution is improved throughout depth.

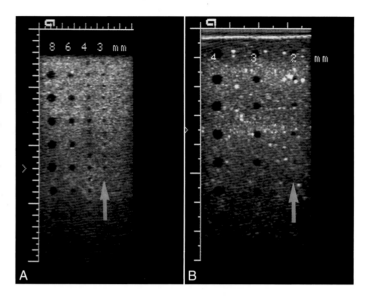

FIGURE 3-34 A, An image of a resolution penetration phantom that contains circular anechoic regions ("cysts") in tissue-equivalent material. From left to right, the cysts are 8, 6, 4, 3, and 2 mm in diameter and occur every 1 or 2 cm in depth of the image. Close examination reveals that the 3-mm cysts are the smallest that can be resolved. This image was produced using a 3.5-MHz transducer. **B,** The same phantom is imaged with a 7.0-MHz transducer. In this instance the 2-mm cysts can be seen. Note the loss of penetration compared with that in **A** (8 cm versus 20 cm). Detail resolution can be improved by increasing the frequency of the ultrasound beam, but at the expense of decreasing the imaging depth.

REVIEW

The key points presented in this chapter are the following:

- Transducers convert energy from one form to another.
- Ultrasound transducers convert electric energy to ultrasound energy, and vice versa.
- Transducers operate on the piezoelectric principle.
- Transducers are operated in pulse-echo mode.
- Operating frequency depends on element thickness.
- Axial resolution is equal to one half the spatial pulse length.
- Pulsed transducers have damping material to shorten spatial pulse length for acceptable resolution.
- Transducers produce sound in the form of beams with near and far zones.
- Lateral resolution is equal to beam width.
- Beam width can be reduced by focusing to improve lateral resolution.
- Detail resolution improves with increasing frequency.
- *Linear* and *convex* are types of array construction.
- *Sequenced*, *phased*, and *vector* are types of array scanning operations.
- Phasing also enables electronic control of focus.

EXERCISES

1. A transducer converts one form of _____ to another.
2. Ultrasound transducers convert _____ energy into _____ energy, and vice versa.
3. Ultrasound transducers operate on the _____ principle.
4. Single-element transducers are in the form of _____.
5. The _____ of a transducer element changes when voltage is applied to its faces.

6. The term *transducer* is used to refer to a transducer _____ or to a transducer _____.
7. A transducer _____ is part of a transducer _____.
8. An electric voltage pulse, when applied to a transducer, produces an ultrasound _____ of a _____ that is equal to that of the voltage pulse.
9. The resonance frequency of an element is determined by its _____.
10. Operating frequency _____ as transducer element thickness is increased.
11. The addition of damping material to a transducer reduces the number of _____ in the pulse, thus improving _____ _____. It increases _____.
12. Damping material reduces the _____ of the transducer and _____ of the diagnostic system.
13. Ultrasound transducers typically generate pulses of _____ or _____ cycles.
14. For a particular transducer element material, if a thickness of 0.4 mm yields an operating frequency of 5 MHz, the thickness required for an operating frequency of 10 MHz is _____ mm.
15. Which of the following transducer frequencies would have the thinnest elements?
    a. 2 MHz
    b. 3 MHz
    c. 5 MHz
    d. 7 MHz
    e. 10 MHz
16. The matching layer on the transducer surface reduces _____ caused by impedance differences.
17. A coupling medium on the skin surface eliminates reflection caused by _____.
18. Damping lengthens the pulse. True or false?
19. Damping increases efficiency. True or false?
20. The damping layer is in front/back of the element.

21. The matching layer is in front/back of the element.
22. The matching layer has _____ impedance.
23. Elements in linear arrays are in the form of _____.
24. Transducer assemblies are also called _____.
    a. transducers
    b. probes
    c. scanheads
    d. scan converters
    e. skinheads
    f. more than one of the above
25. Operating frequency is also called _____.
26. Mixtures of a piezoelectric ceramic and a non-piezoelectric polymer are called _____.
27. To operate a transducer at more than one frequency requires _____ _____.
28. Is it practical to attempt to operate a 5-MHz transducer with a bandwidth of 1 MHz at 6 MHz?
29. Is it practical to attempt to operate a 5-MHz transducer with a bandwidth of 2.5 at 3 and 7 MHz?
30. A beam is divided into two regions, called the _____ zone and the _____ zone.
31. The dividing point between the two regions referred to in Exercise 30 is at a distance from the transducer equal to _____ _____ length.
32. Transducer size is also called _____.
33. Near-zone length increases with increasing source _____ and _____.
34. Which transducer element has the longest near zone?
    a. 6 mm, 5 MHz
    b. 6 mm, 7 MHz
    c. 8 mm, 7 MHz
35. A higher-frequency transducer produces a _____ near-zone length.
36. A smaller transducer produces a _____ near-zone length.
37. A transducer with a near-zone length of 10 cm can be focused at 12 cm. True or false?
38. Which of the following transducer(s) can focus at 6 cm?
    a. 5 MHz, near-zone length of 5 cm
    b. 4 MHz, near-zone length of 6 cm
    c. 4 MHz, near-zone length of 10 cm
    d. b and c
    e. None of the above
39. Sound may be focused by using a _____.
    a. curved element
    b. lens
    c. phased array
    d. more than one of the above
40. Focusing reduces the beam diameter at all distances from the transducer. True or false?
41. The distance from a transducer to the location of the narrowest beam width produced by a focused transducer is called _____.

42. Transducer arrays are transducer assemblies with several transducer _____.
43. Linear arrays scan beams by _____ element groups.
44. A phased linear array with a single line of elements can focus in _____ dimension(s).
45. Focusing in section thickness can be accomplished with _____ elements or a _____.
46. Electronic focusing in section thickness requires multiple rows of _____.
47. Match the following (answers may be used more than once):
    a. Linear array _____.
    b. Phased array _____.
    c. Convex array _____.
    1. Voltage pulses are applied in succession to groups of elements across the face of a transducer.
    2. Voltage pulses are applied to most or all elements as a group, but with small time differences.
48. If the elements of a phased array are pulsed in rapid succession from right to left, the resulting beam is _____.
    a. steered right
    b. steered left
    c. focused
49. If the elements of a phased array are pulsed in rapid succession from outside in, the resulting beam is _____.
    a. steered right
    b. steered left
    c. focused
50. _____ and _____ describe how arrays are constructed.
    a. linear
    b. phased
    c. sequenced
    d. vector
    e. convex
51. _____, _____, and _____ describe how arrays are operated.
    a. linear
    b. phased
    c. sequenced
    d. vector
    e. convex
52. Shorter time delays between elements fired from outside in results in _____ curvature in the emitted pulse and a _____ focus.
    a. no, weak
    b. less, shallower
    c. less, deeper
    d. greater, shallower
    e. greater, deeper

53. A rectangular image is a result of linear scanning of the beam. This means that pulses travel in _____ _____ direction from _____ starting points across the transducer face.

54. A sector image is a result of sector steering of the beam. This means that pulses travel in _____ directions from a common _____ at the transducer face.

55. In _____ and _____ arrays, pulses travel out in different directions from different starting points on the transducer face.

56. Axial resolution is the minimum reflector separation required along the direction of the _____ _____ to produce separate _____.

57. Axial resolution depends directly on _____ _____ _____.

58. Smaller axial resolution is better. True or false?

59. If there are three cycles of a 1-mm wavelength in a pulse, the axial resolution is _____ mm.

60. For pulses traveling through soft tissue in which the frequency is 3 MHz and there are four cycles per pulse, the axial resolution is _____ mm.

61. If there are two cycles per pulse, the axial resolution is equal to the _____. At 5 MHz in soft tissue, this is _____ mm.

62. Doubling the frequency causes axial resolution to be _____.

63. Doubling the number of cycles per pulse causes axial resolution to be _____.

64. When studying an obese subject, a higher frequency likely will be required. True or false?

65. If better resolution is desired, a lower frequency will help. True or false?

66. If frequencies less than _____ MHz are used, axial resolution is not sufficient.

67. If frequencies higher than _____ MHz are used, penetration is not sufficient.

68. Increasing frequency improves resolution because _____ is reduced, thus reducing _____ _____ _____.

69. Increasing frequency decreases penetration because _____ is increased.

70. Lateral resolution is the minimum _____ between two reflectors at the same depth such that when a beam is scanned across them, two separate _____ are produced.

71. Lateral resolution is equal to _____ _____ in the scan plane.

72. Lateral resolution does not depend on _____.
    a. frequency
    b. aperture
    c. phasing
    d. depth
    e. damping

73. For an aperture of a given size, increasing frequency improves lateral resolution. True or false?

74. Lateral resolution varies with distance from the transducer. True or false?

75. For a given frequency, a smaller aperture always yields improved lateral resolution. True or false?

76. Lateral resolution is determined by _____. (more than one correct answer)
    a. damping
    b. frequency
    c. aperture
    d. number of cycles in the pulse
    e. distance from the transducer
    f. focusing

77. Match the following transducer assembly parts with their functions:
    a. Cable _____
    b. Damping material _____
    c. Piezoelectric element _____
    d. Matching layer _____

    1. Reduces reflection at transducer surface
    2. Converts voltage pulses to sound pulses
    3. Reduces pulse duration
    4. Conducts voltage pulses

78. Which of the following improve sound transmission from the transducer element into the tissue? (more than one correct answer)
    a. Matching layer
    b. Doppler effect
    c. Damping material
    d. Coupling medium
    e. Refraction

79. A 5-MHz unfocused transducer with an element thickness of 0.4 mm, an element width of 13 mm, and a near-zone length of 14 cm produces two-cycle pulses. Determine the following:
    a. Operating frequency if thickness is reduced to 0.2 mm: _____ MHz
    b. Axial resolution in the case of (a): _____ mm

    At 5 MHz:
    c. Depth at which lateral resolution is best: _____ cm
    d. Lateral resolution at 14 cm: _____ mm
    e. Lateral resolution at 28 cm: _____ mm
    f. This transducer can be focused at depths less than _____ cm.

80. Lateral resolution is improved by _____.
    a. damping
    b. pulsing
    c. focusing
    d. matching
    e. absorbing

81. For an unfocused transducer, the best lateral resolution (minimum beam width) is _____ the transducer width. This value of lateral resolution is found at a distance from the transducer face that is equal to the _____ _____ length.

82. For a focused transducer, the best lateral resolution (minimum beam width) is found in the _____ region.

83. An unfocused 3.5-MHz, 13-mm transducer will yield a minimum beam width (best lateral resolution) of _____ mm.

84. An unfocused 3.5-MHz, 13-mm transducer produces three-cycle pulses. The axial resolution in soft tissue is _____ mm.

85. In Exercises 83 and 84, axial resolution is better than lateral resolution. True or false?

86. Axial resolution is often not as good as lateral resolution in diagnostic ultrasound. True or false?

87. The two resolutions may be comparable in the _____ region of a strongly focused beam.

88. Beam diameter may be reduced in the near zone by focusing. True or false?

89. Beam diameter may be reduced in the far zone by focusing. True or false?

90. Match each transducer characteristic with the sound beam characteristic it determines (answers may be used more than once):
    a. Element thickness: 1. Axial resolution
       _____, _____   2. Lateral resolution
       and _____   3. Operating frequency
    b. Element width:
       _____
    c. Element shape (flat
       or curved): _____
    d. Damping: _____

91. The principle on which ultrasound transducers operate is the _____
    a. Doppler effect
    b. Acousto-optic effect
    c. Acousto-electric effect
    d. Cause and effect
    e. Piezoelectric effect

92. Which of the following is not decreased by damping?
    a. Refraction
    b. Pulse duration
    c. Spatial pulse length
    d. Efficiency
    e. Sensitivity

93. Which three things determine beam diameter for a disk transducer?
    a. Pulse duration
    b. Frequency
    c. Aperture
    d. Distance from disk face
    e. Efficiency

94. A two-cycle pulse of 5-MHz ultrasound produces separate echoes from reflectors in soft tissue separated by 1 mm. True or false?

95. The lower and upper limits of the frequency range useful in diagnostic ultrasound are determined by _____ and _____ requirements, respectively.

96. The range of frequencies useful for most applications of diagnostic ultrasound is _____ to _____ MHz.

97. Because diagnostic ultrasound pulses are usually two or three cycles long, axial resolution is usually equal to _____ to _____ wavelengths.

98. What is the axial resolution in Figure 3-35, *A-B*?

99. At what depth is the best lateral resolution in Figure 3-14, *C*?

100. Match the transducer type with the display formats in Figure 3-36.
    a. Linear array _____
    b. Convex array _____
    c. Phased array _____
    d. Vector array _____
    e. Phased linear array _____

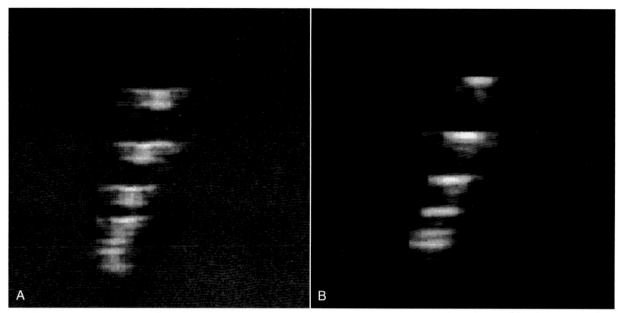

FIGURE 3-35 **Illustration to Accompany Exercise 98. A,** An image of a set of six rods in a test object. They are separated by 5, 4, 3, 2, and 1 mm from top to bottom. This scan was made using a transducer that produces 3.5-MHz ultrasound. The first three rods have been separated, whereas the images of the last three rods have merged. This image also shows small reverberation echoes behind each rod. **B,** The same rods imaged with a 5-MHz transducer. Higher-frequency transducers produce shorter pulse lengths and therefore provide improved axial resolution.

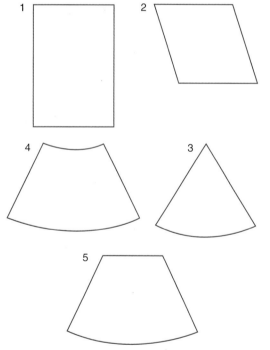

FIGURE 3-36 Illustration to accompany Exercise 100; display formats.

Instruments

Preprocessing
Radio frequency
Real-time
Real-time display
Refresh rate

Scan converter
Scan line
Scanning
Signal
Signal processor

Spatial compounding
Temporal resolution
Time gain compensation
Volume imaging

In the preceding chapters, we discussed the means by which ultrasound is generated and how it interacts with tissues. We now consider the instruments that receive echo voltages from the transducer and display them in the form of anatomic images. Diagnostic ultrasound systems are pulse-echo instruments. They determine echo strengths and locations of echo-generation sites. The directions and arrival times of echoes returning from tissues determine the locations of echo generation sites. This chapter describes how the instrument drives the transducer and what it does with the returning echoes.

Sonographic systems (Figure 4-1) produce visual displays from the echo voltages received from the transducer. Figure 4-1, *A*, presents a diagram of the organization of a pulse-echo sonographic imaging system. The instrument is composed of a **beam former**, a **signal processor**, an **image processor**, and a **display**.

BEAM FORMER

The beam former is where the action originates. The beam former is diagrammed in Figure 4-2. It consists of a pulser, pulse delays, transmit/receive (T/R) switch, amplifiers, analog-to-digital converters, echo delays, and a summer. Box 4-1 lists the functions of a beam former.

Pulser

The pulser produces electric voltages (Figure 4-3) that drive the transducer, forming the beam that sweeps through the tissue to be imaged. The driving voltages are typically in the form of a single cycle of voltage of the desired operating frequency. In response, the transducer produces ultrasound pulses that travel into the patient. The frequency of the voltage pulse determines the frequency of the resulting ultrasound pulse (Figure 4-3, *B-E*). Frequency ranges from 2 to 15 MHz for most applications.

 The pulser generates the voltages that drive the transducer.

Pulse repetition frequency (PRF) is the number of voltage pulses sent to the transducer each second and thus the number of ultrasound pulses produced per second. Pulse repetition frequency ranges from 4 to 15 kHz (5 to 30 kHz for Doppler applications). The ultrasound pulse repetition frequency is equal to the voltage pulse repetition frequency because one ultra-

BOX 4-1	Functions of the Beam Former

- Generating voltages that drive the transducer
- Determining pulse repetition frequency, coding, frequency, and intensity
- Scanning, focusing, and apodizing the transmitted beam
- Amplifying the returning echo voltages
- Compensating for attenuation
- Digitizing the echo voltage stream
- Directing, focusing, and apodizing the reception beam

sound pulse is produced for each voltage pulse. Similarly, the ultrasound pulse repetition period is equal to the voltage pulse repetition period. This is the time from the beginning of one pulse to the beginning of the next. The operator does not normally have direct control of pulse repetition frequency. Rather, the pulser adjusts it appropriately for the current imaging depth. To receive information for display at a rapid rate, a high pulse repetition frequency is desirable. Pulse repetition frequency, however, must be limited to provide proper display of returning echoes. The timing sequence that is initiated by the pulse is shown in Figure 4-4. To avoid echo misplacement, all echoes from one pulse must be received before the next pulse is emitted. For deeper imaging, echoes take longer to return, thus forcing a reduction in pulse repetition frequency and the number of images that are generated each second, called **frame rate**. Imaging depth—that is, penetration (*pen*) in centimeters—multiplied by PRF (in kilohertz) must not exceed 77 if echo misplacement is to be avoided.

$$pen\,(cm) \times PRF\,(kHz) \le 77\,(cm/ms)$$

The symbol $\le$ means "less than or equal to."

The instrument automatically achieves the highest pulse repetition frequency while avoiding echo misplacement. As operating frequency is reduced and penetration increases, pulse repetition frequency is reduced to avoid echo misplacement.

The greater the voltage amplitude produced by the pulser, the greater are the amplitude and intensity of the ultrasound pulse produced by the transducer. Transducer driving–voltage amplitudes range up to about 100 V. Output level is sometimes shown on the display in terms of a percentage or decibels relative to maximum (100% or 0 dB) output (Figure 4-5). Other output indicators account for relevant risk mechanisms.

Reduction of acoustic output reduces received echo amplitude (Figure 4-5, *C*). An increase in amplifier gain

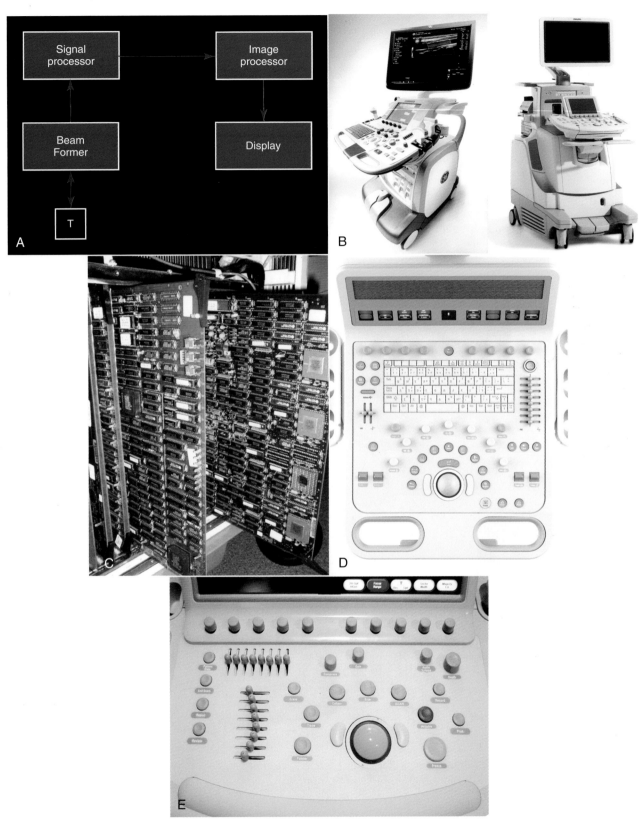

FIGURE 4-1 A, The organization of a pulse-echo imaging system. The beam former produces electric pulses that drive the transducer (T) and performs initial functions on returning echo voltages from the transducer. The transducer produces an ultrasound pulse for each electric pulse applied to it. For each echo received from the tissues, an electric voltage is produced by the transducer. These voltages go through the beam former to the signal processor, where they are processed to a form suitable for input to the image processor. Electric information from the image processor drives the display, which produces a visual image of the cross-sectional anatomy interrogated by the system. **B,** Fully-featured sonographic instruments. **C,** Sonographic instruments contain circuit boards, integrated circuits, and other electronic components. **D-E,** Instrument control panels.

Continued

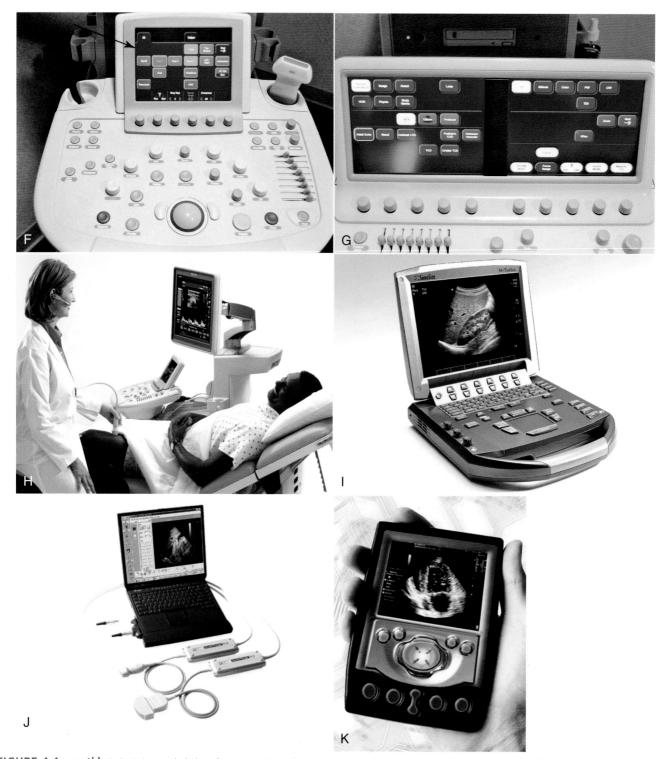

FIGURE 4-1, cont'd F-G, Point-and-click software controls for image control, transducer selection, and other functions. **H,** Some systems have voice-activated controls to allow hands-free operation. **I-K,** Portable systems.

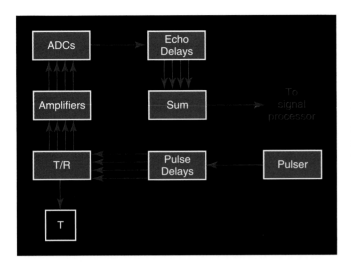

FIGURE 4-2 The beam former consists of a pulser, delays, a transmit/receive (T/R) switch, amplifiers, analog-to-digital converters (ADCs), and a summer. The beam former sends digitized echo-voltage streams to the signal processor. T is the transducer.

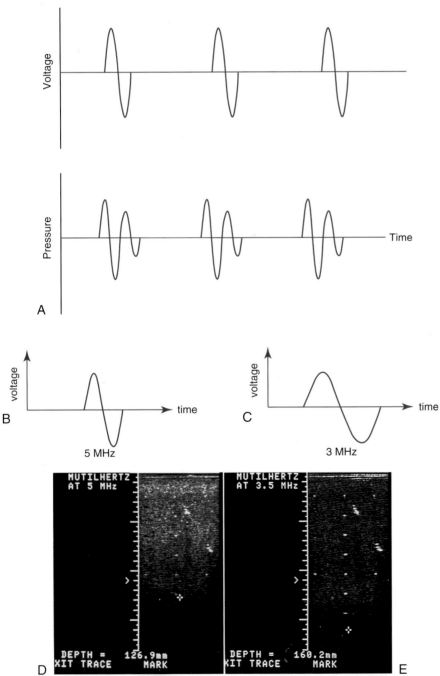

FIGURE 4-3 With every voltage pulse applied **(A)**, an ultrasound pulse is produced by the transducer. Voltage pulses of different frequencies **(B** and **C)** produce ultrasound pulses of different frequencies. The operator can change the operating frequency without changing transducers. **D-E,** Images using 5- and 3.5-MHz frequencies, respectively, with the same transducer.

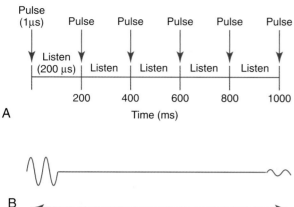

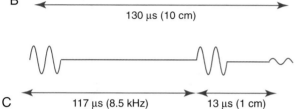

FIGURE 4-4 A, Timing sequence for pulse-echo ultrasound imaging. The sequence is initiated by the production of a 1-μs pulse of ultrasound when the pulser sends a voltage pulse to the transducer. This is followed by a period of up to 250 μs, during which echoes are received from the tissue by the transducer. The length of this time is determined by the maximum depth from which the echoes return. For example, at a frequency of 5 MHz, echoes can return from as deep as 15 cm. The round-trip travel time (13 μs/cm × 15 cm) to this depth is 195 μs. This listening period is followed (5 μs later) by the next pulse. In this illustration, the listening period is 200 μs; that is, the pulse repetition period is 200 μs (pulse repetition frequency [PRF] is 5 kHz). If pulse repetition frequency were greater, pulse repetition period would be decreased, resulting in emission of the next pulse before the reception of all the (deeper) echoes from the previous pulse. This would produce range-ambiguity artifact (see Chapter 6) and thus should be avoided. Pulse repetition frequency is automatically adjusted to avoid this problem: higher pulse repetition frequencies are used for superficial imaging, whereas lower pulse repetition frequencies are used for deep imaging (to allow for the longer time required for the arrival of deeper echoes). The latter causes a reduction in frame rate. **B,** An echo (from a 10-cm depth) arrives 130 μs after pulse emission. **C,** If the pulse repetition period were 117 μs (corresponding to a pulse repetition frequency of 8.5 kHz), the echo in **B** would arrive 13 μs after the next pulse was emitted. The instrument would place this echo at a 1-cm depth rather than the correct value. This is known as *range-ambiguity artifact.*

can compensate for this. A reduction in imaging depth also occurs, but this is surprisingly small. For example, a reduction of 50% in output from a 5-MHz transducer corresponds to only a 5% penetration reduction (from about 12.0 to 11.4 cm).

Pulse Delays

Thus far, the job of the beam former appears simple, but we must remember that with arrays, complicated sequencing and phasing operations are involved. Sequencing, phase delays, and variations in pulse amplitudes, which are necessary for the electronic control of beam **scanning**, steering, transmission focusing, aperture, and apodization must be accomplished. The pulser and pulse delays carry out all of these tasks.

Coded Excitation

Often, more complicated driving voltage–pulse forms called **coded excitation** are used. This approach accomplishes functions such as multiple transmission foci, separation of harmonic echo bandwidth from transmitted pulse bandwidth, increased penetration, reduction of speckle with improved **contrast resolution**, and gray-scale imaging of blood flow (called *B-flow*). In straightforward pulsing, the pulser drives the transducer through the pulse delays with one voltage pulse per **scan line.** In coded excitation, ensembles of pulses drive the transducer to generate a single scan line. For example, instead of a single pulse, a series (such as three pulses followed by a missing pulse [a gap], then two pulses followed by another gap, and then two pulses) could be used. Other examples are shown in Figure 4-6. A decoder in the receiving portion of the beam former recognizes and disassembles the coded sequence in the returning echoes and stacks up the individual pulses in the sequence to make a short, high-intensity echo voltage out of them. The result is equivalent to having a much-higher-intensity driving pulse or a much more sensitive receiving system. Thus, for example, in the case of blood flow, weak echoes from blood are imaged and flow can be seen in **gray scale** along with the much stronger tissue echoes (Figure 4-6, *C*).

 Coded excitation uses a series of pulses and gaps rather than a single driving pulse.

Coded excitation has been applied in radar for decades. A coded pulse is one that has internal amplitude, frequency, or phase modulation used for pulse compression. Pulse compression is the conversion, using a matched **filter**, of a relatively long coded pulse to one of short duration, excellent resolution, and equivalent high intensity and sensitivity. A matched filter maximizes the signal-to-noise ratio of the returning **signal.** The longer the coded pulse, the higher will be the signal-to-noise ratio in matched-filter implementations. Intrapulse coding is chosen to attain adequate axial resolution, and pulse duration is chosen to achieve the desired sensitivity. The matched-filter decoding process can be thought of as a sliding correlation of the parts of the coded pulse with the matched filter. The result of this process is, in effect, a shorter and stronger pulse (Figure 4-7) yielding good resolution and sensitivity while conforming to transmitted pulse amplitude and intensity limitations imposed by technologic and safety considerations. Such

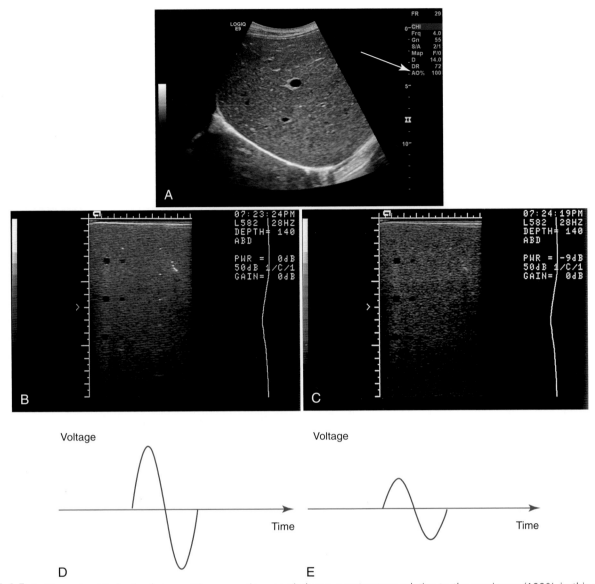

FIGURE 4-5 **A,** The output indicator (*arrow,* AO = acoustic output) shows a percentage relative to the maximum (100% in this example). **B-C,** The output indicator here shows decibels relative to the maximum. An output of 0 dB (100%) is compared with one of -9 dB (12.5%), in which the weaker echoes produce a darker image. **D-E,** Driving voltages from pulser to transducer for 0 and -6 dB, respectively. The voltage amplitude in **E** is half that in **D,** yielding one fourth the power and intensity, thus -6 dB output compared with **D.**

coding schemes are called *Barker codes.* An even better match can be achieved by Golay codes, which use pairs of transmitted pulses with the second being a bipolar sequence in which the latter portion of the pulse is the inverse of the first (Figure 4-7, *J*).

Channels

The pulse delays have a single input from the pulser but multiple outputs to the transducer elements; that is, there are actually many delay paths in the pulse delay circuitry. The reason for this is that each of the many elements in the array needs a different delay to form the ultrasound beam properly. Each independent delay and element combination constitutes a transmission **channel** (Figure 4-8). An increased number of channels allows more precise control of beam characteristics.

On reception, each independent element, **amplifier, analog-to-digital converter,** and delay path constitute a reception channel. Typical numbers of channels in modern sonographic instruments are 64, 128, and 192. Larger numbers are sometimes advertised, but a looser definition (than the one presented here) of the term *channel* is used in such advertisements. Normally, the number of channels does not exceed the number of elements in the transducer.

 A channel is an independent signal path consisting of a transducer element, delay, and possibly other electronic components.

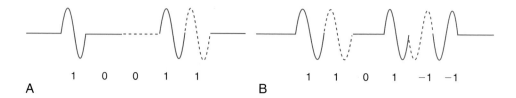

A   1   0   0   1   1   B   1   1   0   1   −1   −1

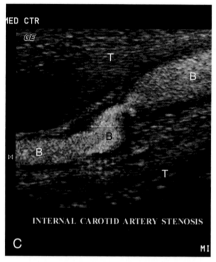

FIGURE 4-6 Examples of coded pulse sequences. Each pulse consists of a cycle of pressure variation. **A,** This sequence includes a pulse, two gaps, and two final pulses. **B,** This sequence includes two pulses, a gap, and one pulse followed by two inverted pulses. **C,** Blood flow imaging, in which weak echoes from flowing blood *(B)* are imaged along with much stronger tissue echoes *(T)*.

Transmit/Receive Switch

The transmit/receive (T/R) switch directs the driving voltages from the pulser and pulse delays to the transducer during transmission and then directs the returning echo voltages from the transducer to the amplifiers during reception (Figure 4-9). The T/R switch protects the sensitive input components of the amplifiers from the large driving voltages from the pulser.

Amplifiers

Amplifiers increase voltage amplitude. The beam former has one amplifier for each channel. **Amplification** is the conversion of the small voltages received from the transducer elements to larger ones suitable for further processing and storage (Figure 4-10). **Gain** is the ratio of amplifier output to electric power input. The power ratio, which is expressed in decibels, is equal to the voltage ratio squared because electric power depends on voltage squared. For example, if the input voltage amplitude to an amplifier is 2 mV and the output voltage amplitude is 200 mV, the voltage ratio is 200/2, or 100. The power ratio is 100^2, or 10,000. As shown in Table 4-1, the gain is 40 dB. Beam former amplifiers typically have 60 to 100 dB of gain. Voltages from transducers to these amplifiers range from a few microvolts (μV; e.g., from blood) to a few hundred millivolts (mV; e.g., from bone

TABLE 4-1	Gain (Expressed in Decibels) and Corresponding Power and Amplitude Ratios*	
Gain (dB)	**Power Ratio**	**Amplitude Ratio**
0	1.0	1.0
1	1.3	1.1
2	1.6	1.3
3	2.0	1.4
4	2.5	1.6
5	3.2	1.8
6	4.0	2.0
7	5.0	2.2
8	6.3	2.5
9	7.9	2.8
10	10	3.2
15	32	5.6
20	100	10
25	320	18
30	1,000	32
35	3,200	56
40	10,000	100
45	32,000	180
50	100,000	320
60	1,000,000	1,000
70	10,000,000	3,200
80	100,000,000	10,000
90	1,000,000,000	32,000
100	10,000,000,000	100,000

*The power (amplitude) ratio is output power (amplitude) divided by input power (amplitude).

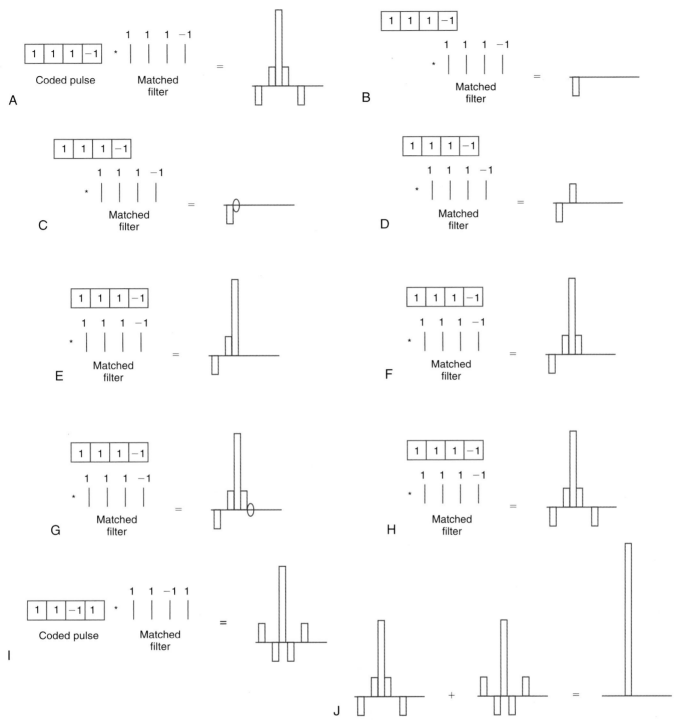

FIGURE 4-7 Matched filter decoding of coded pulse. A, Correlation (*) of the coded pulse with the matched filter yields a result that has a peak amplitude four times (16 times for intensity) that of a comparable uncoded pulse. This is accomplished by sliding the coded pulse in time over the matched filter characteristic and multiplying the two. **B,** Multiplying the first part of the coded pulse (−1) with the first part of the matched filter (+1) yields the result of −1, seen to the right of the equals sign. **C,** With the coded pulse slid more to the right (two portions overlap), there are two multiplications (−1 × +1 and +1 × +1). Summing the results yields 0. **D,** Sliding further to the right yields three multiplications, the sum of which is +1. **E,** The sum of four multiplications [(−1) × (−1), 1 × 1, 1 × 1, 1 × 1] is 4. **F-H,** The next results are +1, 0, and −1. To make the result even stronger and sharper, a pair of codes (called *Golay code pair*) can be used. The appropriate coded sequence to use with **A** is shown in **I. J,** When the two results (**A** and **I**) are summed, there is a sharp, strong result (amplitude 8 compared with the individual amplitudes of 1 in the coded sequence and the amplitude of 4 in the result in **A**).

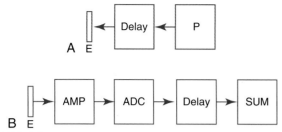

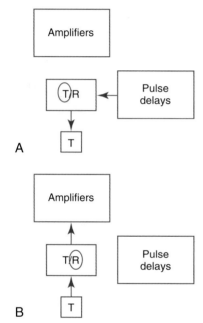

FIGURE 4-8 **A,** A transmission channel consists of an independent delay and transducer element *(E)* combination. Several channels emanate from the pulser *(P)*. **B,** A reception channel consists of an independent element *(E)*, amplifier (AMP), analog-to-digital converter (ADC), and delay. The signals from many channels are combined in the summer (SUM).

FIGURE 4-9 **Transmit/receive (T/R) switch. A,** During transmission (energizing the transducer to send a pulse into the body), the T/R switch opens the path from the pulser to the transducer elements. **B,** During echo reception, the T/R switch opens the path from the elements to the reception amplifiers.

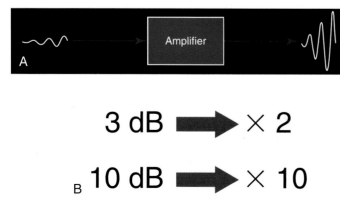

FIGURE 4-10 **Gain. A,** Amplification (gain) increases voltage amplitude and electric power. **B,** A gain of 3 dB corresponds to an output power equivalent to input power × 2; 10 dB corresponds to an input power × 10.

or gas). For a 60-dB gain amplifier, the output power is 1,000,000 times the power input, and the output voltage is 1000 times the input. For a 10-μV voltage input, the output voltage is 10 mV. If the gain of this amplifier is increased to 100 dB, the output voltage increases to 1 V.

> Amplifiers increase voltage amplitudes. This is called *gain*.

Two useful decibel values to remember are 3 and 10 (Figure 4-10, *B*). Whereas 3 dB corresponds to a power gain of ×2, 10 dB corresponds to ×10. Values also can be combined; for example, 6 dB corresponds to two doublings (×4); 20 dB corresponds to ×10×10, or ×100; and 13 dB corresponds to ×10×2, or ×20.

Gain control (Figure 4-11) determines how much amplification is accomplished in the amplifier. Gain control is similar in function to the level control on your sound system at home. With too little gain, weak echoes are not imaged. With too much gain, saturation occurs; that is, most echoes appear bright, and differences in echo strength are lost.

> Gain is set subjectively so that echoes appear with appropriate brightnesses.

The amplifiers must also compensate for the effect of attenuation on the **image. Compensation** (also called **time gain compensation** [TGC] and **depth gain compensation**) equalizes differences in received echo amplitudes caused by different reflector depths. Reflectors with equal reflection coefficients will not result in echoes of equal amplitude arriving at the transducer (Figure 4-12) if their travel distances are different (i.e., if the distances between the transducer and the reflectors are different) because sound weakens as it travels (attenuation). Display of echoes from similar reflectors in a similar way is desirable. As these echoes may not arrive with the same amplitude because of different path lengths, their amplitudes must be adjusted to compensate for differences in attenuation. Longer path lengths result in greater attenuation and later arrival times. Therefore if voltages from echoes arriving later are amplified correctly to a greater degree than are earlier ones, attenuation compensation is accomplished. This is the goal of compensation (Figure 4-13). In other words, the later an echo arrives, the farther it has traveled and the weaker it will be. However, the later it arrives, the more it will be amplified. If this compensation is done properly, the resulting amplitude will be the same as if there had been no attenuation.

The increase of gain with depth is commonly called *time gain compensation slope* because it is sometimes displayed graphically as a line with increasing deflection to the right. This slope can be expressed in decibels of gain per centimeter of depth. When properly adjusted,

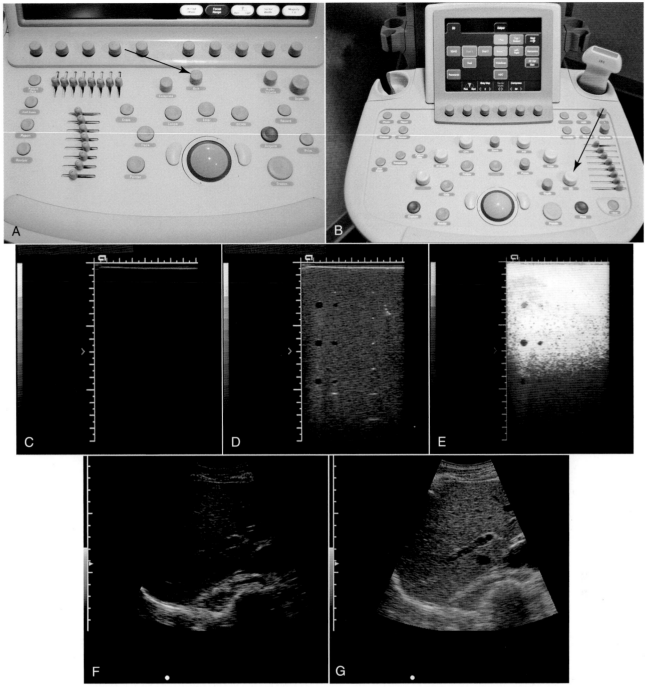

FIGURE 4-11 **A-B,** Gain controls *(arrows).* **C,** Gain is too low. **D,** Proper gain. **E,** Gain is too high, causing saturation. Abdominal scans with low **(F)** and proper **(G)** gain.

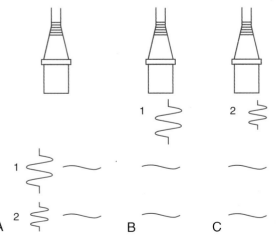

FIGURE 4-12 **Two identical reflectors are located at different distances from the transducer. A,** The echo at the second reflector is weaker because the incident pulse had to travel farther to get there, thereby increasing attenuation. **B,** The echo from the first reflector arrives at the transducer. The echo is weaker than it was in **A** because of attenuation on the return trip. **C,** The echo from the second reflector arrives at the transducer later and in a weaker form than the first one did because of the longer path to the second reflector.

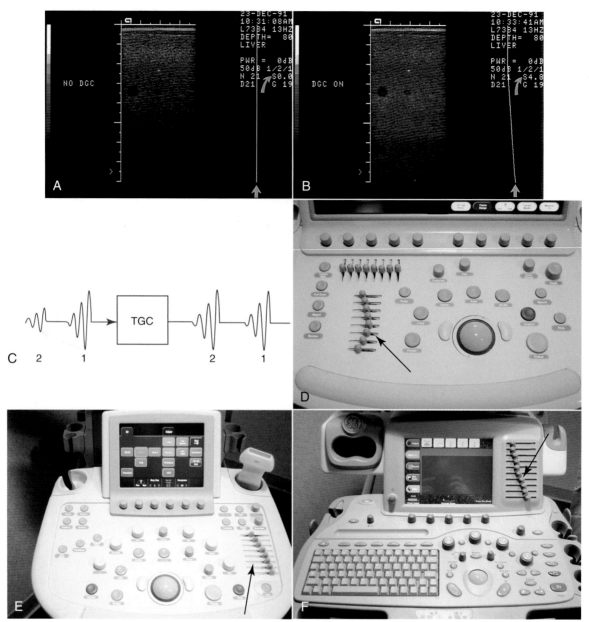

FIGURE 4-13 Time gain compensation (TGC). Two scans of a tissue-equivalent phantom imaged at 7 MHz without **(A)** and with **(B)** depth gain compensation (DGC). Without DGC, the echo brightness (amplitude, intensity, strength) declines with depth (top to bottom). On the display, DGC settings are shown graphically *(straight arrows)*. The slopes *(curved arrows)* are 0 dB/cm **(A)** and 4.8 dB/cm **(B)**. Average tissue attenuation is 0.5 dB/cm-MHz. This is calculated per centimeter of sound propagation. Average attenuation then is 1 dB/cm-MHz when the centimeter value is the distance from the transducer to the reflector. The sound must travel twice this distance (round-trip), so the attenuation number doubles. Typical DGC slopes then will be about 1 dB/cm-MHz. **C,** Uncompensated echoes from identical structures at differing depths enter the TGC amplifier. The second (2) is weaker than the first (1) because it has come from a deeper site and has experienced more attenuation. After TGC, the amplitudes are identical. **D-F,** Time gain compensation controls *(arrows)* on several instruments.

the slope should correspond to the average attenuation coefficient in the tissue, expressed in decibels per centimeter of depth. Remember that each centimeter of depth corresponds to 2 cm of round-trip sound travel, so the resulting slope should be about 1 dB/cm-MHz because average attenuation in soft tissue is 0.5 dB/cm-MHz. The former refers to centimeters of depth, whereas the latter refers to centimeters of travel. Because attenuation depends on the frequency of the ultrasound beam, the operator subjectively adjusts the time gain compensation to compensate for the frequency used and the attenuation of the tissues being imaged. Time gain compensation is set by the operator to achieve, on average, uniform brightness throughout the image. The average attenuation in the tissue cross-section at the operating frequency has been compensated when this is accomplished.

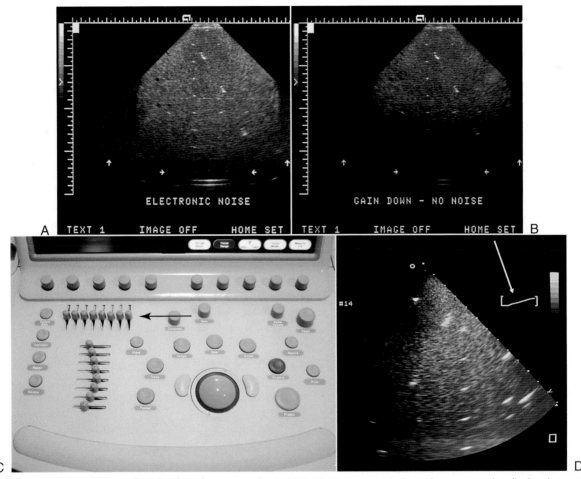

FIGURE 4-14 A, Under conditions of high gain, electronic noise (with its fuzzy appearance) can be seen on the display *(arrows).* **B,** With reduced gain, these weak voltages are not amplified enough to be visualized. **C,** Lateral gain controls *(arrow).* **D,** Lateral gain adjusted to increase gain from left to right.

 Time gain compensates for the effect of attenuation on an image.

Typical time gain compensation amplifiers compensate for about 60 dB of attenuation. At the depth at which maximum gain has been achieved, the echo brightness begins to decrease because the time gain compensation can no longer compensate (the amplifier gain cannot be increased further). Thus attenuation and maximum amplifier gain determine the maximum imaging depth. Maximum amplifier gain is determined by noise. Electronic noise (Figure 4-14, *A-B*) exists in all electronic circuits. High-quality input amplifier circuit noise levels are a few microvolts in amplitude. At maximum gain, the amplifier noise and the weak echoes being amplified have comparable amplitude. Any further increase in gain would only increase the noise, with weaker echoes being lost in the noise and thus being unobservable.

Some instruments have **lateral gain control,** which allows adjustment of gain laterally across the image (Figure 4-14, *C-D*). Regions with different attenuation values located laterally to each other can be compensated to yield similar image brightnesses.

The overall gain control is adjusted first to yield a perceptible image on the display. Then the time gain compensation (and possibly the lateral gain) controls are adjusted to yield on-average uniform brightness over the image. Attenuation variations throughout the image are thus compensated for, yielding a good representation of the tissue cross-section imaged.

Digitizers

After amplification, the echo voltages are digitized; that is, they pass through analog-to-digital converters (ADCs). An ADC (also called *digitizer*) converts the voltage from **analog** to **digital** form (Figure 4-15). The term *analog* means "proportional," and the term *digital* means "in the form of discrete numbers." Thus far in the instrument, the echo voltage has been proportional to the echo pressure. After the ADC, echo voltages are replaced by series of numbers and further manipulation of the echoes is accomplished as digital signal processing (mathematical manipulation of numbers

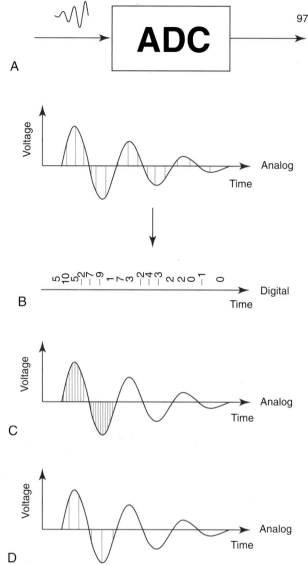

FIGURE 4-15 A, The analog-to-digital converter (ADC) converts **(B)** the analog (proportional) echo voltage into a series of numbers representing the sampled voltage. The higher the sampling rate of the analog-to-digital converter, the better the temporal detail of the voltage is preserved. **C,** High sampling rate. **D,** Low sampling rate.

representing echoes). This is similar to what is done in all digital electronics such as CD and DVD players and digital cellular telephones that handle, store, and process sound and pictures in digital form. The ADC interrogates the incoming voltage at regular intervals and determines its value at each interrogation instant. The interrogation rate must be twice the highest frequency involved in the interrogated voltage to preserve (in the subsequent digital number stream) all the harmonics contained in the interrogated voltage. For example, to digitize a 5-MHz continuous wave voltage properly, the digitizing rate must be at least 10 MHz; that is, the voltage is interrogated 10 million times per second, yielding a stream of 10 million digitized values per second describing the original analog voltage.

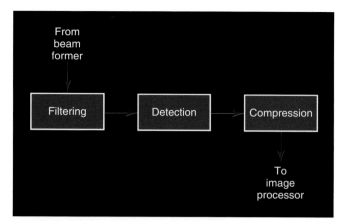

FIGURE 4-16 The signal processor performs filtering, detection, and compression functions. The processor receives digital signals from the beam former and, after processing, sends them on to the image processor.

 Analog-to-digital converters convert the analog voltages representing echoes to numbers for digital signal processing and storage.

Echo Delays

After amplification and digitizing, the echo voltages pass through digital delay lines to accomplish reception dynamic focus and steering functions.

Summer (Adder)

After all the channel signal components are delayed properly to accomplish the focus and steering functions, they are added together in the adder to produce the resulting scan line, which, along with all the others, will be displayed after signal processing and image processing. Reception apodization and dynamic aperture functions are also accomplished as part of this summing process.

The beam former is responsible for electronic beam scanning, steering, focusing, apodization, and aperture functions with arrays.

SIGNAL PROCESSOR

The reception portion of the beam former amplifies and combines the contributions from the individual elements and channels to form the stream of echoes returning from each transmitted pulse and sends them on to the signal processor. Operations carried out here include filtering, **detection**, and **compression**. The signal processor is diagrammed in Figure 4-16. Box 4-2 lists the functions of the signal processor.

Filtering

Tuned amplifiers are used to reduce noise in the electronics. They operate at a specific frequency with a

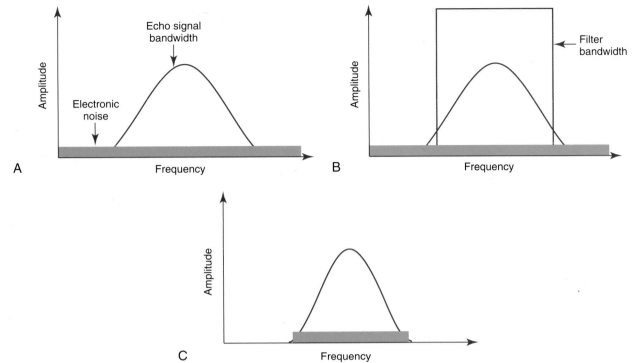

FIGURE 4-17 **A,** Input to filter includes the echo signal bandwidth and the electronic noise with unlimited bandwidth. **B,** The filter bandwidth is designed to accommodate the signal bandwidth. **C,** The output from the filter has the frequencies above and below its bandwidth removed. Only the noise frequencies within the filter bandwidth remain.

BOX 4-2	Functions of the Signal Processor

- Bandpass filtering
- Amplitude detection
- Compression (dynamic range reduction)

bandwidth that includes the frequencies in the returning echoes and eliminates the electronic noise outside that bandwidth. A tuned amplifier is simply an amplifier with an electronic filter called *bandpass filter*. A **bandpass filter** is one that passes a range of frequencies (its bandwidth) and rejects those above and below the acceptance bandwidth (Figure 4-17). Some tuned amplifiers dynamically move the frequency range of the filter to track the bandwidth of the returning series of echoes from a pulse. The echo bandwidth decreases as the echoes return because the higher frequencies in the bandwidth are attenuated more than the lower ones.

Filtering eliminates frequencies outside the echo bandwidth while retaining those that are most useful in a given type of operation.

Harmonic Imaging

A second type of filtering occurs with harmonic imaging, in which the fundamental (transmitted) frequency is filtered out and the second harmonic frequency echoes are passed. (The generation of harmonic frequencies in tissue is discussed in Chapter 2.) At

this point, the bandpass filter is centered at the second harmonic frequency with an appropriate bandwidth to include the bandwidth of the second harmonic echo signal (Figure 4-18, *A-D*). Harmonic imaging improves the image quality in three primary ways (Figure 4-18, *E-F*):

- The primary beam is much narrower, improving lateral resolution, because harmonics are generated only in the highest-intensity portion of the beam.
- Grating lobe artifacts are eliminated because these extra beams are not sufficiently strong to generate the harmonics.
- Because the harmonic beam is generated at a depth beyond where some of the artifactual problems occur (e.g., superficial reverberation), the image degradation that they cause is reduced or eliminated.

Because the fundamental and second harmonic bandwidths must fit within the overall transducer bandwidth (Figure 4-19, *A*), they must be reasonably narrow. This means that the corresponding ultrasound pulses must be somewhat longer than otherwise, causing some degradation in axial resolution. A solution to this degradation in image quality is to use pulse inversion, a technique that uses two pulses per scan line rather than one. The second pulse is the inverse of the first. The echo sequences from the two pulses (Figure 4-19, *B*) are added together to yield the resulting scan line.

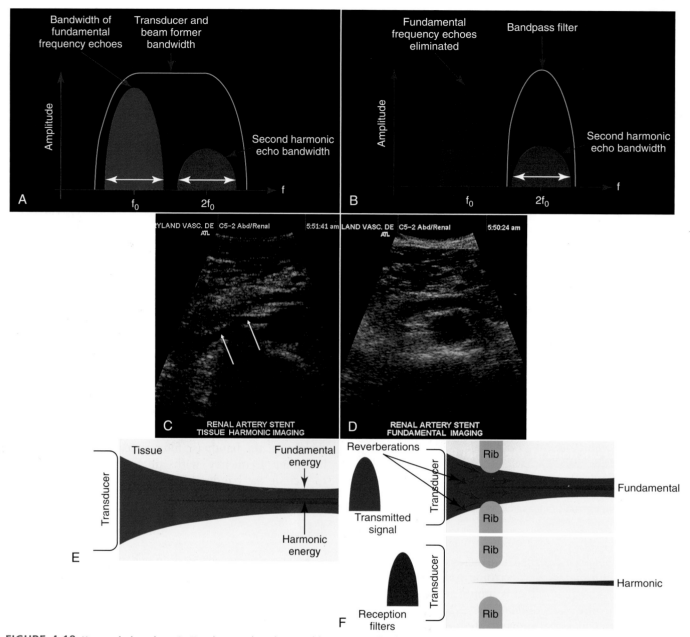

FIGURE 4-18 Harmonic imaging. A, Fundamental and second-harmonic echo bandwidths are shown. The beam former and transducer must pass both to generate the ultrasound beam and to accomplish harmonic imaging. **B,** For harmonic imaging, the bandpass filter eliminates the fundamental frequency echoes and passes the second harmonic echoes. The harmonic image **(C)** has improved quality compared with the fundamental-frequency image **(D). E,** The harmonic beam is much narrower than the fundamental. **F,** Reverberations are reduced with the harmonic beam.

Fundamental frequency echoes are cancelled (Figure 4-19, *C*), and the second harmonic echoes remain (Figure 4-19, *D*). This technique allows broad-bandwidth, short pulses to be used so that detail resolution is not degraded (Figure 4-19, *E*). Instead, the frame rate is reduced, with some degradation of **temporal resolution.**

Detection

Detection (also called **demodulation**) is the conversion of echo voltages from **radio frequency** form to amplitude form (Figure 4-20). This is done by detecting and connecting together the maxima of the cyclic variations. The cyclic voltage form is called *radio frequency* because it is similar to voltages found in a radio receiver, and the frequencies are similar to those in the low end of the shortwave radio band. The detected form retains the amplitudes. Because diagnostic ultrasound pulses do not have constant amplitude, when demodulated, they do not have the simplified blocked appearance shown in Figure 4-20. Detection is not an operator-controllable function.

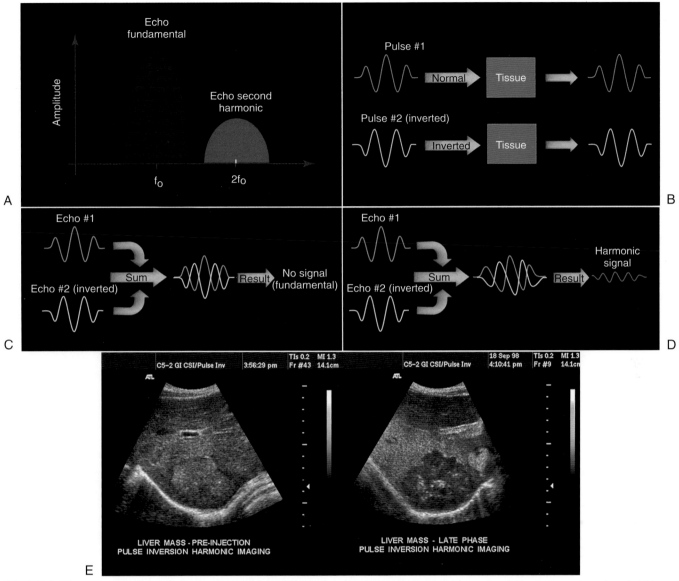

FIGURE 4-19 **A,** In harmonic imaging, two bandwidths (fundamental and second harmonic) must fit within the transducer bandwidth and not overlap so that the fundamental frequency echoes can be eliminated from the second harmonic image. **B,** In pulse inversion harmonic imaging, a normal pulse of ultrasound is followed by an inverted pulse. Two series of echoes return from these two pulses (only one echo is shown for each pulse in this drawing). When the echoes from the two pulses are summed, the fundamental frequency echoes cancel **(C),** whereas the second harmonic echoes are not canceled **(D). E,** Pre- and postinjection abdominal images using a contrast agent and pulse inversion harmonic imaging.

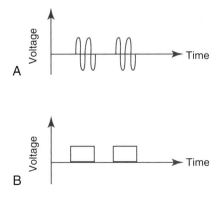

FIGURE 4-20 Echo voltages are produced in a complicated cyclic form **(A)** called *radio frequency* (RF), which would be difficult to store and display. Furthermore, only the amplitude of each echo is needed for a gray-scale display of anatomy. Thus the radio frequency form is converted to amplitude form **(B),** which retains the amplitude of each echo voltage.

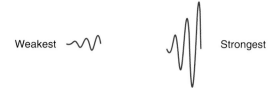

Weakest ~~~∿∿∧~~~   ~~~∿∿∿~~~ Strongest

FIGURE 4-21 Dynamic range is the relationship between the weakest and strongest echoes and is expressed in decibels.

 Detection is the conversion of echo voltages from radio frequency form to video form. The video form retains amplitudes of the echo voltages.

Compression

The ratio of the largest to the smallest amplitude or power that a system can handle is called **dynamic range** (Figure 4-21). Dynamic range is expressed in decibels. For example, if an amplifier is insensitive to voltage amplitudes of less than 0.01 mV (because they are buried in the electronic noise) and cannot properly handle voltage amplitudes of greater than 1000 mV, the ratio of usable voltage extremes is 1000/0.01, or 100,000. The power ratio is equal to the square of the voltage ratio: $100,000^2$, or 10,000,000,000. According to Table 4-1, the dynamic range of the amplifier is 100 dB. Amplifiers have typical dynamic ranges of 100 to 120 dB. System dynamic ranges are claimed to be as high as 170 dB. Greater values indicate the ability to detect weaker echoes, that is, greater sensitivity. The higher dynamic ranges assume some bandwidth reduction (to reduce electronic noise) and improvement yielded by the reception beam–forming process with several reception channels. Other portions of the electronics (especially the display) have much smaller dynamic range capability. Displays have dynamic ranges of up to 30 dB. Furthermore, human vision is limited to a dynamic range of about 20 dB. The largest power (brightness) can be only about 100 times the smallest for our viewing of the display. Thus the largest voltage amplitude can be only about 10 times the smallest. The echo dynamic range remaining after compensation is typically 50 to 100 dB. Compression is the process of decreasing the differences between the smallest and the largest echo amplitudes to a usable range (Figure 4-22). Amplifiers that amplify weak inputs more than strong ones accomplish this. A compressor would have to compress the intensity ratio (100,000) corresponding to 50 dB to an intensity ratio of 100 (acceptable for the display).

 Compression reduces dynamic range with selective amplification.

Compression is operator adjustable as a dynamic range control (Figure 4-23). This control reduces dynamic

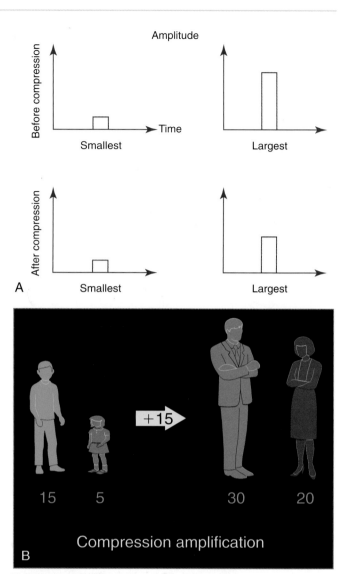

FIGURE 4-22 Compression decreases the difference between the smallest and largest amplitudes passing through the system. A, In this example, the ratio of largest to smallest amplitudes before compression is 5. After compression, the ratio is 3. **B,** A family illustration of compression amplification. Big brother (age 15 years) is twice as tall (large dynamic range) as his little sister (age 5 years). Fifteen years later, the brother (age 30 years) is just slightly taller than the sister (age 20 years). Both have grown (amplification), but the shorter child grew more than the taller one, reducing the difference between them (compression).

range by assigning some weak echo amplitude values to zero or by assigning some of the strongest to maximum. Reassigned echoes may be at either end of the dynamic range or at both ends (Figure 4-23, *J-L*). A smaller dynamic range setting presents a higher-contrast image. Gain control moves the dynamic range curve to the left or right (down or up the dynamic range) as gain is increased or decreased (Figure 4-23, *M-N*).

 Signal processing includes digital filtering, detection, and compression of echo data.

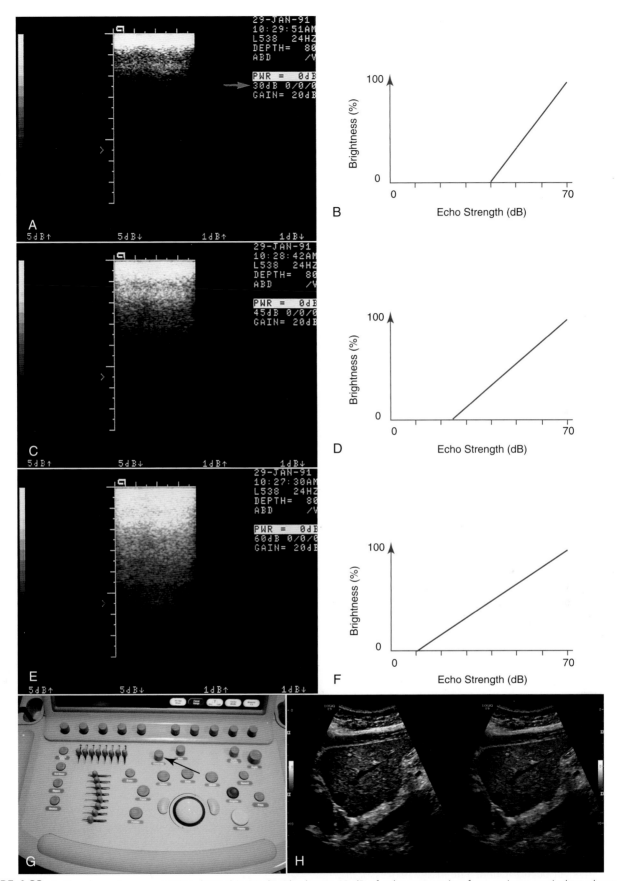

FIGURE 4-23 A, The dynamic range setting *(arrow)* is 30 dB. The lower 40 dB of echoes returning from a tissue-equivalent phantom are set to 0 *(black portion)*. The remainder show high contrast, with brightness progressing from black for 40-dB echoes to white for 70-dB echoes. **B,** A 30-dB dynamic range setting assigns the weakest 40 dB of echo dynamic range to zero *(black)* and the remaining 30 dB of dynamic range to linearly higher brightnesses. **C,** A display with a dynamic range of 45 dB. **D,** Brightness assignment for a 45-dB dynamic range. **E,** A display with a dynamic range of 60 dB. **F,** Brightness assignment for a 60-dB dynamic range. **G,** Compression control *(arrow)*. **H,** Dynamic range 54 dB *(left)* and 72 dB *(right)*.

Continued

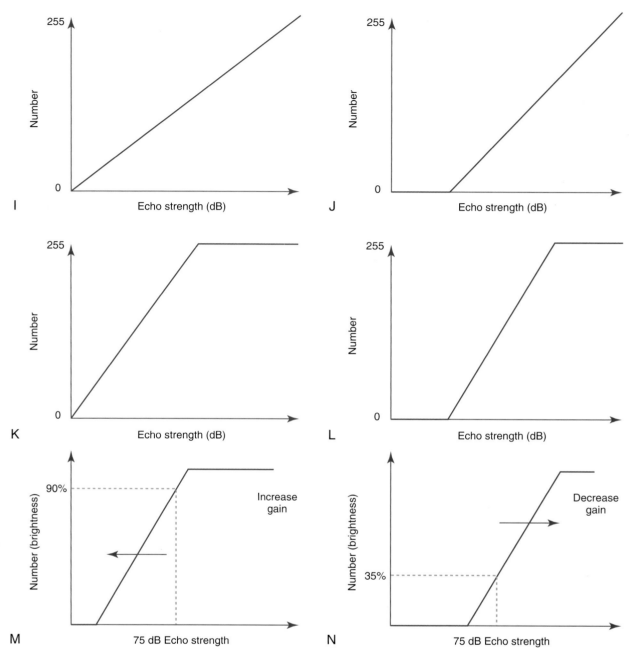

FIGURE 4-23, cont'd I, Full system dynamic range displayed. **J,** Dynamic range reduced by setting a weaker portion to 0 *(black).* **K,** Dynamic range reduced by setting a stronger portion to maximum *(white).* **L,** Dynamic range reduced by setting weaker and stronger portions to black and white, respectively. **M,** This curve of brightness versus echo strength moves to the left as gain is increased. A midrange echo appears bright. **N,** The curve moves to the right for decreasing gain. The midrange echo appears dark.

IMAGE PROCESSOR

Up to this point (through the beam former and signal processor), the echo data are traveling in scan-line form serially through the system, that is, one scan line at a time. No image has yet been formed. The image processor converts the digitized, filtered, detected, and compressed serial scan-line data into images that are processed before and after storage in **image memory,** all in preparation for presentation on the instrument display. Following detection of the echo voltage amplitudes in the signal proces-

sor, the scan-line data enter the image processor, where they are converted into image form by scan conversion and then are processed in image form (Figure 4-24). Box 4-3 lists the functions of the image processor.

Scan Conversion

Using a computer-monitor scan format, digital scan converters provide means for displaying the acquired information in a linear or sector ultrasound scan-line format. Information about the direction of each scan line and the

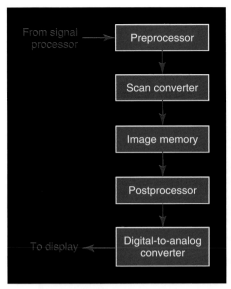

FIGURE 4-24 The image processor converts scan-line data into images, processes the images before storing them in the image memory, processes them as they come out of the memory, converts them from digital form to analog form, and sends them on to the display.

BOX 4-3	Functions of the Image Processor

- Scan conversion
- Preprocessing
- Persistence
- Panoramic imaging
- Spatial compounding
- Three-dimensional acquisition
- Storing image frames
- Cine loop
- Postprocessing
- Gray scale
- Color scale
- Three-dimensional presentation
- Digital-to-analog conversion

location of echoes in depth down each scan line is used to determine the proper location in the memory (and thus on the display) for each echo. For example, a pulse emitted from the transducer straight down into the body will result in a series of echoes that are located in appropriate memory locations straight down a column in memory at various depths, that is, various row locations (Figure 4-25, *A*). A pulse emitted in an off-vertical direction will result in a series of echoes that must be located in various rows and columns (Figure 4-25, *B*). The **scan converter** properly locates each series of echoes corresponding to each scan line for each pulse emitted from the transducer, filling up the memory with echo information. This is accomplished in a fraction of a second, yielding one scan or **frame** of image information. This process is repeated several times per second to produce a rapid sequence of frames stored in the memory and

presented on the display. This rapid-sequence presentation is called **real-time display**, and the entire process is called *real-time sonography*. Image depth control (Figure 4-25, *C*) determines the depth to be displayed and thus the depth range covered by the image memory in the scan conversion process.

 The scan converter formats echo data into image form for image processing, storage, and display.

Preprocessing

Prior to the scan conversion process (scan-line information going into the image memory), various processing functions may be performed on the image. This is called **preprocessing** because it occurs before the echo data are stored in the image memory. Examples of preprocessing include edge enhancement (a function that sharpens boundaries to make them more detectable and measurements more precise), pixel interpolation, **persistence**, **panoramic imaging**, **spatial compounding**, and three-dimensional (3D) acquisition.

 Preprocessing is signal and image processing done before echo data are stored in the memory.

Pixel Interpolation

Image improvement can be accomplished by filling in missing pixels. A common situation where this occurs is in sector scans in which scan lines have increasing separation with distance from the transducer and intervening pixels are left out. Interpolation assigns a brightness value to a missed **pixel** based on an average of brightnesses of adjacent pixels (Figure 4-25, *D*).

Persistence

Persistence is the averaging of sequential frames for providing a smoother image appearance and for reduction of noise (Figure 4-26). Noise, primarily speckle, is reduced because it is a random process. When several frames containing random content are averaged, the random content is reduced. Speckle reduction improves dynamic range and contrast resolution. But frame averaging, in effect, reduces frame rate because averaged frames are no longer independent. Operator control permits averaging of a selectable number of sequential frames from zero up to some maximum. Lower levels of persistence, or none at all, are appropriate for following rapidly moving structures. Higher levels are appropriate for slower-moving structures.

 Persistence reduces noise and smoothes the image by frame averaging.

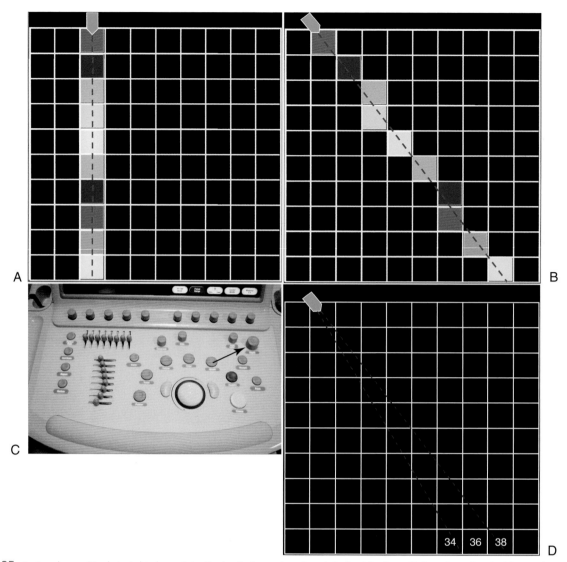

FIGURE 4-25 **A,** A pulse emitted straight down into the body *(arrowhead and dashed line)* results in echoes located in a column of memory locations. **B,** A pulse emitted in another direction results in echoes located in various rows and columns. **C,** Image depth control. **D,** Pixel interpolation. Part of the image memory pixel grid is shown along with the paths of two pulses. At the bottom of the grid, the paths have separated sufficiently so that the pixel between them is missed. The interpolation calculation determines the mean value of the two adjacent pixels (34 and 38), which is 36. That value then is entered in the intervening pixel.

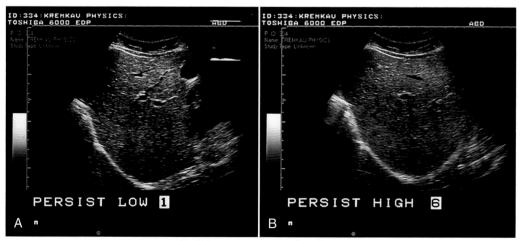

FIGURE 4-26 **A,** Persistence off. **B,** Persistence on.

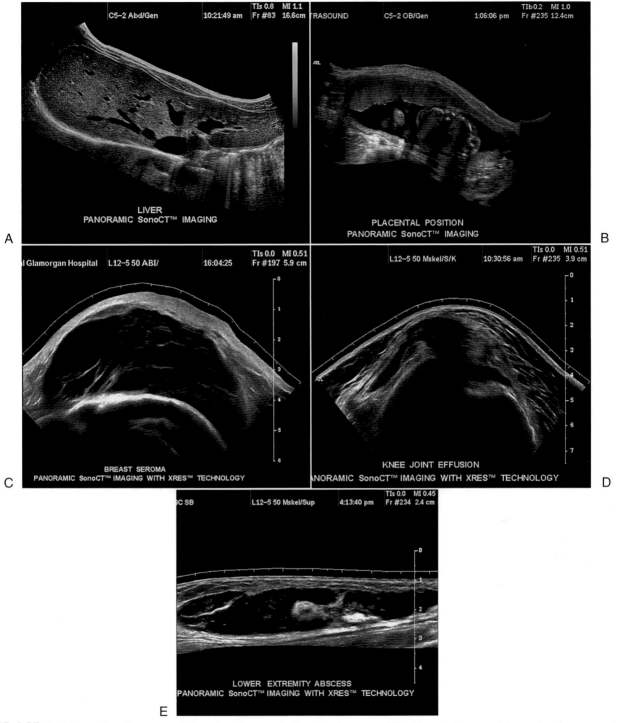

FIGURE 4-27 **A-E,** Examples of panoramic imaging. Panoramic imaging is accomplished by adding new information to one end of an image, spatially correlating the overlapping old echoes to properly locate the new ones.

Continued

Panoramic Imaging

Panoramic imaging provides a way to produce an image that has a wider field of view than what is available on an individual frame from a transducer. Panoramic imaging is achieved by manually sliding the transducer in a direction parallel to the scan plane, thus extending

the scan plane. At the same time, the old echo information from previous frames is retained, while the new echoes are added to the image in the direction in which the scan plane is moving. The result is a larger field of view allowing presentation of large organs and regions of anatomy on one image (Figure 4-27). During the addition of new echoes, as the transducer is moved, it is

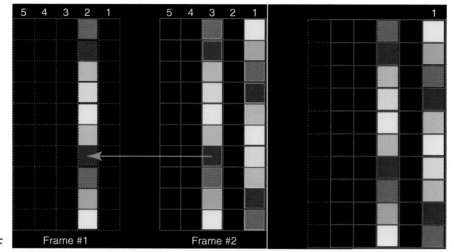

FIGURE 4-27, cont'd F, Two sequential frames are shown; frame No. 2 temporally follows frame No. 1. Frame No. 2 is located slightly to the right of frame No. 1 in the anatomy by manual movement of the transducer by the sonographer. Thus a new scan line is added to frame No. 2. Scan line No. 3 in the new frame corresponds to scan line No. 2 in the previous frame. A spatial correlation process in the image processor identifies the equality of these two scan lines. Frame No. 2 then is slid to the left over the top of frame No. 1 so that the identical scan lines in the two frames overlap. **G,** The new scan line is thus added properly to the old frame. This process is repeated many times as the transducer is moved in a direction parallel to the scan plane. The old scan lines are retained as the new ones are added to the image.

important to properly locate the new echoes relative to the existing image. This is accomplished by correlating locations of echoes common to adjacent frames (i.e., the overlap) so that the new information on the new frame is located properly (Figure 4-27, *F-G*).

 Panoramic imaging expands the image beyond the normal limits of the field of view of the transducer.

Spatial Compounding

Spatial compounding is a technique in which scan lines are directed in multiple directions by phasing so that structures are interrogated more than once by the ultrasound beam (Figure 4-28). Averaging sequential frames spatially, up to nine typically, improves the quality of the image in several ways:

- As in persistence (which is temporal averaging), speckle is reduced.
- Clutter caused by artifacts is reduced.
- Smooth (specular) surfaces are presented more completely because they are interrogated at more than one angle, increasing the probability that close to 90-degree incidence is achieved (which is necessary to receive echoes from them).
- Structures previously hidden beneath highly attenuating objects can be visualized.

 Spatial compounding is the averaging of frames that view the anatomy from different angles.

Elastography

For several years, an ultrasound imaging mode termed *elastography*[3] has been studied. It has now become commercially available. By subjecting tissues to a small push (by the sonographer using a push on the transducer or a high-amplitude ultrasound pulse) and then tracking the movement of tissues, it is possible to estimate and depict tissue stiffness since soft tissues will move more than hard ones. Essentially, **elastography** is the imaging version of palpation. It is commonly shown as a color overlay on top of the gray-scale image (Figure 4-29) and has been used clinically for cancer detection, for characterization of small parts (breast, thyroid, and prostate), for assessing the viability of the myocardium, and for monitoring therapies that alter tissue composition, such as ablation procedures.

Volume Imaging

Three-dimensional imaging (**volume imaging**) is accomplished by acquiring many parallel two-dimensional (2D-slice imaging) scans (Figure 4-30, *A*) and then processing this 3D volume of echo information in appropriate ways for presentation on 2D displays. The multiple 2D frames are obtained by (1) manual scanning of the transducer, with position-sensing devices keeping track of scan-plane location and orientation; (2) automated mechanically scanned transducers; or (3) electronic scanning with 2D element-array transducers. Common ways of presenting the 3D echo data include surface renderings (Figure 4-30, *B*), 2D slices through the 3D volume, and transparent views. The advantage of the 2D slice presentation is that it is possible to present image-plane orientations that are impossible to obtain with conventional 2D scanning.

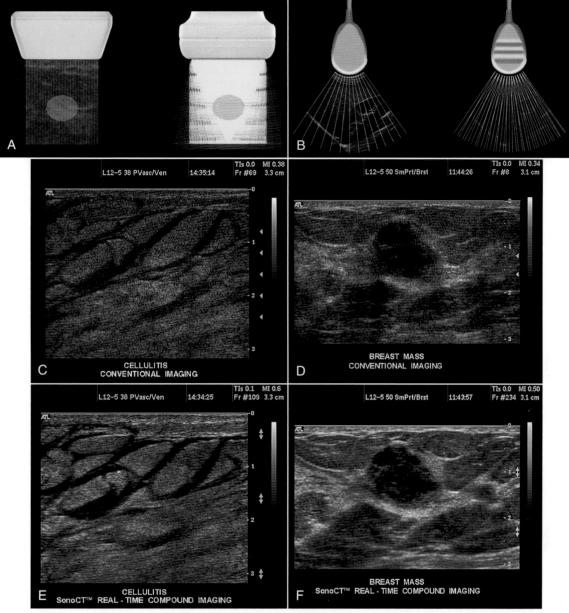

FIGURE 4-28 Conventional scan lines and spatial compounding with **(A)** linear array and **(B)** convex array. A comparison of conventional imaging **(C-D)** with compound imaging **(E-F)** shows improvement in image quality.

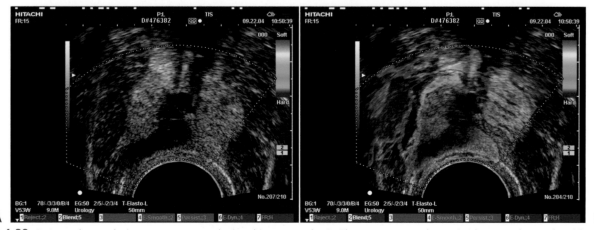

FIGURE 4-29 A, Large hypoechoic prostate tumor depicted in gray-scale. **B,** The same tumor shown in elastography mode with red colors signifying soft tissues and blue colors signifying hard tissue. The designations as "soft" and "hard" are relative to the maximum stiffness found in the image. Note the soft edges of the gland and the harder tumor.

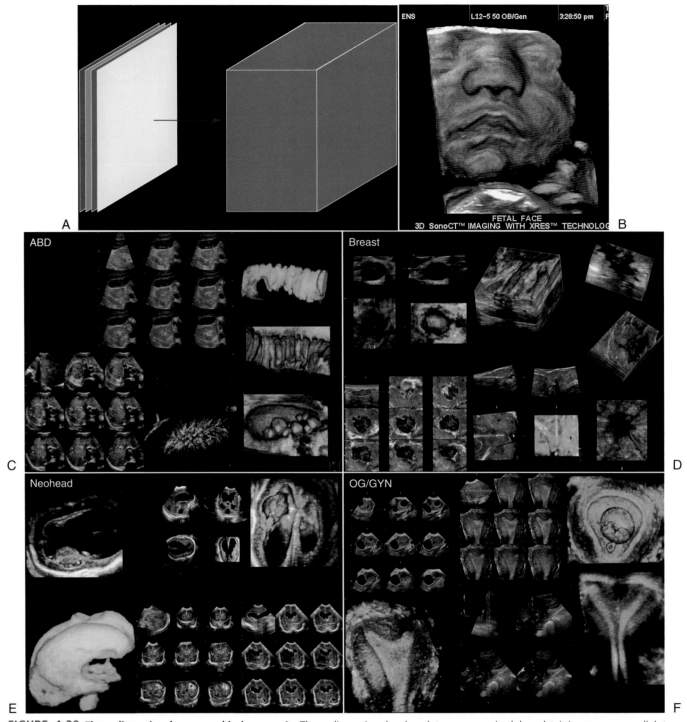

FIGURE 4-30 Three-dimensional sonographic images. A, Three-dimensional echo data are acquired by obtaining many parallel two-dimensional sections of echo information from the imaged anatomy yielding **(B)** a three-dimensional fetal surface-rendered image. **C-H,** Various presentations of volume imaging of the abdomen, breast, neonatal head, obstetric/gynecologic cases, testicle, and blood vessel.

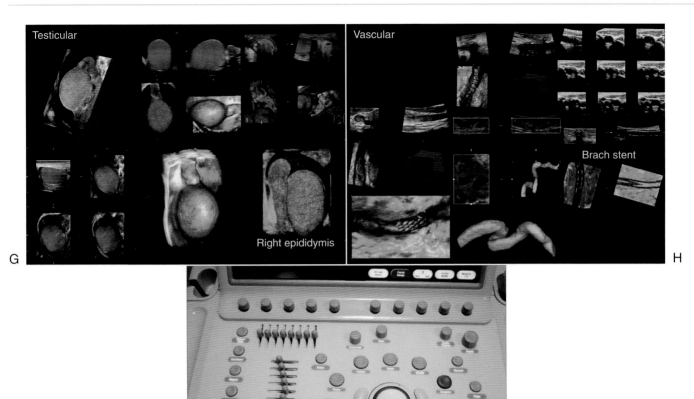

Testicular

Right epididymis

G

Vascular

Brach stent

H

I

FIGURE 4-30, cont'd I, The freeze button *(arrow)* stops the scanning and saves the last several image frames in the image memory.

Serial slice presentations like those in other imaging modes (magnetic resonance imaging [MRI] and computed tomography [CT]) can be presented (Figure 4-30, *C-H*). Surface renderings are popular in obstetric imaging. Transparent views allow "see-through" imaging of the anatomy as with plain film radiographs.

 Three-dimensional images are acquired by assembling several 2D scans into a 3D volume of echo information in the image memory.

Three-dimensional images can be acquired at rates of up to 30 volumes per second and thus are considered "live" or real-time presentations. The current tendency is to call this *4D imaging,* where the fourth dimension is time. Although this term sounds fashionable for marketing purposes, it is inconsistent with previous terminology; that is, real-time 2D imaging is not called 3D. Nevertheless, the moniker has, to some extent, caught on.

Image Memory

After echo data are preprocessed and scan-converted into image form, the image frames are stored in the image memory. Storing each image in the memory as the sound beam is scanned through the anatomy permits display of a single image (frame) out of the rapid sequence of several frames acquired each second in real-time sonographic instruments. Holding and displaying one frame out of the sequence is known as **freeze-frame** (Figure 4-30, *I*). Most instruments store the last several frames acquired before freezing. This is called **cine loop,** cine review, or image review feature.

Pixels and Bits

Image memories used in sonographic instruments are digital; that is, they are computer memories that store numbers (digits) as digital cameras do (Figure 4-31, *A*). The 2D image plane is divided like a checkerboard (Figure 4-31, *B*) into squares called *pixels* (picture elements), in a rectangular matrix, for example, 1024×768 or 512×384. The pixels number several thousands (786,432 and 196,608 in the previous examples), so they are tiny and not normally noticed unless magnified sufficiently. A number that corresponds to the echo strength received from the location within the anatomy corresponding to that memory position (Figure 4-31, *C*) is stored in each of the pixel locations in the memory. The more pixels there are, the finer is the spatial detail in the stored image

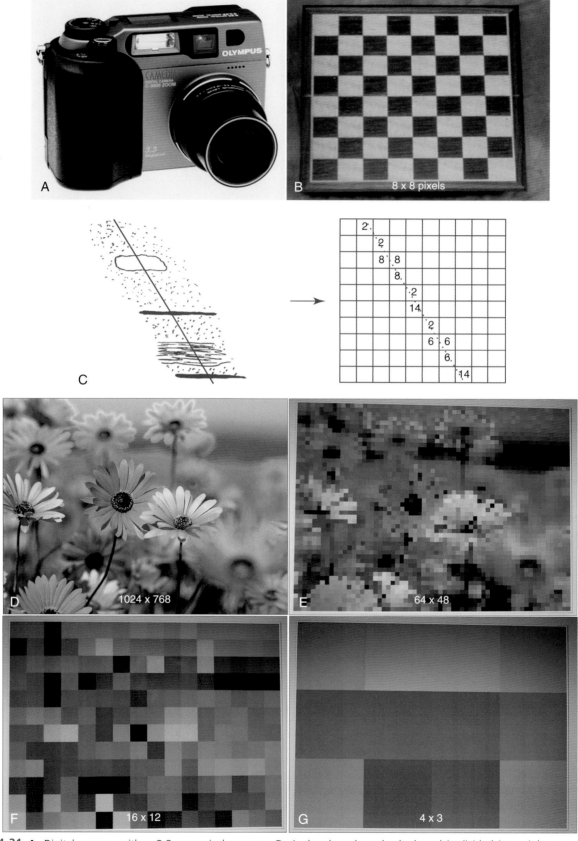

FIGURE 4-31 A, Digital camera with a 3.3 megapixel memory. **B,** A chessboard or checkerboard is divided into eight rows and eight columns of squares, for a total of 64 "pixels." **C,** Anatomic cross-section to be scanned, and the front view of a portion of the image memory. Numbers are stored in the memory elements according to the intensity of the echoes received from corresponding anatomic locations as an ultrasound pulse passes through them. **D-G,** Digital photos at pixel resolutions of 1024 × 768, 64 × 48, 16 × 12, 4 × 3, respectively.

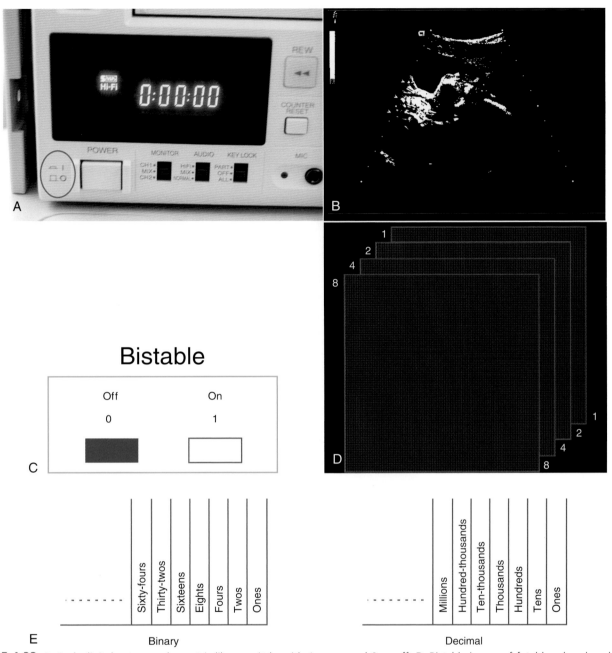

Bistable

FIGURE 4-32 **A,** Each digital memory element is like a switch, with 1 as on and 0 as off. **B,** Bistable image of fetal head and neck. **C,** In bistable imaging, only two values are used: memory element off represents 0 and is presented as black; memory element on represents 1 and is presented as white. **D,** A 10 × 10-pixel, 4-bit-deep (4 bits per pixel) digital memory. **E,** Columns in decimal numbers represent multiples of 10, whereas those in binary numbers represent multiples of 2. *Continued*

(Figure 4-31, *D-G*). If the digital memory were composed of a single-layer matrix checkerboard, each pixel location could store only one of two numbers: a zero or a one. The reason is that the memory element assigned to each pixel is an electronic device that is binary (*bi* meaning "two"), like an on–off switch (Figure 4-32, *A*) and so can operate only in two conditions corresponding to one or zero. This would allow only **bistable** (black-and-white) imaging (Figure 4-32, *B-C*). To image gray scale (several shades of gray or brightness, in addition to black and white), storage of one of several possible numbers in each memory location is necessary. This requires the memory

to have more than one matrix. These "checkerboards" can be thought of as being layered back to back. In a four-binary-digit memory, there are four checkerboards back to back (Figure 4-32, *D*) so that each pixel has 4 bits (binary digits) associated with it. In the binary numbering system, this allows numbers from 0 to 15 to be stored (a 16-shade system). Thus a 4-bit memory is a 16-shade memory. A 4-bit memory has four binary digits assigned to each pixel, that is, four layers of memory.

 The memory divides the image into pixels, such as a matrix of 512 × 384.

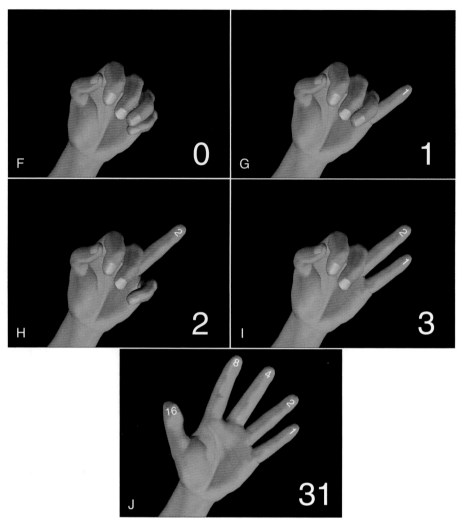

FIGURE 4-32, cont'd F-J, Conventional counting with fingers assigns the value 1 to each finger. Counting is much more efficient if different values are assigned to different fingers. Using the binary assignment procedure, each finger represents double the value of the previous finger. Normally we count only to 5 on one hand, but in this manner we can count to 31 (1 + 2 + 4 + 8 + 16) and to 1023 on two hands.

Binary Numbers

Because the memory elements are binary, digital memories use the binary numbering system to store echo information in the image memory. Computer memories and processors use binary numbers in carrying out their functions because they contain electronic components that operate in only two states, representing the numbers 0 and 1.

Binary digits (**bits**) consist of only zeros and ones, represented by their respective numeric symbols, 0 and 1. Other values must be represented by moving these symbols to different positions (columns). In the decimal system, in which there are 10 different symbols, 0 through 9, there is no single symbol for the number 10 (9 is the largest number for which there is a single symbol). To represent 10 in symbolic form then, the symbol for one is used, but it is moved to the left, to the second column. A 0 is placed in the right column to clarify this, resulting

in the symbol 10. The same symbol used to represent one is used, but in such a way—that is, in the second column—that it no longer represents one but rather ten.

A similar procedure is used in the binary numbering system. The symbol 1 represents the largest number (one) for which there is a symbol in this system. To represent the next number (two), the same thing is done as in the decimal system; that is, the symbol 1 is placed in the next column to represent the number 2. In this case, a 1 in the second column represents a value of 2 rather than 10, as in the decimal system. Columns in the two systems represent values as shown in Figure 4-32, *D-J*. In the decimal system, each column represents 10 times the column to its right. In the binary system, each column represents 2 times the column to its right.

Table 4-2 lists the binary forms of the decimal numbers 0 to 63. Numbers 64 to 127 would have one additional digit (representing the "sixty-fours" column), and so forth with higher multiples of 2.

Binary numbers use only the digits 0 and 1. Each column of a binary number represents double the column to its right.

Table 4-3 gives several examples of digital memories. Figure 4-32, *D*, shows a 4-bit (per pixel) memory. Table 4-4 gives the total number of memory elements in various digital memories. A group of 8 bits is called *byte*, and 1024 bytes (8192 bits) are called *kilobyte*. In today's ultrasound instruments, 6-, 7-, and 8-bit memories are present. Human vision can differentiate about 100 gray levels. More than the 256 shades of an 8-bit system are not directly perceived by human vision.

In summary, then, the procedure for entering the echo information required for display of the 2D cross-sectional image into a digital memory is as follows:

- The beam is scanned through the patient in such a way that it "cuts," like a knife, through the tissue cross-section.
- Echoes received from all points on this cross-section are converted to numbers that are stored at corresponding pixel locations in the digital memory.
- All the information necessary for displaying this cross-sectional image now is stored in the memory.
- The information then can be taken out of the memory and presented on a 2D display and in such a way that the numbers coming out of the memory are displayed with corresponding pixel brightnesses on the face of the display (Figure 4-33).

Figure 4-34 shows examples of such presentations. To enlarge the pixels, read magnification (sometimes called *zoom*) is used. In this presentation, rather than viewing all the pixels in the memory, the monitor shows a smaller group of pixels in expanded (magnified) fashion. This increases pixel size, making the pixel composition of the image more obvious. Read zoom is a postprocessing function. Write magnification is also available on some

TABLE 4-2	Binary and Decimal Number Equivalents		
Decimal	Binary	Decimal	Binary
0	000000	32	100000
1	000001	33	100001
2	000010	34	100010
3	000011	35	100011
4	000100	36	100100
5	000101	37	100101
6	000110	38	100110
7	000111	39	100111
8	001000	40	101000
9	001001	41	101001
10	001010	42	101010
11	001011	43	101011
12	001100	44	101100
13	001101	45	101101
14	001110	46	101110
15	001111	47	101111
16	010000	48	110000
17	010001	49	110001
18	010010	50	110010
19	010011	51	110011
20	010100	52	110100
21	010101	53	110101
22	010110	54	110110
23	010111	55	110111
24	011000	56	111000
25	011001	57	111001
26	011010	58	111010
27	011011	59	111011
28	011100	60	111100
29	011101	61	111101
30	011110	62	111110
31	011111	63	111111

TABLE 4-4	Bits (Binary Digits or Memory Elements) in Digital Memories With 512 × 512 (262,144) Pixels	
Bits per Pixel	Total Bits	Total Kilobytes*
4	1,048,576	128
5	1,310,720	160
6	1,572,864	192
7	1,835,008	224
8	2,097,152	256

*1 byte = 8 bits; 1 kilobyte = 1024 bytes, or 8192 bits.

TABLE 4-3	Characteristics of Digital Memories					
	Lowest Number Stored			Highest Number Stored		
Bits per Pixel	Decimal	Binary		Decimal	Binary	Number of Shades
4	0	0000		15	1111	16
5	0	00000		31	11111	32
6	0	000000		63	111111	64
7	0	0000000		127	1111111	128
8	0	00000000		255	11111111	256

FIGURE 4-33 For display of scanned anatomic structures, numbers are read out of pixel locations in digital memory **(A)** and applied to the display in such a way that pixel brightness corresponds to those stored numbers **(B)**. The display for the scan line acquired in Figure 4-31, *C*, is shown.

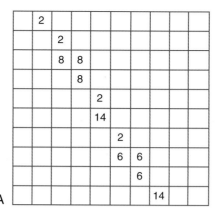

A

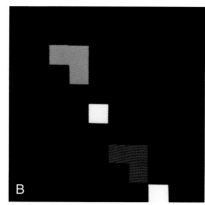

B

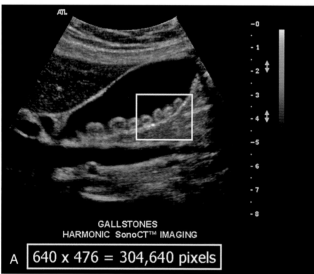

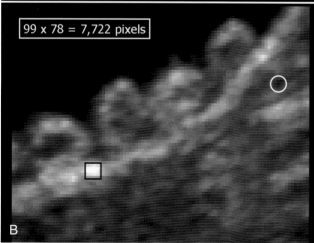

FIGURE 4-34 **Displays of pixels of various brightnesses representing various numbers in the corresponding memory locations.** The display is magnified *(zoom)* here to make the square pixels more easily discernible. Normally, the pixels are too small and numerous to be noticed individually. **A,** Unmagnified abdominal image containing 304,640 unresolved pixels. The box encloses the region magnified in **B.** Magnification reveals the 7722 pixels included within the box in **A.** The circle and the box enclose regions of small and large numbers in the image memory, respectively.

instruments. This allows a smaller anatomic field of view to be written into the entire memory, thereby enlarging the image without enlarging pixel size (Figure 4-35). Write zoom is a preprocessing function.

Digital (derived from the Latin term *digitus*, meaning "finger" or "toe") memories are discrete rather than continuous, which means that they can store only whole numbers in each pixel location. These numbers range from zero to a maximum that is determined by the number of bits per pixel (see Table 4-3).

For a 256 × 512 matrix in which the represented anatomic width and depth are 10 and 20 cm, respectively, each pixel represents an anatomic dimension of 0.4 mm. This represents the spatial (detail) resolution of the memory matrix. If the width and depth are 5 and 10 cm, then the memory spatial resolution is 0.2 mm. Detail resolution is usually limited by spatial pulse length and beam width rather than by pixel density in the memory.

Contrast Resolution

For linear assignment of echo intensities to numbers in the memory, the echo dynamic range is equally divided throughout the gray levels of the system. Table 4-5 gives, for 4- to 8-bit systems, the number of decibels of dynamic range covered by each shade (for two different echo dynamic range values, 40 dB and 60 dB, after attenuation compensation) and the average intensity difference between two echoes for them to be assigned to different shades (different numbers) in the memory. This relates to contrast resolution, which is the ability visually to observe subtle echo strength differences between adjacent tissues. Increasing the number of bits per pixel (more gray shades) improves contrast resolution. For a 4-bit, 40-dB dynamic range system, an echo must have nearly twice the intensity of another one for it to be assigned a different shade. With a 60-dB dynamic range, more than twice the intensity would be required. For a 6-bit, 40-dB system, only a 15% difference is required. For an 8-bit, 60-dB system, a 5% difference is sufficient. Table 4-5 and Figure 4-36

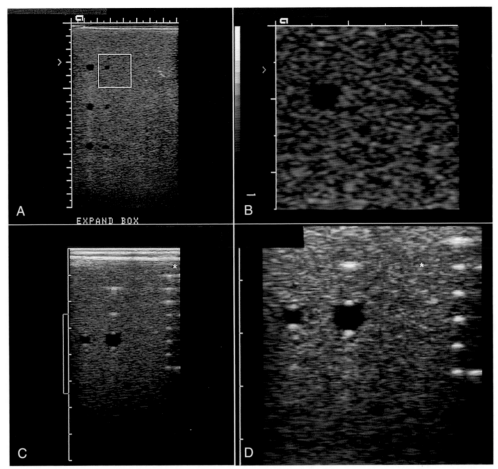

FIGURE 4-35 Write and read zoom or magnification. A, A scan of a phantom without write magnification. **B,** A scan using write magnification. Included are 4- and 2-mm simulated cysts. Read magnification, or zoom, when applied to an "unzoomed" image **(C),** magnifies the stored pixels **(D).**

TABLE 4-5	**Contrast Resolution of Digital Memories**				
	40-dB Dynamic Range		**60-dB Dynamic Range**		
Bits per Pixel	**Decibels per Shade**	**Intensity Difference (%)***	**Decibels per Shade**	**Intensity Difference (%)***	
4	2.5	78	3.8	140	
5	1.2	32	1.9	55	
6	0.6	15	0.9	23	
7	0.3	7	0.5	12	
8	0.2	5	0.2	5	

* The average difference required between two echoes for the echoes to be assigned different shades.

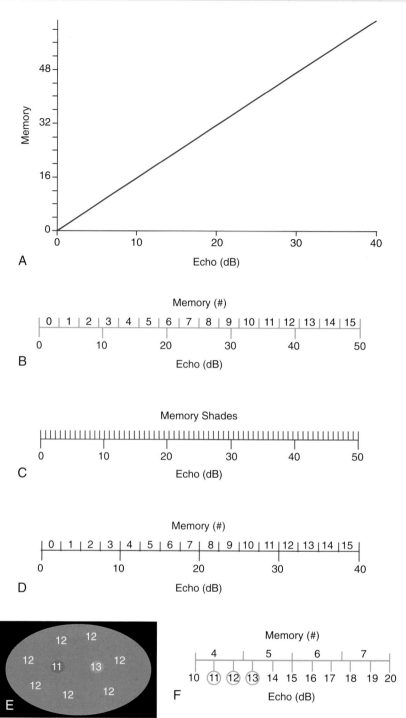

FIGURE 4-36 **A,** Assignment of numbers (to be stored in the memory) to echo intensities. Echo intensity is expressed in decibels in the form of a straight-line assignment (relative to the weakest echo, which is represented as 0 dB; the strongest echo is 40 dB, which is 10,000 times the intensity of the weakest). An instrument dynamic range of 40 dB and a 6-bit (64-shade) memory are assumed. **B,** With a 4-bit memory, a 50-dB dynamic range is divided into 16 regions (shades). **C,** With a 6-bit memory, a 50-dB dynamic range is divided into 64 regions, which are numbered 0 to 63. **D,** With a 4-bit memory, a 40-dB dynamic range is divided into 16 regions. **E,** Liver echoes are 12 dB in strength on the dynamic range scale, whereas two metastasic regions have strengths 11 and 13 dB, respectively. These regions should be displayed slightly darker and lighter as shown. **F,** The 10- to 20-dB dynamic range portion of **D** is expanded. If normal liver echoes were 12 dB (assigned 4 in the memory) and metastases were 13 dB (slightly hyperechoic; assigned 5), the normal and abnormal would be different in the memory and would appear with different brightness on the display. If the metastases were 11 dB (slightly hypoechoic), they would be assigned 4 in the memory, just as would the normal echoes, and the difference would be lost (identical displayed brightnesses).

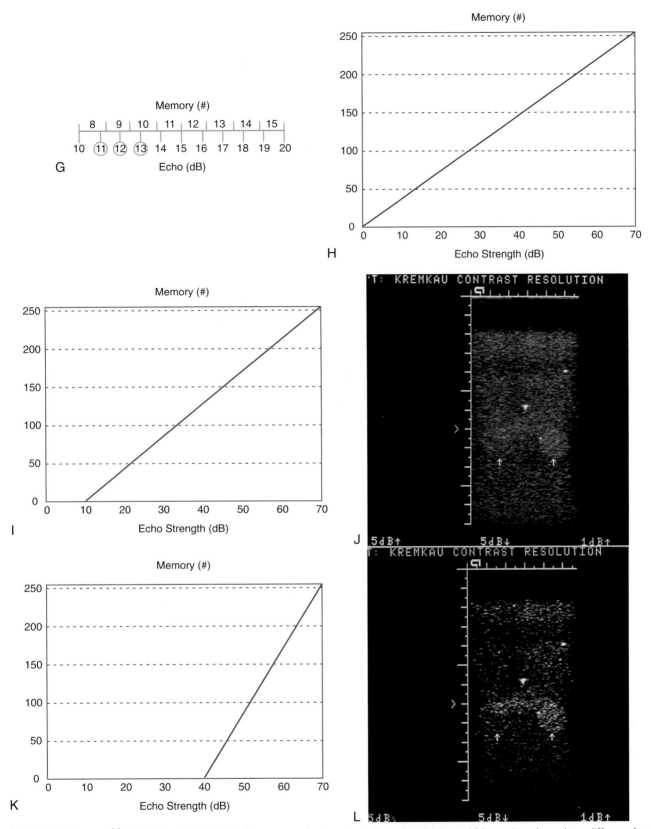

FIGURE 4-36, cont'd G, With a 5-bit (32-shade) memory, both metastatic regions in **E** would be assigned numbers different from those for normal liver and different from each other; that is, contrast resolution would be maintained for both. A dynamic range or compression (preprocessing) control reassigns echo intensities in memory, with the weaker portion as zeros and the remainder in linear fashion. The compression control is set at maximum (70 dB; **H**), 60 dB **(I-J),** and 30 dB **(K-L).** With decreasing dynamic range, more of the weaker portion is assigned to zero in memory (black on the display), and the contrast of the remainder (displayed) is enhanced with improved contrast resolution.

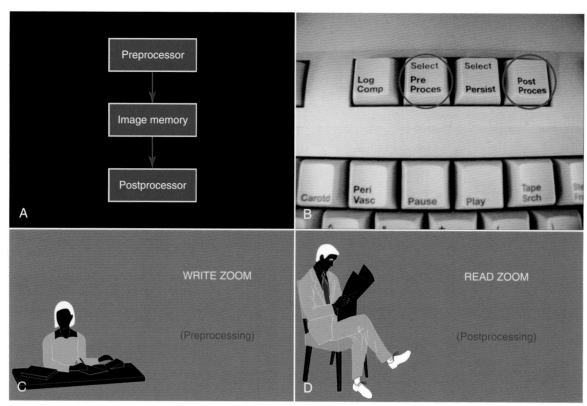

FIGURE 4-37 A, Preprocessing *(red circle in B)* includes operations performed on echoes before storage in memory. **B,** Postprocessing *(blue circle)* includes operations performed after information is stored in memory. Write (**C;** see Figure 4-35, *B*) and read (**D;** see Figure 4-35, *D*) magnification are examples of preprocessing and postprocessing, respectively.

show how a greater number of shades or a reduced dynamic range improves contrast resolution.

 Contrast resolution is the ability of a gray-scale display to distinguish between echoes of slightly different intensities. Contrast resolution depends on the number of bits per pixel in the image memory.

Postprocessing

Signal processing and image processing done before storing of the echo information in the image memory are called *preprocessing*. In general, preprocessing includes all that is done to echoes before they are stored in the memory (Figure 4-37). Image processing that is accomplished after the echoes are stored in the memory is called **postprocessing**. In general, postprocessing includes everything done with echoes as they are brought out of the memory in order to be displayed. Read magnification is an example. Postprocessing is the assignment of specific display brightnesses to numbers retrieved from the memory (Figure 4-38). Some aspects of preprocessing such as persistence and spatial compounding are operator controllable. Postprocessing is also an operator-controllable operation.

 Postprocessing is image processing performed on image data retrieved from the memory. Postprocessing determines how echo data stored in the memory will appear on the display.

On most instruments, preprogrammed postprocessing brightness assignment schemes are selectable by the operator. A linear assignment (Figure 4-38) equally divides the display brightness range among the stored gray levels of the system. This can be in white-echo (Figure 4-38, *D*) or black-echo (Figure 4-38, *E*) form although the latter is seldom used. The assignment rules for these two schemes are the inverse of each other (Figure 4-38, *A-B*). Other schemes (Figure 4-39) that allow assignment of more of the brightness range to certain portions of the stored number range capability of the system may also be used. This can improve the presentation and perception of small echo strength differences stored in the memory (improved contrast resolution). Liver metastases (Figure 4-40) illustrate the importance of contrast resolution because they can be slightly more or less echogenic than the surrounding normal liver tissue. The less difference in echogenicity, the more difficult it is to detect the masses. First, more

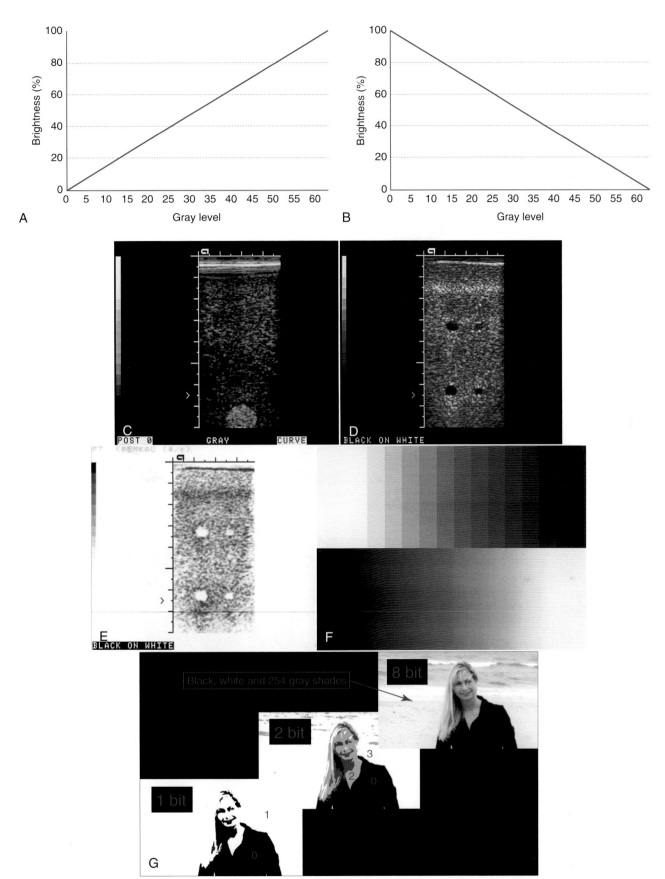

FIGURE 4-38 Postprocessing is the assignment of specific display brightnesses to numbers derived from specific pixel locations in memory.
A, Brightness increases with increasing echo intensity (i.e., gray level stored in the memory). This is called *white-echo display*. **B,** Brightness increases with decreasing echo intensity *(black-echo display)*. Both forms of display were common in the early days of gray-scale imaging. The latter is now seldom used because the white-echo display has been shown to be superior. **C-D,** Examples of the numerical assignment shown in **A. E,** Example of the numerical assignment shown in **B. F,** The upper portion shows 16 shades using a numerical assignment similar to that of **B.** The lower portion shows 256 shades and uses a numerical assignment similar to that of **A.** In both cases, echo strength increases to the right. **G,** Digital photographs with 1-, 2-, and 8-bit gray-scale resolutions. They yield 2 (black and white), 4 (black, white, and two grays) and 256 shades, respectively.

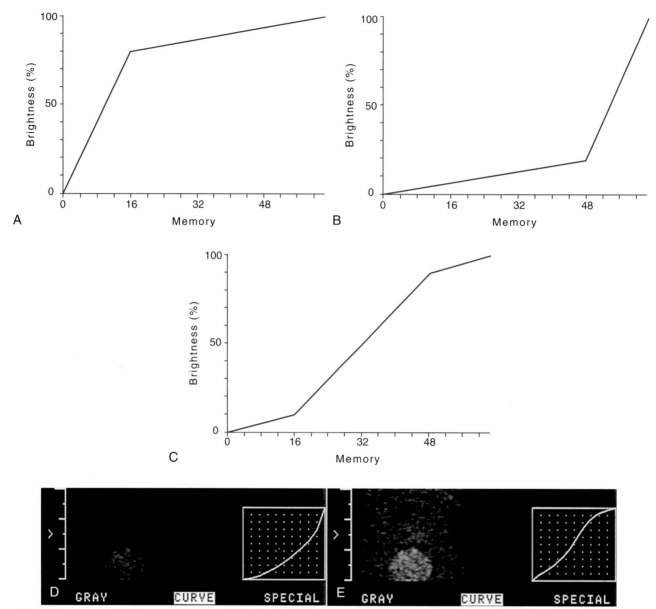

FIGURE 4-39 **Nonlinear postprocessing assignment schemes.** A large brightness range is reserved for weak **(A)**, strong **(B)**, and intermediate-strength **(C)** echoes. Each area has improved contrast resolution at the expense of poorer contrast resolution in the remainder of the dynamic range. **D,** A display using a postprocessing curve similar to that in **B, E,** A display using a postprocessing curve similar to that in **C,** Compare **D** and **E** with the linear case in Figure 4-38, C.

gray shades (more bits per pixel) will be required to store the echoes emanating from metastases with different numbers in the memory than those for the surrounding liver. Even then, if a linear postprocessing assignment is used, these small number differences in the memory may not be observed in the display. For example, in Figure 4-40, E, in which more gray-scale range is assigned to the weaker echoes, if normal and abnormal tissue echoes differed by one digit in the memory (e.g., normal = 40; abnormal = 41), there would be a 1.2% difference in brightness (gray level) between the two on the display. This difference could be observed. However, with linear postprocessing (see Figure 4-40, D), there would be only a 0.4% brightness difference, which would go unnoticed.

In Figure 4-40, E, the improvement in contrast resolution for weaker echoes (because of the steeper slope for echoes assigned values 0 to 64 in the memory) is accomplished at the cost of degraded contrast resolution for the remainder of the dynamic range (shallow slope for echoes assigned values 65 to 255 in the memory). Figure 4-41, A-B, shows a hemangioma, the presentation of which is enhanced by using a specially crafted, steep postprocessing assignment at the echo level corresponding to the echogenicity of the hemangioma. The contrast between abnormal and normal tissues is greatly increased. If the mass were not obvious with linear postprocessing, the steep slope assignment likely would have made it visible.

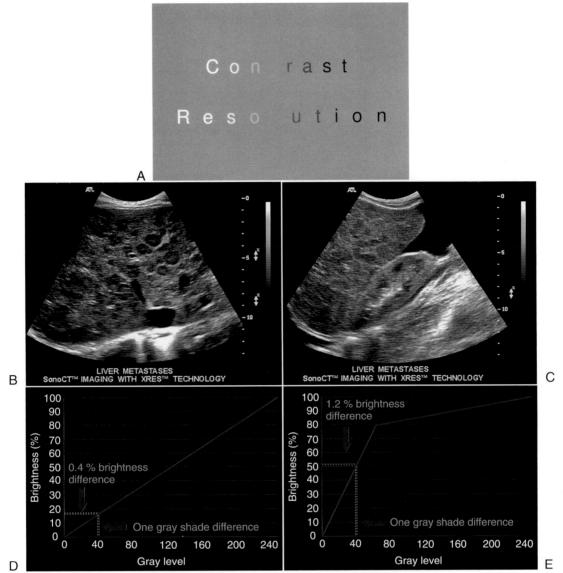

FIGURE 4-40 A, Contrast resolution is the ability of a gray-scale display to distinguish between echoes of slightly different amplitudes or intensities. **B,** Liver metastases that are less echogenic (and therefore darker) than the surrounding liver tissue. **C,** Liver metastases that are not easily visualized because they are only slightly hypoechoic compared with normal liver. Two tissue regions with slightly different echogenicities require good contrast resolution to be observed with different brightnesses. This requires enough gray levels so that echoes from the two regions are stored in the memory with different numbers to indicate their different strengths (echogenicities). Even then, the differences may not be observed on the display if they are minimal. **D,** In this example, one tissue region has echoes stored as gray level 40, whereas an adjacent region has echoes stored at gray level 41. These two regions would differ in brightness by 0.4% using a linear postprocessing assignment. This difference would not be noticed by a human observer. **E,** Using a different postprocessing choice, the brightness difference is 1.2%, which could be observed.

B Color

Some instruments have the postprocessing ability to present different echo intensities in various colors rather than in gray shades, that is, the ability to colorize echoes. In this case, different colors, rather than gray levels, are assigned to various echo intensities. Because the eye can differentiate more color tints than gray shades, color displays offer improved contrast resolution capability. This process is called *B color* or *color scale* (compared with gray scale). A color bar is included in such displays to show how colors are assigned to various echo strengths. Figure 4-41, *C-E*, provides some examples.

 B color is a form of postprocessing that improves contrast resolution by assigning colors, rather than gray shades, to different echo strengths.

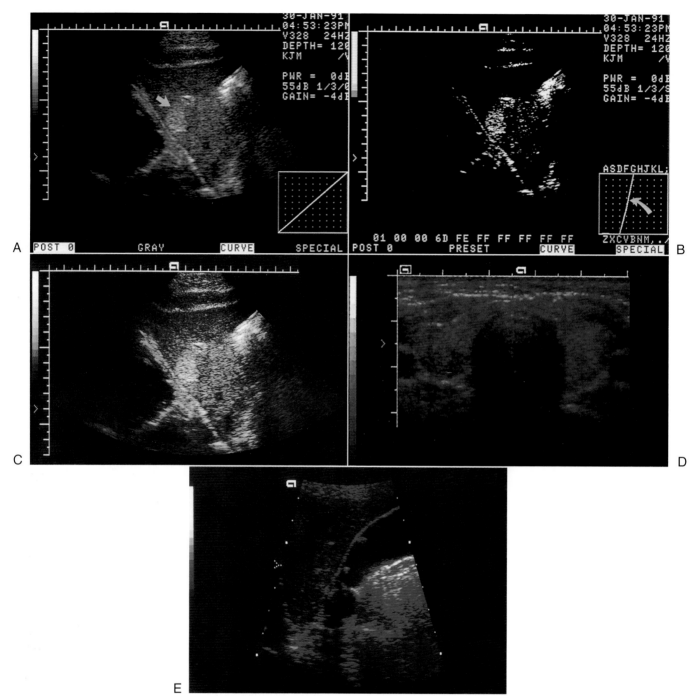

FIGURE 4-41 A, An image of a hemangioma *(arrow)* obtained using linear postprocessing. **B,** An image of a hemangioma with a steep postprocessing assignment *(curved arrow)* designed to produce a great contrast between these normal and abnormal tissue echoes. **C-E,** Color displays of a hemangioma (**C;** compare with **A** and **B**), thyroid **(D),** and gallbladder **(E).** Color assignments, shown in the color bars on the left, are designated as follows: **(C)** temperature (increasing intensity assigned dark orange through yellow to white), **(D)** magenta (dark magenta through light magenta to white), and **(E)** rainbow (dark violet through various colors to white).

Volume Presentation

Common ways of presenting 3D echo data (volume imaging) (Figure 4-42) include surface renderings, 2D slices through the 3D volume, and transparent views. The advantage of 2D slice presentation is that it is possible to present image-plane orientations that are difficult or impossible to obtain with conventional 2D scanning. Surface renderings are popular in obstetric and cardiac imaging. Transparent views allow "see-through" imaging of the anatomy as with plain-film radiographs. These presentation forms are postprocessing choices that present the stored 3D volume of echo information in different ways on the display.

 A 3D volume of echo data can be displayed in several ways, including 2D slices, surface renderings, and transparent views.

Digital-to-Analog Converter

After numbers are retrieved from the memory and postprocessed, they are converted into voltages that determine the brightnesses of echoes on the display. This task is accomplished by the **digital-to-analog converter**. The digital-to-analog converter converts the digital data received from the image memory to analog voltages that are fed to the display to determine the echo brightnesses displayed (Figure 4-43).

DISPLAY

The chain of events covered thus far in this chapter is illustrated in Figure 4-44. Gray-scale operation causes a brightening of the spot for each echo in memory. The brightness (gray scale) is proportional to the echo strength. The memory is filled with echoes from many pulses as the beam is scanned through the anatomy to be imaged. The 2D gray-scale scan is a brightness image that represents an anatomic cross-section in the scanning plane, as if the sound beam cuts a section through the tissue like a knife. Each individual image is called a *frame*. Because several frames can be acquired and presented every second, this is called *real-time display*. Several 2D scans can also be acquired to form a 3D volume of stored echo information.

Frame rate is the number of sonographic 2D or 3D images entered into the image memory per second, whereas **refresh rate** is the number of times per second that images are retrieved from the memory and presented on the display. These two rates can be, but are not necessarily, equal.

The information delivered to the display can be presented in several ways. Common to all clinical applications is brightness mode, also called **B mode, B scan,** or *gray-scale sonography*. Gray-scale anatomic displays can be in 2D or 3D forms. In echocardiography, motion mode (**M mode**) is also used. In ophthalmology, amplitude mode (**A mode**) is used as well.

Formerly, the commonly used display device was the **cathode-ray tube** (CRT). The CRT generated a display with an electron beam that painted the image in horizontal lines, each corresponding to a row of echo information in the image memory. In recent years, CRTs have been replaced by flat-panel displays, as has occurred with computers and television sets.

Flat-Panel Display

Sonographic images are presented on computer displays because they represent the digital information stored in the image (computer) memory. Computer displays present image information in the form of horizontal lines (Figure 4-45, *A*). Each horizontal display scan line corresponds to a row of digital data in the image memory. The information is read out of the memory, row by row (much as we read a page of text), and is written on the display, line by line, like writing on a lined sheet of paper. Because the display includes more than the sonographic image (such as alphanumeric data, icons, and Doppler spectral display), the data in the memory are of various types. But whatever is stored in a given pixel in the memory (whether it be part of a gray-scale anatomic image, part of an alphabetic letter, or anything else) will appear at the corresponding pixel location on the display with the appropriate brightness and color. Because color is used in some cases, such as B color and color Doppler, color displays are common in sonographic instruments.

 The display is a flat-panel display that presents an image in horizontal lines from top to bottom.

Various standards are used in computer displays. An example is the SVGA (super-video-graphics array) standard, in which the pixel matrix can be, among other values, 1024×768 and the display refresh rate (the number of images per second extracted from image) is 60 Hz.

 A computer monitor is a display that presents data retrieved from the memory in a 2D pixel matrix, refreshing the display often (e.g., 60 times per second).

Because we want to display pixels with proportional brightnesses, not the numbers that represent the echo intensities in the image memory, these numbers must be converted by the digital-to-analog converter to proportional voltages that control the brightness.

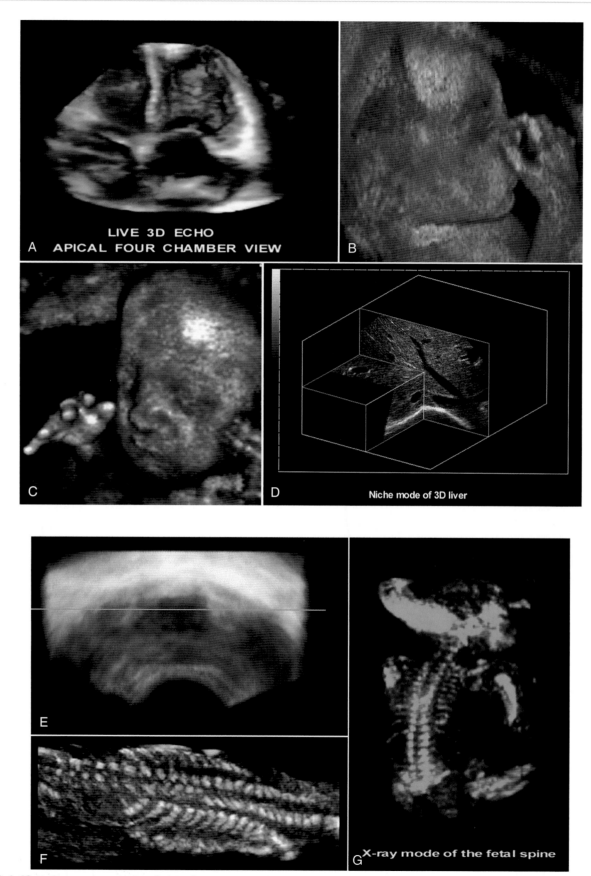

FIGURE 4-42 Various postprocessing choices for presenting three-dimensional images. Three-dimensional surface renderings. **A,** Cardiac image. **B,** Fetus holding nose. **C,** Fetal head and hands. **D,** Three orthogonal two-dimensional slices through the three-dimensional liver echo volume. **E-G,** Transparent (X-ray) mode. **E,** All echoes in the volume can be included, as in this image of the prostate, or **(F-G)** only the strongest ones.

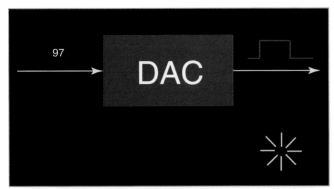

FIGURE 4-43 The digital-to-analog converter (DAC) converts the numbers (digital) stored in the memory to proportional (analog) voltages that control the brightness of each echo on the display.

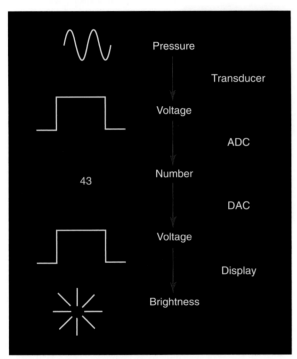

FIGURE 4-44 **Information chain from the echo (pressure), through the transducer and electronics, to the display.** The analog-to-digital converter (ADC) is part of the beam former. An echo is stored as a number in the image memory (part of the image processor). The digital-to-analog converter (DAC) is part of the image processor.

Flat-panel displays have been on notebook (laptop) computers from the start and are now common on desktop computers, television sets, and sonographic instruments (Figure 4-45, *B-C*). Advantages include lighter weight, slim profile (i.e., less bulky), and less power consumption and heat generation. A **flat-panel display** is a back-lighted liquid crystal display (LCD). Such a display is composed of a rectangular matrix of thousands of LCD elements (e.g., a 1024 × 768 matrix contains 786,432 LCD elements). These elements can be electrically turned on or off individually and act as tiny light valves for blocking or passing the light from the light

source underneath the matrix. More specifically, the elements can be turned on partially to allow a measured amount of light through, usually in 256 steps of luminance, that is, 256 displayed gray levels from black to white. Groups of red, green, and blue elements allow what is called *24-bit color* (8 bits or 256 luminance values for each primary color element) yielding 16,777,216 possible colors presented at each pixel location. Red, green, and blue (RGB) are known as *primary additive colors* because various combinations of them can produce nearly any color desired. For example, red and green, mixed equally, produce yellow. Green and blue produce *cyan*, the technical term for aqua. Red and blue produce magenta. Red, green, and blue, equally mixed, produce white (or gray, depending on brightness).

Temporal Resolution

Sonographic instruments store several frames of echo information in the image memory per second. The number of sonographic images stored per second is called *frame rate*. This is the rate at which the sound beam is scanned through the tissue cross-section by the transducer. A rapid sequence of frames yields what appears to be a continuously changing image. The effective frame rate observed on the display is limited by the refresh rate. For example, the echo information may be entering the image memory at a frame rate of 100 Hz, but if the refresh rate is 75 Hz, echo information is retrieved from the memory 75 times per second, and only 75 images per second are then viewed on the display. However, there is an advantage to storing a frame rate that is higher than the refresh rate. When a frozen cine loop is displayed, the individual frames retain the temporal resolution achieved with the frame rate.

When the freeze-frame mode is activated, ultrasound beam scanning and echo data entry into the memory are halted, and the last frame entered is shown continuously on the display. Although the display continues to present what is in the memory at the refresh rate, it is the same image every time, so it appears as a static, unchanging image.

Real-time imaging affords rapid and convenient acquisition of the desired image (with the display changing continuously as the scan plane is moved through tissues) and two-dimensional imaging of the motion of moving structures (with the display changing continuously as the structures move). Temporal resolution is the ability of a display to distinguish closely spaced events in time and to present rapidly moving structures correctly. Temporal resolution is expressed in milliseconds, which is the time from the beginning of one frame to the beginning of the next one. This is also the time required to generate one complete frame. Temporal resolution improves as the frame rate increases (Figure 4-46) because less time elapses from one frame to the next.

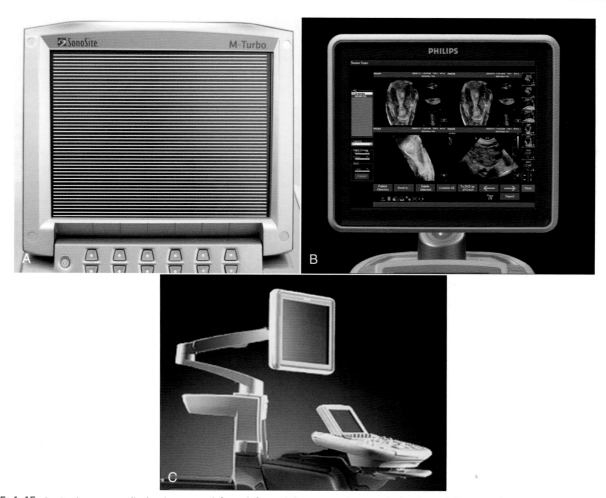

FIGURE 4-45 **A,** An image on display is scanned from left to right, top to bottom in horizontal lines, each corresponding to a row of echo-amplitude numbers in image memory. **B-C,** Flat-panel displays.

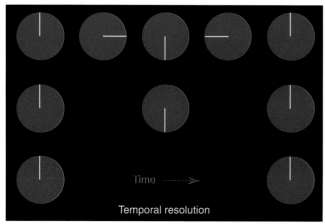

Temporal resolution

FIGURE 4-46 **Temporal resolution improves with frame rate.** *(Top row))* A wheel is rotated in a clockwise direction. Four images are taken during one revolution; thus the frame rate is four per revolution. *(Middle row)* With a frame rate of two per revolution, it can be seen that the wheel is rotating, but the direction is ambiguous: it could be clockwise or counterclockwise. *(Bottom row)* The frame rate is one per revolution. The motion of the wheel is not observed; indeed, it appears to be stationary. A similar result would occur in echocardiography if one frame per cardiac cycle were acquired. The heart would appear to be inactive.

Each frame is made up of many scan lines and may have more than one focus. For each focus on each scan line in each frame, a pulse is required. The required pulse repetition frequency (*PRF*), therefore, is determined by the required number of foci (*n*), lines per frame (*LPF*), and the frame rate (*FR*) in frames per second, that is, hertz (*Hz*). Indeed, pulse repetition frequency is equal to these three quantities multiplied together.

 For each focus on each scan line in each frame, a pulse is required.

$$PRF\,(Hz) = n \times LPF \times FR\,(Hz)$$

 To increase the number of foci, pulse repetition frequency must increase.

 To increase the number of lines per frame, pulse repetition frequency must increase.

 To increase the frame rate, pulse repetition frequency must increase.

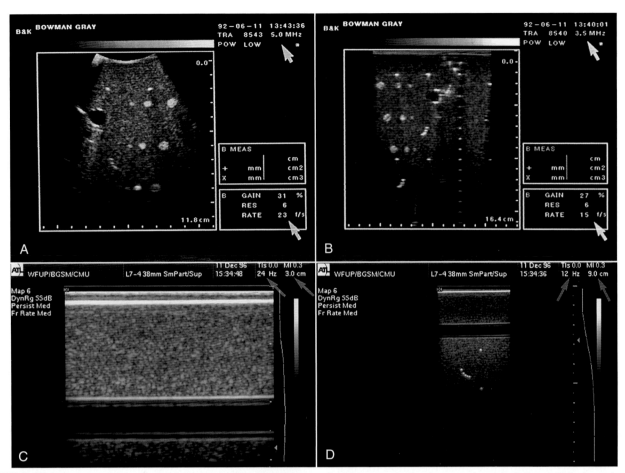

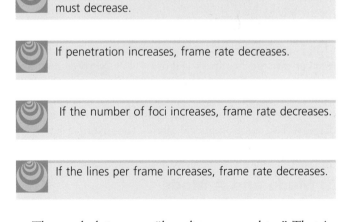

FIGURE 4-47 **A lower operating frequency allows greater penetration, thereby necessitating longer echo arrival time, which slows down the frame rate. A,** 5 MHz, penetration of 9 cm, 23 frames per second. **B,** 3.5 MHz, penetration of 13 cm, 15 frames per second. **C,** With a displayed depth of 3 cm, the frame rate is 24 frames per second (hertz; *arrow*). **D,** A displayed depth increase to 9 cm reduces the frame rate to 12 Hz. At first this seems surprising because the operating frequency (5.5 MHz), and therefore the penetration are the same in both cases. However, the effective penetration is reduced with the reduced displayed depth in **C** by increasing pulse repetition frequency. The echoes from beyond the displayed depth are weaker because of attenuation. When the next pulse is sent, the amplifier gain drops with the restarting of the time gain control. Thus the deeper echoes are not amplified enough to be seen (in incorrect locations, that is, range ambiguity artifact).

However, time is required for echoes to return while a pulse travels into the tissue. The greater the penetration, the longer it takes for all of the echoes to return (remember the *13 µs/cm rule*). To avoid misplacement of echoes on the display because of the late arrival of echoes, all echoes from one pulse must be received before the next pulse is emitted. To accomplish this, pulse repetition frequency must decrease as penetration increases. That is, if a lower operating frequency is used, penetration is increased and pulse repetition frequency must decrease to avoid echo misplacement. This will occur as a frame rate reduction (Figure 4-47) for lower operating frequencies. Frame rate decreases when displayed depth is increased (Figure 4-47, *C-D*). Likewise, wider images (requiring more scan lines) and multiple foci also reduce frame rate (Figure 4-48) because more time is required, in both cases, to generate each frame. The relationship between these competing variables is as follows:

$$\text{pen (cm)} \times n \times \text{LPF} \times \text{FR (Hz)} \le 77,000 \text{ cm/s}$$

If penetration increases, pulse repetition frequency must decrease.

If penetration increases, frame rate decreases.

If the number of foci increases, frame rate decreases.

If the lines per frame increases, frame rate decreases.

The symbol ≤ means "less than or equal to." That is, when penetration is multiplied by the number of foci, the number of scan lines per frame, and the frame rate, the result must not exceed 77,000. Otherwise, the required pulse repetition frequency would not allow the

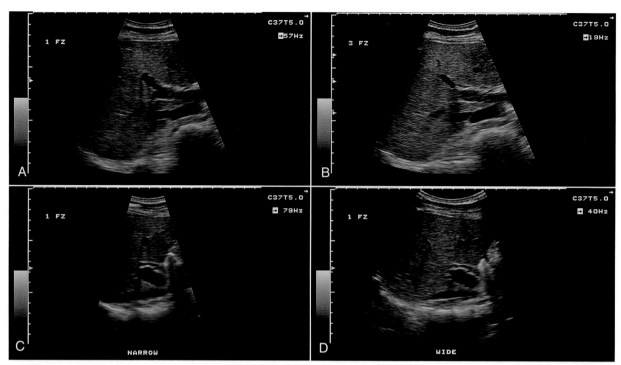

FIGURE 4-48 A, One focus; frame rate of 57. **B,** Multiple foci (3) reduce the frame rate to 19. **C,** Frame rate of 79. **D,** An increased frame width (doubling the number of scan lines) reduces the frame rate to 40.

return of all of the echoes before the emission of the next pulse (resulting in echo misplacement).

Table 4-6 lists the allowable pulse repetition frequencies and frame rates for various penetration and lines-per-frame values. Multiple foci reduce permitted frame rates inversely (e.g., two foci with a penetration of 20 cm and 100 lines per frame are equivalent to ½ × 38, or 19 frames per second).

 Temporal resolution is the ability to follow moving structures in temporal detail. Temporal resolution depends on frame rate, which depends on depth, lines per frame, and number of foci.

TABLE 4-6	Pulse Repetition Frequencies (PRF) and Frame Rates (FR) Permitted for Various Single-Focus Imaging Depths (Penetration) and 100 or 200 Scan Lines per Frame

		FR	
Penetration (cm)	PRF (Hz)	100 Lines	200 Lines
20	3850	38	19
15	5133	51	25
10	7700	77	38
5	15,400	154	77

For measurement purposes, displays include range marker dots and calipers (Figure 4-49). Marker dots are presented as a series of dots in a line with a given separation (e.g., 1 cm). Calipers are two plus signs (or some other symbol) that can be placed anywhere on the display. The instrument calculates the distance between them and shows it on the display.

M Mode and A Mode

Another display mode (*M mode*) is used to show the motion of cardiac structures (Figure 4-50). M mode is a display form that presents depth (vertical axis) versus time (horizontal). An uncommon display, except in ophthalmologic sonography, shows the amplitudes of echoes and is called *A mode*. (Figure 4-51). A mode

is a depth versus amplitude display. Temporal resolution in M and A modes is equal to pulse repetition period because each pulse produces a new line of echo information on these displays. The sound beam is stationary in these presentations. Ultrasound pulses travel down the same path over and over. In the M mode display, the vertical scan lines are written next to each other across the horizontal time axis.

Output Devices

External recording devices (Figure 4-52) have been provided to allow videotaping of real-time scanning or to produce hard copies of frozen images. These devices include video cassette recorders (VCRs), printers, and digital devices. Figure 4-53 shows a diagram of the

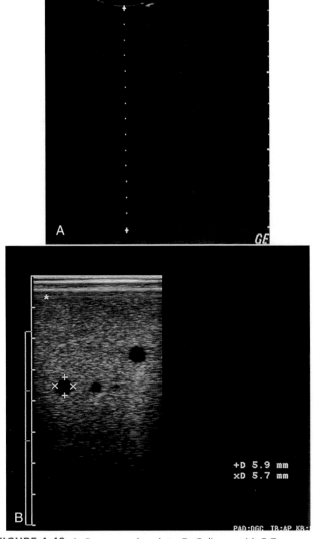

FIGURE 4-49 **A,** Range marker dots. **B,** Calipers with 5.7-mm and 5.9-mm separations.

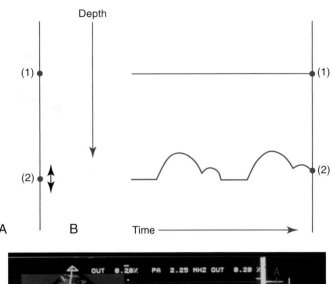

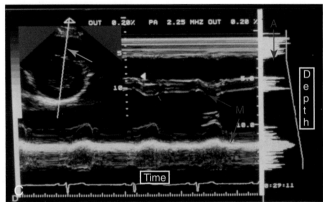

FIGURE 4-50 **A,** B mode presentation of echo depth with echoes from both a stationary structure (1) and a moving one (2). **B,** If pulses are sent down the same path repeatedly, and vertical scan lines are placed next to each other, a display of depth-versus-time results. The pattern of motion of moving structures (2) is traced out on the display for evaluation. This is called *M mode display.* **C,** A mode and M mode presentations of moving cardiac structures. Depth is the vertical axis in both cases. For M mode, time increases to the right. The two-dimensional real-time anatomic cross-sectional image also is shown *(upper left).* The green arrow indicates the repeating path of the ultrasound pulses used to generate the A and M mode displays.

instrument with input and output devices. An internal hard disk in the instrument stores images in digital form. Images also can be sent to a computer via a CD or DVD drive (Figure 4-52, *C*) or a USB connection (Figure 4-52, *D*). Various standard protocols are used for communicating and storing digital images (e.g., JPEG [joint photographic experts group] and TIFF [tagged image file format]) and video clips (e.g., AVI [audio-video interweave] and MPEG [moving picture experts group]). Quality depends on the number of pixels per image and the amount of compression used (image compression is a process that reduces digital file size while retaining the data essential for acceptable image quality). Because sonographic images are not collections of random echo data, their repeating patterns allow shortened coding, called *lossless compression,* to reduce file size. Lossless compression reduces file size to about one half its usual size without altering the image. *Lossy compression* involves visually similar, but not identical, images. The

JPEG file is a compressed image file (file extension .jpg). File size is a trade-off with quality. The TIFF file (file extension .tif) has better quality than JPEG but has larger files. The same is true for MPEG (file extension .mpg) compared with AVI (file extension .avi). A single 8-bit (1 byte; 256 shade) uncompressed gray scale image with 1024×768 pixels requires 768 kilobytes (kB) of memory for the image data. Including the remaining data for proper handling of the image, the TIFF file size is 779 kB. A moderately compressed JPEG file size for the same image is 83 kB. A comparable color image would have a TIFF file size of 2.26 megabytes (MB) (three times the gray-scale file because data on three primary colors [red, green, blue] are stored rather than data on just one color, [i.e., gray]). The compressed JPEG color file size is 95 kB. Communicating an uncompressed 256 gray-shade video clip of 30, 1024×768 pixel frames per second requires data transfer at 189 megabits per second (Mb/s) or 24

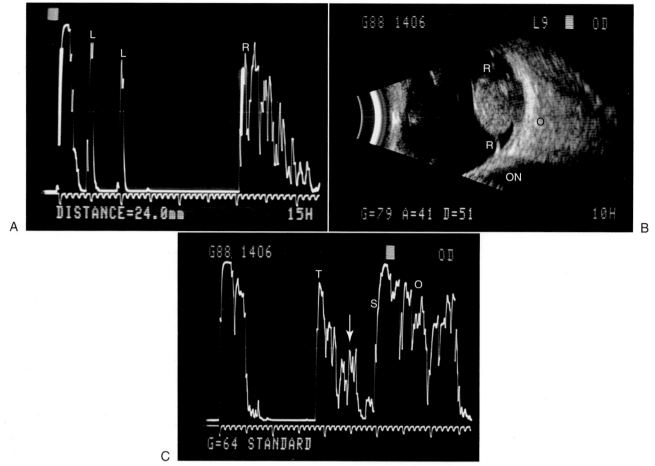

FIGURE 4-51 A, A normal ophthalmologic A mode presentation, where *L* represents lens echoes and *R* represents the retina. A longitudinal B scan **(B)** and standardized A mode presentation **(C)** demonstrate the typical acoustic appearance of a choroidal melanoma. The B scan shows a mushroom-shaped mass with exudative retinal detachment *(R)* at the tumor margins *(O,* orbital fat; *ON,* optic nerve). The A mode scan demonstrates a high spike from the tumor surface *(T)* and low to medium echogenicity within the lesion *(arrow)* *(S,* sclera; *O,* orbital fat). In this figure, the horizontal axis represents depth.

megabytes per second (MB/s). Compression, such as MPEG, reduces this requirement to a more manageable value.

Picture Archiving and Communications Systems (PACS)

Picture archiving and communications systems provide means for electronically communicating images and associated information to workstations (Figure 4-52, *E*) and devices external to the sonographic instrument, the examining room, and even the building in which the scanning is done. Indeed, through the Internet, these files can be transmitted to virtually anywhere in the world. Picture archiving and communications systems are used

with all digital imaging modes, including ultrasound. The protocols for communicating images and associated information between imaging devices and workstations have been standardized in the Digital Imaging and Communications in Medicine (DICOM) standard.[4] This standard specifies a hardware interface, a minimum set of software commands, and a consistent set of data formats. This standard promotes communication of information, regardless of manufacturers of the linked devices, including the sonographic instrument, the picture archiving and communications systems reading station, and other hospital/clinic information systems. The DICOM standard also enables the creation of diagnostic information bases that can be interrogated by a wide variety of devices geographically distributed.

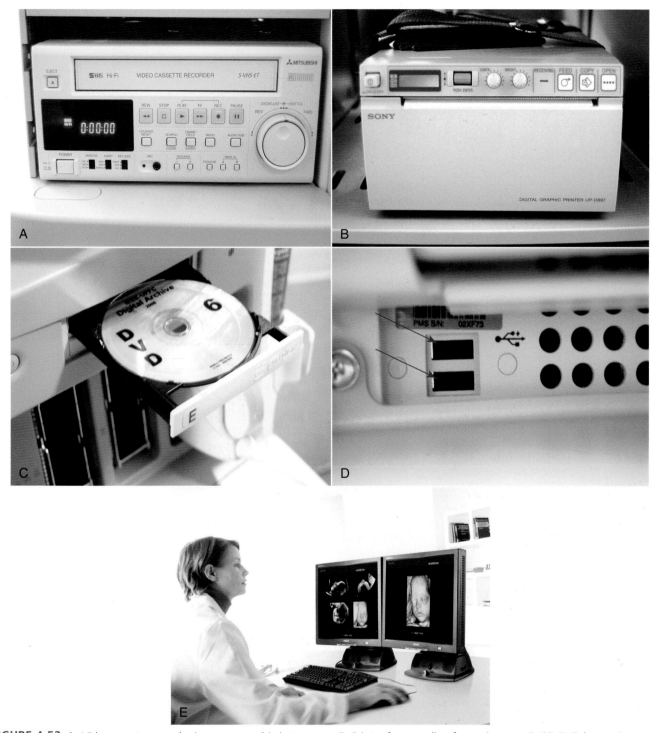

FIGURE 4-52 A, Videocassette recorder in a sonographic instrument. **B,** Printer for recording frozen images. **C,** CD-DVD burner in a sonographic instrument. **D,** USB (universal serial bus) ports *(arrows)* for connection to a flash memory device, other digital device, or a computer. **E,** Picture archiving and communications system (PACS) workstation.

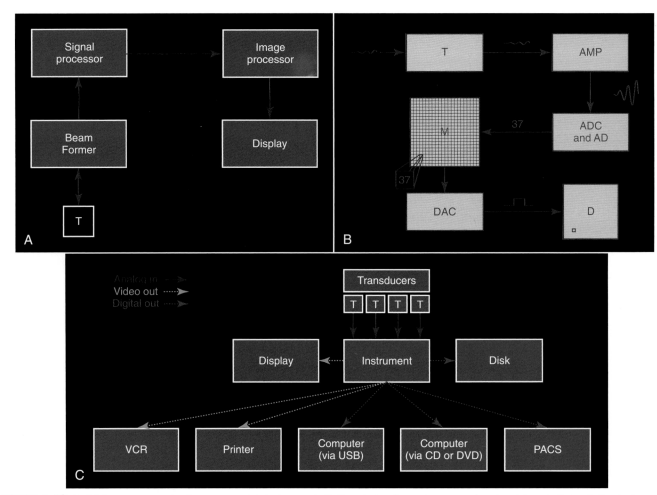

FIGURE 4-53 A, Major components of a sonographic instrument. **B,** The chain of events as an echo signal travels through the instrument. The transducer (T) converts the echo pressure variation to a voltage variation. The amplifier (AMP) increases the amplitude of the echo voltage. The analog-to-digital converter (ADC) converts the echo to a series of numbers, and the amplitude detector (AD) converts this series from radio frequency (RF) form to amplitude form. The echo amplitude is stored as a number in the image memory (M). The echo amplitude is retrieved from its pixel location in the memory. The digital-to-analog converter (DAC) converts the number to a corresponding voltage. The voltage determines the brightness of the echo presented on the display *(D)*. **C,** Echo information enters the instrument from the transducers in analog form. Image information flows in video form to the internal display and externally to a VCR and printer. Image information flows in digital form (numbers) to an internal disk and externally to a computer (via CD, DVD, or USB connection) and picture archiving and communications system (PACS) to be stored in digital format, just as it is in the image memory of the instrument. Such storage involves no loss of quality and allows postprocessing, measurements and any other function that can be applied to a stored (frozen) image in the instrument memory.

REVIEW

The key points presented in this chapter are the following:

- Sonographic instruments are of the pulse-echo type.
- These instruments use the strength, direction, and arrival time of received echoes to generate A, B, and M mode displays.
- Sonographic instruments include the beam former, signal processor, image processor, and display, and often these are attached to peripheral recording and display devices.
- The beam former is responsible for directing, focusing, and apodizing the ultrasound beam on transmission and reception. The beam former also amplifies

the echo voltages, compensates for attenuation using time gain compensation, and digitizes the voltages.

- The signal processor filters, detects, and compresses the echo signal.
- The scan converter converts the echo data in scan-line format to image format for storage and display.
- A mode presents depth-versus-echo amplitude display.
- B and M modes use a display of echo strength as brightness.
- M mode shows reflector motion in time. M mode is a presentation of echo depth versus time.
- B mode scans show anatomic cross-sections through the scanning plane.

- Image memories store echo intensity information as binary numbers in memory elements.
- Contrast resolution improves with increasing bits per pixel.
- Real-time imaging is the rapid sequential display of ultrasound images (frames), resulting in a moving presentation.
- Real-time imaging requires rapid, repeatable, sequential scanning of the sound beam through the tissue. This is accomplished with electronic transducer arrays.
- Increasing frame rate improves temporal resolution.

EXERCISES

1. The ultrasound pulse repetition frequency is equal to the voltage _____ repetition frequency of the pulser.
2. Increased voltage amplitude produced by the pulser increases the _____ and _____ of ultrasound pulses produced by the transducer.
3. If a 6-MHz transducer images to a depth of 10 cm, to avoid range ambiguity, the maximum pulse repetition frequency permitted is _____.
   a. 7.7 kHz
   b. 6.0 kHz
   c. 10.0 kHz
   d. 1.54 MHz
   e. 13.0 MHz
4. Functions performed by the signal processor include _____, _____, and _____.
5. Match the following functions with what they accomplish:
   a. Amplification:
   b. Compensation:
   c. Filtering:
   d. Detection:
   e. Compression:
      1. Converts pulses from radio frequency to amplitude form
      2. Increases all amplitudes
      3. Decreases dynamic range
      4. Corrects for tissue attenuation
      5. Reduces noise
6. If the input voltage to an amplifier is 1 mV and the output voltage is 10 mV, the voltage amplification ratio is _____. The power ratio is _____. The gain is _____ dB.
7. An amplifier with a gain of 60 dB has 1 μW of power applied to the input. The output power is _____ W.
8. An amplifier with a gain of 60 dB has 10 μV of voltage applied to the input. The output voltage is _____ mV.

9. Time gain compensation is accomplished in the _____.
   a. pulser
   b. beam former
   c. signal processor
   d. scan converter
   e. image processor
10. Compensation takes into account reflector _____.
11. Compensation amplifies echoes differently, according to their arrival _____.
12. Compression decreases the _____ range to a range that the _____ and human _____ can handle.
13. If a display has a dynamic range of 20 dB and the smallest voltage it can handle is 200 mV, then the largest voltage it can handle is _____ V.
14. Detection converts voltage pulses from _____ form to _____ form.
15. Filtering widens bandwidth. True or false?
16. Filtering is accomplished in the _____.
    a. pulser
    b. beam former
    c. signal processor
    d. scan converter
    e. image processor
17. The compression or dynamic range control reduces the range of echo amplitudes displayed by reducing the weakest to _____ and/or the strongest ones to the _____ value and assigning the others to increasing _____. This produces a _____ contrast image with elimination of _____ and maximizing of _____ echoes.
18. An amplifier has a power output of 100 mW when the input power is 0.1 mW. The amplifier gain is _____ dB.
19. If the beam-former output to the transducer is reduced by 3, 6, and 9 dB, the ultrasound pulse output intensity is reduced by _____%, _____%, and _____%, respectively.
20. One watt is _____ dB below 100 W.
21. One watt is _____ dB above 100 mW.
22. If the input power is 1 mW and the output is 10,000 mW, the gain is _____ dB.
23. If an amplifier has a gain of 15 dB, the ratio of output power to input power is _____. (Use Table 4-1.)
24. If the output of a 22-dB gain amplifier is connected to the input of a 23-dB gain amplifier, the total gain is _____ dB. The overall power ratio is _____. (Use Table 4-1.)
25. If a 17-dB electric attenuator is connected to a 15-dB amplifier, the net gain is _____ dB. The net attenuation is _____ dB. For a 1-W input, the output is _____ W. (Use Table 2-3.)

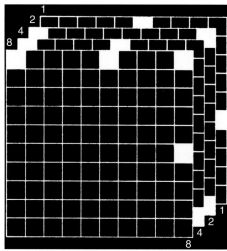

FIGURE 4-54 Digital memory description to accompany Exercise 26. The white color indicates that the memory device is on.

26. For the digital memory shown in Figure 4-54, enter the number stored in each pixel location:
    a. Lower right: _____
    b. Middle right: _____
    c. Upper right: _____
    d. Upper middle: _____
    e. Upper left: _____
27. The contrast resolution for an instrument that has an echo dynamic range of 43 dB and 32 shades is _____ dB per shade.
    a. 1.3
    b. 3.2
    c. 4.3
    d. 32
    e. 43
28. The contrast resolution for an instrument that has a 6-bit memory and a 45-dB echo dynamic range is _____ dB per shade.
    a. 0.3
    b. 0.5
    c. 0.7
    d. 0.9
    e. 6
29. Match the following:
    a. Analog:
    b. Digital:
    c. Preprocessing:
    d. Postprocessing:
    e. Pixel:
    f. Bit:
       1. Picture element
       2. Assignment of stored numbers
       3. Discrete
       4. Binary digit
       5. Proportional
       6. Assignment of displayed brightness

30. Typical image pixel dimensions are _____.
    a. 640 × 128
    b. 16 × 64
    c. 100 × 100
    d. 512 × 1540
    e. 512 × 384
31. How many bits per pixel are required for each number of shades?
    a. 16: _____
    b. 32: _____
    c. 64: _____
    d. 128: _____
    e. 256: _____
32. _____ total memory elements are required for a 100 × 100-pixel, 5-bit digital memory.
33. Memories of _____ bits per pixel are common in ultrasound today.
    a. 4–8
    b. 4–6
    c. 6–8
    d. 5–7
    e. 4–5
34. Digital memories store _____.
    a. logarithms
    b. electric magnetism
    c. electric current
    d. electric charge
    e. numbers
35. _____ is commonly controllable by the operator.
    a. Postprocessing
    b. Pixel matrix
    c. Bits per pixel
    d. Digitization
    e. All of the above
36. In binary numbers, how many symbols are used?
37. The term *binary digit* is commonly shortened into the single word _____.
38. Each binary digit in a binary number is represented in the memory by a memory element, which, at any time, is in one of _____ states that are _____ or _____.
39. Match the following (See Fig. 4-32, *E*)
    Column in an 8-bit binary number hgfedcba:
    Decimal number represented by a 1 in the column:
    a. _____   1. 64
    b. _____   2. 32
    c. _____   3. 1
    d. _____   4. 16
    e. _____   5. 8
    f. _____   6. 128
    g. _____   7. 2
    h. _____   8. 4

40. The binary number 10110 represents zero 1, one 2, one 4, zero 8, and one 16; that is, the decimal number $0 + 2 + 4 + 0 + 16 = $ **22**. What decimal number does the binary number 11001 represent?

41. The decimal number 13 is made up of one 1, zero 2, one 4, and one 8 ($8 + 4 + 0 + 1 = 13$). The number therefore is represented by the binary number _____.

42. Match the following:
Decimal Number Binary Number
   a. 1 _____   1. 0001111
   b. 5 _____   2. 0011001
   c. 10 _____   3. 0001010
   d. 15 _____   4. 0110010
   e. 20 _____   5. 0000001
   f. 25 _____   6. 1100100
   g. 30 _____   7. 0101000
   h. 40 _____   8. 0011110
   i. 50 _____   9. 0010100
   j. 100 _____   10. 0000101

43. How many binary digits are required in the binary numbers representing the following decimal numbers?
   a. 0 _____
   b. 1 _____
   c. 5 _____
   d. 10 _____
   e. 25 _____
   f. 30 _____
   g. 63 _____
   h. 64 _____
   i. 75 _____
   j. 100 _____

44. How many bits are required to represent each decimal number in binary form?
   a. 7 _____
   b. 15 _____
   c. 3 _____
   d. 511 _____
   e. 1023 _____
   f. 63 _____
   g. 255 _____
   h. 1 _____
   i. 127 _____
   j. 31 _____

45. How many bits are required to store numbers representing each number of different gray shades?
   a. 2 _____
   b. 4 _____
   c. 8 _____
   d. 15 _____
   e. 16 _____
   f. 25 _____
   g. 32 _____
   h. 64 _____

   i. 65 _____
   j. 128 _____

46. The primary formats of image presentation are called _____ *mode*, _____ *mode*, and _____ *mode*. They are used in _____, _____, and _____ types of clinical imaging, respectively.

47. _____ mode is used for studying the motion of a structure such as a heart valve.

48. A B scan presents a cross-section through the _____ plane.

49. A display that shows various echo strengths as different brightnesses is called a _____-_____ or _____ _____ *display*.

50. The _____ _____ stores the gray-scale image and allows it to be displayed on a computer monitor.

51. Match the following:
   Transducer   Display
   a. Linear array _____   1. Rectangular
   b. Convex array _____   2. Sector
   c. Phased array _____
   d. Vector array _____

52. If the pulse repetition frequency of an instrument is 1 kHz and it displays (single focus) 25 frames per second, there are _____ lines per frame.

53. The pulse repetition frequency is _____ Hz if 30 frames (40 lines each) are displayed per second (single focus).

54. Imaging involving 10-cm penetration, a single focus, 100 scan lines per frame, and 30 frames per second can be accomplished without range ambiguity. True or false?

55. The maximum frame rate permitted for 15-cm penetration, three foci, and 200 scan lines per frame is _____.
   a. 3.0
   b. 5.5
   c. 8.5
   d. 15
   e. 30

56. The primary components of a diagnostic ultrasound imaging system are the _____, _____ _____, _____ _____, _____ _____, and _____.

57. The information that can be obtained from an M mode display includes _____.
   a. distance and motion pattern
   b. transducer frequency, reflection coefficient, and distance
   c. acoustic impedances, attenuation, and motion pattern
   d. none of the above

58. The time gain compensation control compensates for _____.
    a. machine instability in the warm-up time
    b. attenuation
    c. transducer aging
    d. the ambient light in the examining area
    e. patient examination time

59. A gray-scale display shows _____.
    a. gray color on a white background
    b. echoes with one brightness level
    c. white color on a gray background
    d. a range of echo amplitudes

60. The dynamic range of an ultrasound system is _____.
    a. the speed with which ultrasound examination can be performed
    b. the range over which the transducer can be manipulated while an examination is performed
    c. the ratio of the maximum amplitude to the minimum echo strength that can be displayed
    d. the range of voltages applied to the transducer

61. A _____ _____ formats scan line data to image form.

62. Which of the following is *not* performed by a signal processor?
    a. Detection
    b. Filtering
    c. Digital-to-analog conversion
    d. Radio frequency–to–amplitude conversion
    e. Compression

63. In a digital memory, echo intensity is represented by _____.
    a. positive charge distribution
    b. a number stored in the memory
    c. electron density of the scan converter writing beam
    d. a and c
    e. all of the above

64. If there were no attenuation in tissue, _____ would not be needed.
    a. filtering
    b. compression
    c. detection
    d. time gain compensation

65. Echo imaging includes ultrasound generation, propagation and reflection in tissues, and reception of returning _____.

66. The diagnostic ultrasound systems in common clinical use today are of the _____-_____ type.

67. Gray-scale instruments show echo amplitude as _____ on the display.

68. Pulse-echo instruments look for three things: the _____, _____, and arrival _____ of echoes returning from tissues.

69. An image memory stores image information in the form of _____ numbers.
    a. electric charge
    b. binary
    c. decimal
    d. impedance
    e. none of the above

70. Imaging systems produce a visual _____ from the electric _____ received from the transducer.

71. The transducer is connected to the signal processor through the _____ _____.

72. The transducer receives voltages from the _____ _____ in pulse-echo systems.

73. The _____ _____ receives digitized echo voltages from the beam former.

74. Increasing gain generally produces the same effect as _____.
    a. decreasing attenuation
    b. increasing attenuation
    c. increasing compression
    d. increasing rectification
    e. b and c

75. The analog-to-digital converter is part of the _____.
    a. beam former
    b. signal processor
    c. image processor
    d. display
    e. a and b
    f. c and e

76. Voltage pulses from the pulser are applied through delays to the _____.

77. Detection is a function of the _____.
    a. beam former
    b. signal processor
    c. image processor
    d. display
    e. a and b

78. If gain is reduced by one half, with input power unchanged, the output power is _____ what it was before.
    a. equal to
    b. twice
    c. one half
    d. none of the above

79. If gain is 30 dB and output power is reduced by one half, the new gain is _____ dB.
    a. 15
    b. 60
    c. 33
    d. 27
    e. none of the above

80. If four shades of gray are shown on a display, each twice the brightness of the preceding one, the brightest shade is _____ times the brightness of the dimmest shade.
   a. 2
   b. 4
   c. 8
   d. 16
   e. 32
81. The dynamic range displayed in Exercise 80 is _____ dB.
   a. 10
   b. 9
   c. 5
   d. 2
   e. 0
82. In which units are gain and attenuation usually expressed?
   a. dB
   b. dB/cm
   c. cm
   d. cm/3 dB
   e. None of the above
83. Time gain compensation makes up for the fact that reflections from deeper reflectors arrive at the transducer with greater amplitude. True or false?
84. The modes that show one-dimensional (depth) real-time images are _____ and _____ mode.
85. The mode that shows two-dimensional real-time images is _____ mode.
86. A real-time B mode display may be produced by rapid _____ scanning of a transducer array.
87. Each complete scan of the sound beam produces an image on the display that is called a _____.
88. For a single focus, the number of lines in each frame is equal to the number of times the transducer is _____ while the frame is produced; that is, while the sound beam is scanned.
89. In real-time scanning, pulse repetition frequency depends on the number of _____ per frame and _____ rate.

90. Increasing the number of foci reduces _____ _____.
91. To correct for attenuation, time gain compensation must _____ the gain for increasing depth.
92. If a higher frequency is used, resolution is _____, imaging depth _____, and the time gain compensation slope must be _____.
93. For pixel dimensions 256 × 512 and 512 × 512, calculate the number of image pixels.
94. Which type of array gives a wide view close to the transducer? _____ Which of the following produce(s) a sector format image? _____
   a. Vector
   b. Linear
   c. Phased
   d. Convex
   e. More than one of the above
95. If a single-focus ultrasound instrument produces 1000 pulses per second and 20 frames per second, how many scan lines make up each frame?
96. In Figure 4-55, if two foci were used, the frame rate would be _____.
   a. 33
   b. 22
   c. 11
   d. 6
   e. 1

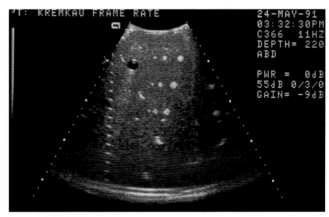

FIGURE 4-55 Illustration to accompany Exercise 96.

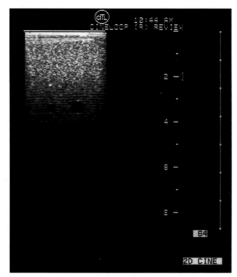

FIGURE 4-56 Illustration to accompany Exercise 97.

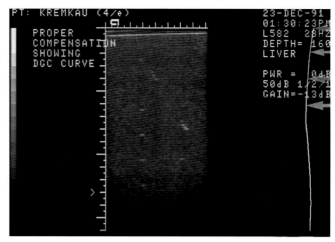

FIGURE 4-57 Illustration to accompany Exercise 98.

97. What is adjusted improperly in Figure 4-56?
   a. Gain
   b. Time gain compensation
   c. Compression
   d. Frame rate
   e. Rejection

98. The decreasing gain of the time gain compensation curve (*arrows*) in Figure 4-57 is caused by _____.
   a. weak attenuation
   b. refraction
   c. strong attenuation
   d. beam broadening
   e. beam narrowing

99. In the linear amplifier of Figure 4-58, the gain is _____ dB.
   a. 1000
   b. 300
   c. 100
   d. 60
   e. 10

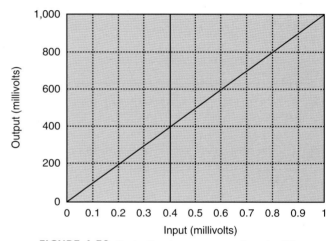

FIGURE 4-58 Illustration to accompany Exercise 99.

100. Compression is a function of the _____.
   a. beam former
   b. signal processor
   c. image processor
   d. scan converter
   e. image memory

5

Doppler Principles

LEARNING OBJECTIVES

After reading this chapter, the student should be able to do the following:

- List and compare the various kinds of flow encountered in blood circulation
- Explain how a stenosis affects flow
- Define and discuss the Doppler effect, the Doppler shift, and the Doppler angle
- Explain how two-dimensional flow information is color encoded on a sonographic display
- Compare Doppler-shift and Doppler-power displays
- Explain how flow detection is localized to a specific site in tissue using pulsed Doppler techniques
- Describe spectral analysis
- Discuss examples of how spectral analysis is applied to evaluate flow conditions at the site of measurement and elsewhere

OUTLINE

Flow
   Fluid
   Pressure, Resistance, and Volumetric Flow Rate
   Poiseuille's Equation
   Types of Flow
   Pulsatile Flow
   Continuity Rule
   Bernoulli Effect
Doppler Effect
   Doppler Shift
   Doppler Ultrasound
   Operating Frequency
   Doppler Angle
   Angle Accuracy

Color-Doppler Displays
   Color-Doppler Principle
   Instruments
   Doppler-Shift Detection
   Color Controls
   Color-Doppler Limitation
   Doppler Shift Displays
   Angle
   Doppler Power Displays
   Advantages and Disadvantages
Spectral-Doppler Displays
   Continuous-Wave Operation
   Components of a Continuous-Wave Doppler System
   Continuous-Wave Sample Volume

Angle Incorporation or Correction
Wall Filter
Pulsed-Wave Operation
Range Gate
Duplex Instrument
Spectral Analysis
Frequency Spectrum
Fast Fourier Transform
Spectral Displays
Spectral Broadening
Downstream (Distal) and Upstream (Proximal) Conditions
Review
Exercises

KEY TERMS

Autocorrelation
Baseline shift
Bernoulli effect
Bidirectional
Clutter
Color Doppler display
Compliance
Continuous wave Doppler
Cosine

Disturbed flow
Doppler angle
Doppler effect
Doppler equation
Doppler-power display
Doppler shift
Doppler spectrum
Duplex instrument
Eddies

Ensemble length
Fast Fourier transform
Filter
Flow
Fluid
Frequency spectrum
Gate
Hue
Inertia

FLOW

The circulatory system consists of the heart, arteries, arterioles, capillaries, venules, and veins, altogether containing about 5 liters (L) of blood. The heart is the pump that produces blood flow through the circulatory system. It is a contracting and relaxing muscle (the myocardium) with four chambers: two atria and two ventricles. Flow is from the superior and inferior vena cava and pulmonary veins into the right and left atria, respectively, and from there into the ventricles. From the left and right ventricles flow is into the aorta and pulmonary artery, respectively. When the heart contracts, the intended result is forward flow into the aorta and pulmonary artery. Valves are present in the heart to permit forward flow and prevent reverse flow. Malfunctioning valves can restrict forward flow by not opening sufficiently (**stenosis**) or allow reverse flow by not closing completely (insufficiency or regurgitation). Doppler ultrasound is useful for detecting both these conditions.

Flow in the heart, arteries, and veins can be detected with Doppler ultrasound. The capillaries are the tiniest vessels, measuring a few micrometers in diameter. The human body has approximately one billion capillaries. Across the capillary walls, the exchange of gases, nutrients, and waste products with the cells takes place, sustaining their life (this is the purpose of the circulatory system).

Fluid

Matter generally is classified into three categories: gas, liquid, and solid. Gases and liquids are **fluids**; that is, they are substances that **flow** and conform to the shape of their containers. To flow is to move in a stream, continually changing position and, possibly, direction. Rivers flow downstream. Water flows through a garden hose. Air flows through a fan. Blood flows through the heart, arteries, capillaries, and veins.

Gases and liquids are materials that flow.

Viscosity is the **resistance** to flow offered by a fluid in motion. Viscosity is given in units of **poise** or kilogram per meter-second (kg/m-s). One poise is 1 g/cm-s or 0.1 kg/m-s. Water has a relatively low viscosity compared with molasses, for example, which has a high viscosity. The viscosity of blood plasma is about 50% greater than that of water. The viscosity of normal blood is 0.035 poise at 37° C, approximately five times that of water. Blood viscosity (poise) can vary from about 0.02 (with anemia) to about 0.10 (with polycythemia). Blood viscosity also varies with flow speed.

Viscosity is the resistance of a fluid to flow.

Pressure, Resistance, and Volumetric Flow Rate

Pressure is the driving force behind fluid flow. Pressure is force per unit area. Pressure is equally distributed throughout a static fluid and exerts its force in all directions (Figure 5-1). A pressure difference is required for flow to occur. Equal pressures applied at both ends of a liquid-filled tube will result in no flow. If the pressure is greater at one end than at the other, the liquid will flow from the higher-pressure end to the lower-pressure end. This pressure difference can be generated by a pump (e.g., the heart in the circulatory system) or by the force of gravity (i.e., by raising one end of a tube higher than the other). (Because this is the situation in the lower-extremity veins in a standing person, these vessels have valves in them to prevent reverse flow.) The greater the pressure difference, the greater will be the flow rate. This pressure difference is sometimes called *pressure gradient*, although, strictly defined, pressure gradient is pressure difference *divided by distance between the two pressure locations*. The term *gradient* comes from the Latin *gradus* and refers to the upward or downward sloping of something. As the pressure decreases from one end of the tube to the other, this decrease can be thought of as a slope (i.e., pressure difference divided by distance over which the pressure drop occurs; Figure 5-2). A constant driving

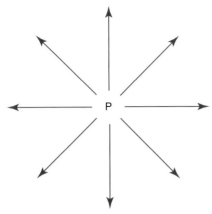

FIGURE 5-1 Pressure *(P)* is distributed uniformly throughout a static fluid and exerts its force in all directions.

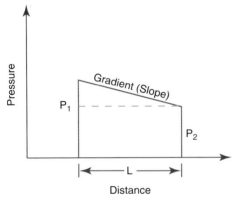

FIGURE 5-2 The pressure gradient or slope is the pressure difference *(P₁ − P₂)* divided by the separation *(L)* between the two pressure locations.

pressure produces steady (unchanging with time) flow. The driving pressure produced by the heart varies with time. This concept is considered later in this section.

 Fluid flows in a tube in response to a pressure difference at the ends.

Volumetric flow rate (*Q*) (sometimes simply called *flow,* although that term is used in other ways also) is the volume of blood passing a point per unit of time. Volumetric flow rate is usually expressed in milliliters (mL) per minute or per second. The total adult blood flow rate (cardiac output) is about 5000 mL/min (i.e., the total blood volume circulates in about 1 minute). The volumetric flow rate in a long straight tube is determined not only by the pressure difference (*ΔP*) but also by the resistance *(R)* to flow.

$$Q\,(mL/s) = \frac{\Delta P\,(dyne/cm^2)}{R\,(poise)}$$

 If pressure difference increases, volumetric flow rate increases.

 If flow resistance increases, volumetric flow rate decreases.

The flow resistance in a long, straight tube depends on the fluid viscosity (η) and the tube length (L) and radius (r), as follows:

$$R\,(g/cm^4\text{-}s) = 8 \times L\,(cm) \times \frac{\eta\,(poise)}{\pi \times [r^4\,(cm^4)]}$$

 If tube length increases, flow resistance increases.

 If tube radius increases, flow resistance decreases.

 If viscosity increases, flow resistance increases.

As expected, an increase in viscosity or tube length increases resistance, whereas an increase in the radius or diameter of the tube decreases resistance. The latter effect is particularly strong, with resistance depending on radius to the fourth power (r⁴). Thus doubling the radius of a tube decreases its resistance to one sixteenth its original value. From experience, we know that a longer- or smaller-diameter garden hose reduces water flow rate. And we can presume that if we tried to force molasses through a hose, we would not get nearly the flow rate we would get with water.

Poiseuille's Equation

Using the flow resistance equation in the flow rate equation and tube diameter (d) instead of radius yields **Poiseuille's equation** for volumetric flow rate:

$$Q\,(mL/s) = \frac{\Delta P\,(dyne/cm^2) \times \pi \times d^4\,(cm^4)}{128 \times L\,(cm) \times \eta\,(poise)}$$

Recall that this equation is for steady flow in long, straight tubes. Thus the equation serves only as a rough approximation of the conditions in blood circulation. The equation is useful, however, in making qualitative conclusions and predictions, as follows:

 If pressure difference increases, flow rate increases.

 If diameter increases, flow rate increases.

If length increases, flow rate decreases.

 If viscosity increases, flow rate decreases.

The resistance of the arterioles accounts for about half the total resistance in systemic circulation. The muscular walls of arterioles can constrict or relax, producing dramatic changes in flow resistance. The walls thus can control blood flow to specific tissues and organs in response to their needs.

 The volumetric flow rate in a tube depends on the pressure difference, the length and diameter of the tube, and the viscosity of the fluid.

Types of Flow

Flow can be divided into five spatial categories: (1) plug, (2) laminar, (3) parabolic, (4) disturbed, and (5) turbulent. At the entrance to a tube, the speed of the fluid is essentially constant across the tube (Figure 5-3). This is called **plug flow** because it is similar to the motion of a solid object (a plug, for example) that does not flow but moves as a unit. As the fluid flows down the tube, laminar (from the Latin term for "layer") flow develops. **Laminar flow** is a flow condition in which **streamlines** (which describe the motion of fluid particles) are straight and parallel to each other. Flow speed is maximum at the center of the tube and minimum or zero at the tube walls. A decreasing profile of flow speeds from the center to the wall is present. Successive layers of fluid slide on each other with relative motion. The pressure difference at each end of the tube overcomes the viscous resistance of the layers sliding over each other, maintaining the laminar flow through the tube. Steady flow in a long, straight tube results in a **parabolic flow** profile (Figure 5-4). Parabolic flow is a particular pattern of laminar flow in which varying flow speeds across the tube are described by a parabola (the curved dashed line in Figure

5-4). In the case of parabolic flow, the average flow speed across the vessel is equal to one half the maximum flow speed (at the center). Parabolic flow is not commonly seen in blood circulation because blood vessels generally are not long and straight. However, nonparabolic laminar flow is commonly seen; indeed, its absence is often an indicator of abnormal flow conditions at a site where there is vascular or cardiac-valvular disease.

 Laminar flow is flow where layers of fluid slide over each other.

Disturbed flow occurs when the parallel streamlines describing the flow (see Figure 5-3) are altered from their straight form (Figure 5-5). This occurs, for example, in the region of a stenosis or at a bifurcation (the point at which a vessel splits into two). In disturbed flow, particles of fluid still flow in the forward direction. Parabolic and disturbed flows are forms of laminar flow.

In the final category, turbulent flow, or **turbulence**, the flow pattern is random and chaotic, with particles moving at different speeds in many directions, even in circles called **eddies**, with forward *net* flow still maintained. As flow speed increases in a tube, turbulent flow eventually will occur (Figure 5-6). Turbulence also occurs in the transition from high flow speed in a narrow channel to slow flow in a broad stream (Figure 5-7).

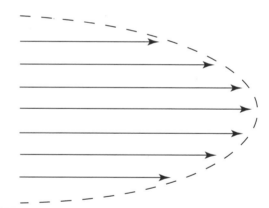

FIGURE 5-4 Parabolic flow profile. The dashed line is a parabola.

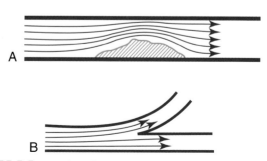

FIGURE 5-5 Disturbed flow at a stenosis **(A)** and at a bifurcation **(B)**.

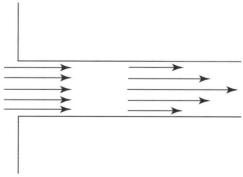

FIGURE 5-3 At the entrance to a tube or vessel, plug flow exists. After some distance, laminar flow is achieved.

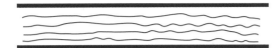

FIGURE 5-6 Turbulent flow in a vessel may result from too great a flow speed.

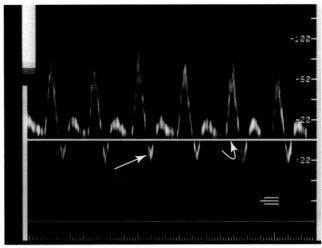

FIGURE 5-8 Flow reversal *(straight arrow)* below the baseline *(curved arrow)* is seen in the superficial femoral artery in diastole.

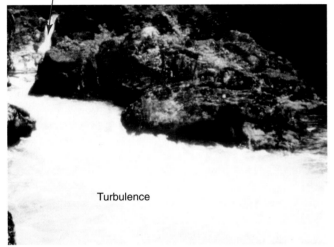

Fast flow in stenosis

Turbulence

FIGURE 5-7 In a narrow gorge, flow speeds are high. Beyond the narrow region there is abundant turbulence.

 Disturbed flow is a form of laminar flow in which streamlines are not straight. *Turbulent flow* is nonlaminar flow with random and chaotic speeds and directions.

Pulsatile Flow

Thus far, we have considered steady flow in which pressures, flow speeds, and flow patterns do not change with time. This is generally the situation on the venous side of the circulatory system, although cardiac pulsations or respiratory cycles can influence venous flow in some locations. However, in the heart and in arterial circulation, flow is pulsatile, being directly influenced by the effects of the beating heart with pulsatile variations of increasing and decreasing pressure and flow speed. For steady flow, volumetric flow rate is simply related to pressure difference and flow resistance. With **pulsatile flow**, the relationship between the varying pressure and flow rate depends on flow impedance, which includes resistance, as discussed earlier; the **inertia** of the fluid as it accelerates and decelerates; and the **compliance** (expansion and contraction) of the nonrigid vessel walls. The mathematical analysis is complex and is not presented here. Two dominant characteristics of interest in this type of flow are the Windkessel effect and flow reversal. When the pressure pulse forces a fluid into a compliant vessel, such as the aorta, the vessel expands and increases the volume within it. (This is why it is easy to feel the

pulse on the wrist or neck.) Later in the cycle, when the driving pressure is reduced, the compliant vessel is able to contract, producing extended flow later in the pressure cycle. This is known as the *Windkessel effect.* In the aorta, the Windkessel effect results in continued flow in the forward direction because aortic valve closure prevents backward flow into the heart. In the distal circulation, the expansion of distensible vessels results in the reversal of flow in diastole as the pressure decreases and the distended vessels contract. Flow reversal occurs where there are no valves to prevent it (Figure 5-8). This is a normal occurrence in these locations. Pulsatile flow in compliant vessels thus includes added forward flow and/or flow reversal in diastole, depending on location within arterial circulation. Arterial diastolic flow (absence, presence, direction, quantity) reveals much concerning the state of downstream arterioles, where flow cannot be measured directly with ultrasound.

 Pulsatile flow is nonsteady flow, with acceleration and deceleration over the cardiac cycle.

 Pulsatile flow in distensible vessels includes added forward flow and/or flow reversal over the cardiac cycle in some locations in circulation.

Continuity Rule

A narrowing of the lumen of a vessel, or **stenosis**, produces disturbed (see Figure 5-5, *A*) and possibly turbulent flow (see Figure 5-7). The average flow speed in the stenosis must be greater than the average flow speed proximal and distal to the stenosis so that the volumetric flow rate is constant throughout the vessel. Examples of increased flow speed at a stenosis and turbulence beyond it are given later in this chapter. Volumetric flow rate must be constant in all three regions—proximal to the stenosis, at the stenosis, and distal to the stenosis—because blood is neither created nor destroyed as it flows through a vessel. This is called the *continuity rule*. Volumetric flow rate is equal to average flow speed across the vessel multiplied by the cross-sectional area of the vessel. Therefore, if the stenosis has an area measuring one half the area of the proximal and distal vessel, the average flow speed within the stenosis is twice the average flow speed proximal and distal to the stenosis. If a stenosis has a diameter that is one half the diameter of the adjacent area, the area at the stenosis is one fourth that of the adjacent area, so the average flow speed in the stenosis must quadruple.

 Flow speed increases at a stenosis, and turbulence can occur distal to it.

It is sometimes puzzling to students that Poiseuille's law and the continuity rule for a stenosis seem contradictory. One states that flow speed decreases with smaller diameters (Poiseuille's law), whereas the other says that flow speed increases with smaller diameters (continuity rule). How can this be so? The answer is that the two situations are different. Poiseuille's law deals with a long, straight vessel with no stenosis. The diameter in Poiseuille's law refers to the diameter of the *entire vessel*.

By contrast, the diameter in the continuity rule refers to the diameter of a short portion of a vessel (the stenosis). If the diameter of the entire vessel is reduced (as in vasoconstriction), flow speed is reduced. If the diameter of only a short segment of a vessel is reduced (stenosis), the flow speed in the vessel is unaffected, except at the stenosis, where it is increased. Flow speed increases because the stenosis has little effect on the overall flow resistance of the entire vessel if the stenosis length is small compared with the vessel length and if the lumen in the stenosis is not too small (does not approach occlusion). Figure 5-9 illustrates these dependencies of volumetric flow rate and flow speed at the stenosis with increasing stenosis. The maximum normal flow speed in circulation is about 100 cm/s. However, in stenotic regions, flow speeds can increase to a few meters per second. Doppler ultrasound is useful for detecting flow speed increases associated with vascular disease.

The increased flow speed within a stenosis can cause turbulence distal to it. Sounds produced by turbulence, which can be heard with a stethoscope, are called *bruits*. The ultimate stenosis is called an *occlusion*, where the vessel is blocked and there is no flow. Using our garden hose analogy again, we can compress the hose (not near the nozzle) and see little effect on the flow at the nozzle until the hose is compressed to near-occlusion. At that point, turbulence may occur, and vibration can be felt on the surface of the hose.

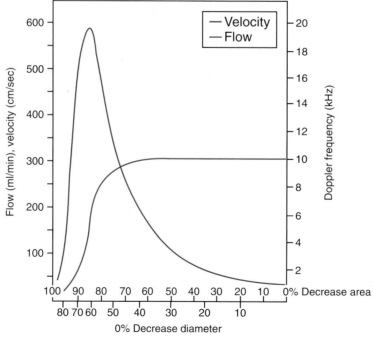

FIGURE 5-9 As the diameter of the stenosis is reduced (moving to the left on the horizontal axis; tighter stenosis), volumetric flow rate (*Q*) is unaffected initially because the stenosis does not contribute substantially to the total vessel resistance. As the diameter continues to decrease, however, the vessel resistance increases, reducing the volumetric flow rate (eventually to zero at occlusion). Flow rate and, thus, distal pressure begin to drop significantly beyond a diameter reduction of about 50% (area reduction of 75%). As the diameter of the stenosis decreases, flow speed increases (because of the flow continuity requirement), reaches a maximum, and then decreases to zero as the increasing flow resistance effect dominates. *(Modified from Spencer MP, Reid JM: Quantitation of carotid stenosis with continuous-wave (C-W) Doppler ultrasound,* Stroke *10:326–330, 1979. Reprinted with permission. Copyright 1979 American Heart Association.)*

Bernoulli Effect

At the stenosis, the pressure is less than it is proximal and distal to the stenotic area (Figure 5-10). This pressure difference is necessary to allow the fluid to accelerate into the stenosis and decelerate out of it and also to maintain energy balance. (Pressure energy is converted to flow energy upon entry, and then vice versa upon exit.) This decreased pressure in regions of high flow speed is known as the **Bernoulli effect** and is described by Bernoulli's equation, a description of the constant energy of the fluid flow through a stenosis, ignoring viscous loss. As flow energy increases, pressure energy decreases. The magnitude of the decrease in pressure (ΔP) that results from the increasing flow speed (v) at the stenosis can be found from Bernoulli's equation. In a simplified form of the equation, the flow speed proximal to the stenosis is assumed to be small enough, compared with the flow speed in the stenosis, to be ignored. Pressure drop from a stenotic heart valve can reduce cardiac output. For calculating pressure drop across a stenotic valve, the following form of the equation is used in Doppler echocardiography:

$$\Delta P = 4(v_2)^2$$

In this equation, v_2 is the flow speed (meters/second) in the jet and ΔP (millimeters of mercury) is the pressure drop across the valve. For example, if the flow speed in the jet is 5 m/s, the pressure drop is 100 mm Hg. Thus pressure drop can be calculated from a measurement of flow speed at the stenotic valve using Doppler ultrasound.

 If flow speed increases, the magnitude of the pressure drop increases.

 The Bernoulli effect is a drop in pressure associated with high flow speed at a stenosis.

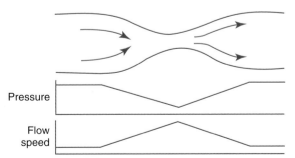

FIGURE 5-10 To maintain flow continuity, flow speed must increase through a stenosis. In conjunction with this, the pressure drops (the Bernoulli effect) in the stenosis. (*From Kremkau FW:* Fluid Flow III, *J Vasc Technol 17:153–154, 1993. Reprinted with permission.*)

DOPPLER EFFECT

The **Doppler effect** is a change in frequency (and wavelength) caused by the motion of a sound source, receiver, or reflector. If a reflector is moving toward the source and receiver, the received echo has a higher frequency than would occur without the motion. Conversely, if the motion is away (recedes), the received echo has a lower frequency. The amount of increase or decrease in frequency depends on the speed of reflector motion, the angle between the wave propagation direction and the motion direction, and the frequency of the wave emitted by the source.

A quantitative description of the Doppler effect is provided by the **Doppler equation**. The Doppler equation can deal with any of three situations: (1) moving source, (2) receiver, or (3) reflector. Only the moving reflector result will be given because it is the relevant situation of interest for diagnostic Doppler ultrasound.

A moving reflector (Figure 5-11) or scatterer of a wave is a combination of a moving receiver and a source. For a moving reflector approaching a stationary source, more cycles of a wave are encountered in 1 second than would be if the reflector were stationary. Additionally, the reflected cycles are compressed in front of the reflector as it moves into its own reflected wave. Both effects increase the frequency of the reflected wave (echo).

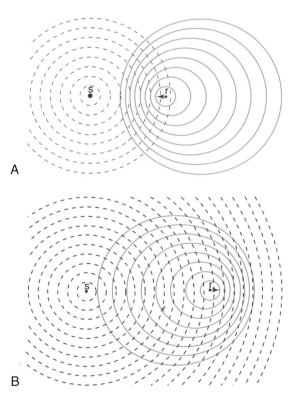

FIGURE 5-11 A moving reflector *(r)* returns a higher frequency echo if it is approaching the source *(s)* and receiver *(s)* **(A)** and a lower frequency echo if it is moving away from the source and receiver **(B).**

Doppler Shift

The change in frequency caused by motion is called the *Doppler-shift frequency* or, more commonly, the **Doppler shift** (f_D). The Doppler shift is equal to the received frequency (f_R) minus the source frequency (f_0). For an approaching reflector (scatterer), the Doppler shift is positive; that is, the received frequency is greater than the source frequency. For a receding reflector, the Doppler shift is negative; that is, the received frequency is smaller than the source frequency. The relationship between the Doppler shift and the reflector speed (v) is given by the Doppler equation:

$$f_D(kHz) = f_R(kHz) - f_0(kHz) = f_0(kHz) \times \frac{[2 \times v(cm/s)]}{c(cm/s)}$$

If scatterer speed increases, the Doppler shift increases. If source frequency increases, the Doppler shift increases.

The Doppler shift is the difference between the emitted frequency and the echo frequency returning from moving scatterers.

Take, for example, a source frequency of 5 MHz, a scatterer speed of 50 cm/s (0.5 m/s), and a propagation (sound) speed of 1540 m/s. The scatterer is approaching the source, so the received frequency is greater than the source frequency, with a positive Doppler shift of 0.0032 MHz or 3.2 kHz. For a scatterer moving away from a receiver, the Doppler shift is –3.2 kHz. Other examples using various source frequencies and scatterer speeds are given in Table 5-1.

The Doppler shift is detected by the instruments described in this chapter. However, we are interested in the speed of tissue motion or blood flow, not the Doppler shift itself. To facilitate this, the Doppler equation is rearranged to place the speed of motion alone on the left side of the equation. Substituting the speed of sound in tissues (154,000 cm/s) and using units as indicated for the various quantities yield the equation in the following form:

$$v(cm/s) = \frac{77(cm/ms) \times f_D(kHz)}{f_0(MHz)}$$

The Doppler equation relates the Doppler shift to flow speed and frequency.

The fact that the Doppler shift is proportional to the blood flow speed explains why the Doppler effect is so useful in medical diagnosis. Doppler instruments measure the Doppler shift. Blood flow is what interests us. The measured shifts are proportional to flow speed, which is the information we seek. The Doppler shift is measured by the instrument and the Doppler equation is solved to yield calculated flow-speed information.

Doppler Ultrasound

With diagnostic medical ultrasound, stationary transducers are used to emit and receive the ultrasound. The Doppler effect is a result of the motion of blood, the flow of which we wish to measure, or the motion of tissue that we wish to evaluate. Physiologic flow speeds, even in highly stenotic jets, do not exceed a few meters per second. Table 5-1 gives Doppler shifts resulting from typical physiologic flow speeds. The minimum detectable blood flow speed with Doppler ultrasound is a few millimeters per second. The maximum is determined by *aliasing* (discussed in Chapter 6).

The Doppler shift is proportional to flow speed.

Operating Frequency

For a given flow in a vessel, the Doppler shift measured by an instrument is proportional to the operating frequency of the instrument (Figure 5-12; also see Table 5-1). Thus measurement of Doppler shifts from flow in the same vessel using two transducers operating at 2 MHz and 4 MHz will yield two Doppler shifts. The higher-frequency transducer will have a Doppler shift that is twice that of the lower-frequency transducer. Therefore, when comparing Doppler shifts, one must consider the frequency of the devices. The operating frequency is incorporated into the calculation of flow speed using the Doppler equation. Thus comparisons of flow speeds between different instruments have taken this variable into account.

TABLE 5-1	Doppler Frequency Shifts for Various Scatterer Speeds Toward* the Sound Source at a Zero Doppler Angle		
Incident Frequency (MHz)	Scatterer Speed (cm/s)	Reflected Frequency (MHz)	Doppler Shift (kHz)
2	50	2.0013	1.3
5	50	5.0032	3.2
10	50	10.0065	6.5
2	200	2.0052	5.2
5	200	5.013	13.0
10	200	10.026	26.0

*Motion away from the source would yield negative Doppler shifts.

The Doppler shift is proportional to the operating frequency.

Doppler frequencies used in vascular studies are slightly less than those used for anatomic imaging

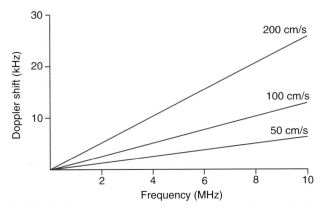

FIGURE 5-12 The Doppler shift as a function of operating frequency, as determined by the Doppler equation for various flow speeds (at a zero Doppler angle).

because echoes from blood are weaker than those from soft tissues.

Doppler Angle

If the direction of sound propagation is exactly opposite the flow direction, the maximum positive Doppler shift is obtained. If the flow speed and propagation speed directions are the same (parallel), the maximum negative Doppler shift is obtained. If the angle between these two directions (Figure 5-13) is nonzero (non-parallel), lesser Doppler shifts will occur. The Doppler shift depends on the **cosine** of the **Doppler angle (θ)**.

$$f_D(kHz) = \frac{[f_o(kHz) \times 2 \times v(cm/s) \times (\cos\theta)]}{c(cm/s)}$$

$$v(cm/s) = \frac{[77(cm/ms) \times f_D(kHz)]}{[f_o(MHz) \times \cos\theta]}$$

Table 5-2 gives cosine values for various angles. Only the portion of the motion direction that is parallel to the sound beam contributes to the Doppler effect. The cosine gives the component of the flow velocity vector that is

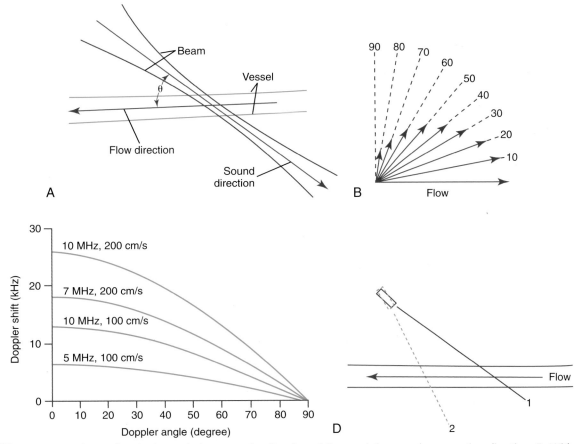

FIGURE 5-13 A, The Doppler angle θ is the angle between the direction of flow and the sound propagation direction. **B,** With constant flow, as the Doppler angle increases, echo Doppler shift frequency decreases. The direction of the arrows indicates the beam direction. The length of the arrows indicates the magnitude of the Doppler shift. **C,** The Doppler shift as a function of angle, as determined by the Doppler equation for various incident frequencies and scatterer speeds. **D,** The same flow in a vessel, viewed at different angles, yields different Doppler shifts.

TABLE 5-2	Cosines for Various Angles
Angle A (degrees)	Cos A
0	1.000
5	0.996
10	0.980
15	0.970
20	0.940
25	0.910
30	0.870
35	0.820
40	0.770
45	0.710
50	0.640
55	0.570
60	0.500
65	0.420
70	0.34
75	0.26
80	0.17
85	0.09
90	0.00

parallel to the sound beam (Figure 5-14). For a given flow, the larger the Doppler angle, the less is the Doppler shift (see Figure 5-13, *B–C*). Table 5-3 lists examples of Doppler shifts for various angles.

 If the Doppler shift increases, the calculated scatterer speed increases.

 If the source frequency increases, the calculated scatterer speed decreases.

 If cosine increases, the calculated scatterer speed decreases.

 If the Doppler angle increases, the calculated scatterer speed increases.

Angle Accuracy

Flow speed calculations based on Doppler shift measurements can be accomplished correctly only with proper incorporation of the Doppler angle. The calculations, therefore, are only as good as the accuracy of the measurement, estimate, or guess of that angle. Estimation of the angle is usually done by orienting an indicator line on the anatomic display so that it is parallel to the presumed direction of flow (e.g., parallel to the vessel wall for a straight vessel with no flow obstruction). This is a subjective operation performed by the instrument operator. Error in this estimation of the Doppler angle is more

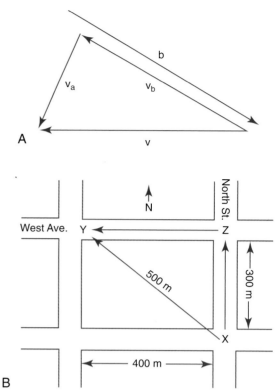

FIGURE 5-14 A, The flow velocity vector *(v)* can be broken into two components: one *(v_b)* that is parallel to the sound beam *(b)* direction and one *(v_a)* that is perpendicular to the sound beam direction. Only the component parallel to the beam contributes to the Doppler effect. **B,** A city block can be used as an analogy to the vector components in **A.** To get from point X to point Y, one could walk diagonally across the block, a distance of 500 m. However, if buildings blocked that path, an alternative route would be 300 m north on North Street and then 400 m west on West Avenue. The 500-m northwest vector from X to Y is equivalent to a 300-m north vector plus a 400-m west vector (i.e., the result is the same: depart from X and arrive at Y). In this example, the component of the XY vector parallel to North Street is the XZ vector and the component parallel to West Avenue is the ZY vector.

TABLE 5-3	Doppler Frequency Shifts for Various Angles and Scatterer Speeds Toward the Sound Source of Frequency 5 MHz	
Scatterer Speed (cm/s)	Angle (degrees)	Doppler Shift (kHz)
100	0	6.5
100	30	5.6
100	60	3.2
100	90	0.0
300	0	19.0
300	30	17.0
300	60	9.7
300	0	0.0

| TABLE 5-4 | Cosine and Calculated-Speed Errors for Angle Errors of 2 and 5 Degrees | | | |

True Angle (degrees)	Cosine Error (%)		Speed Error (%)	
	+2 Degrees	+5 Degrees	+2 Degrees	+5 Degrees
0	−0.1	−0.4	+0.1	+0.4
10	−0.7	−1.9	+0.7	+2.0
20	−1.3	−3.6	+1.3	+3.7
30	−2.1	−5.4	+2.1	+5.7
40	−3.0	−7.7	+3.1	+8.3
50	−4.2	−10.8	+4.4	+12.1
60	−6.1	−15.5	+6.5	+18.3
70	−9.6	−24.3	+10.7	+32.1
80	−19.9	−49.8	+24.8	+99.2

| TABLE 5-5 | Doppler Shifts (for 4 MHz) at Various Doppler Angles for the Same Flow Yielding a Consistent Calculated Flow Speed | |

Calculated Flow Doppler Shift (kHz)	Angle (degrees)	Speed (cm/s)
2.25	30	50
1.99	40	50
1.84	45	50
1.67	50	50
1.30	60	50

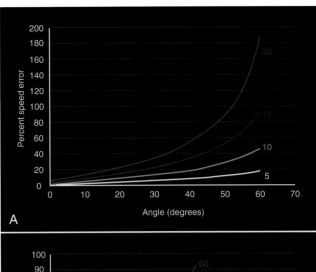
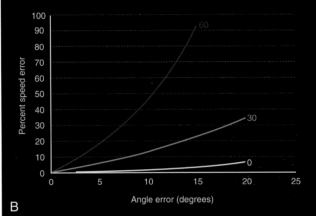

FIGURE 5-15 A, Percent calculated speed error versus correct Doppler angle for 5-, 10-, 15-, and 20-degree angle errors. B, Percent calculated speed error versus angle error for three values (0, 30, and 60 degrees) of the correct Doppler angle.

critical at large angles than at small ones because the cosine changes rapidly at large angles. Table 5-4 gives error values for various angles. For example, if the correct Doppler angle is 60 degrees but the estimation is 5 degrees in error (the angle estimate is 55 or 65 degrees), the error in the cosine value is about 15%, yielding a calculated speed that is in error by about 18%. Figure 5-15 shows how the error in the calculated flow speed increases with angle. For this reason, and because Doppler shift frequencies become very small at large angles, thereby reducing the system sensitivity, Doppler measurements (and particularly the calculated flow speeds) are not reliably achieved at Doppler angles greater than about 60 degrees. In principle, if the angle is incorporated correctly, the calculated flow speed in the vessel should be the same, regardless of what the Doppler angle is; that is, the actual flow speed is certainly not altered by the Doppler angle used in detecting it (Table 5-5). Not surprisingly, however, inaccuracies in angle estimation do occur. Flow is also often not parallel to vessel walls, even in unobstructed vessels.

At Doppler angles less than about 30 degrees, the sound no longer enters the blood at all but is reflected totally at the wall–blood boundary. One generally achieves success, then, at angles greater than this. However, in Doppler echocardiography, Doppler angles of near-zero are useful, and zero is commonly assumed (i.e., angle correction is not incorporated in this application, as it is in vascular work). The angle between the beam and the heart wall is large, which avoids the total reflection problem (Figure 5-16).

In this discussion, we have considered the Doppler angle only in the scan plane. One must remember that the flow may not be parallel to the imaging scan plane, which includes the Doppler beam, so there may be a component of Doppler angle between flow direction and scan plane. Thus one must keep in mind the three-dimensional character of the components involved in the process (vessel anatomy, flow direction, and ultrasound image scan plane).

COLOR-DOPPLER DISPLAYS

Doppler instruments present information on the presence, direction, speed, and character of blood flow (Box 5-1) and on the presence, direction, and speed of tissue

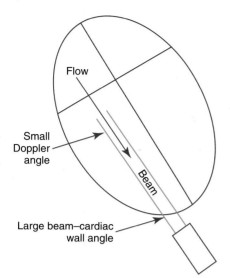

FIGURE 5-16 In cardiac Doppler work, Doppler angles are usually small, whereas the angle between the beam and the cardiac wall is usually large.

BOX 5-1	Types of Flow Information Provided by Doppler Ultrasound

- Presence of flow
  - Yes
  - No
- Direction of flow
  - →
  - ←
- Speed of flow
  - Slow
  - Fast
- Character of flow
  - Laminar
  - Turbulent

BOX 5-2	Various Forms of Presentation of Doppler Information

- Audible sounds
- Strip-chart recording
- Spectral display
- Color-Doppler display

motion. This information is present in audible, color Doppler, and spectral Doppler forms (Box 5-2). Color Doppler imaging presents two-dimensional, cross-sectional, real-time blood flow or tissue motion information along with two-dimensional, cross-sectional, gray-scale anatomic imaging. Two-dimensional real-time presentations of flow information allow the observer to readily locate regions of abnormal flow for further evaluation using **spectral analysis**. The direction of flow is appreciated readily, and disturbed or turbulent flow is presented dramatically in two-dimensional form. Color

Doppler presents anatomic information in the conventional gray-scale form but also rapidly detects Doppler shift frequencies at several locations along each scan line, presenting them in color at appropriate locations in the cross-sectional image.

Color-Doppler Principle

Color-Doppler imaging (sometimes called *color-flow imaging*) extends the use of the pulse-echo imaging principle to include Doppler-shifted echoes that indicate blood flow or tissue motion. Echoes returning from stationary tissues are detected and presented in gray scale in appropriate locations along scan lines. Depth is determined by echo arrival time, and brightness is determined by echo intensity. If a returning echo has a different frequency from that of what was emitted, a Doppler shift has occurred because the echo-generating object was moving. Depending on whether the motion is toward or away from the transducer, the Doppler shift is positive or negative. At locations along scan lines where Doppler shifts are detected, appropriate colors are assigned to the display pixels.

Doppler-shifted echoes can be recorded and presented in color at many locations along each scan line (Figure 5-17, A–B). As in all sonography, many such scan lines make up one cross-sectional image (see Figure 5-17, C–D). Several of these images (frames) are presented each second, yielding real-time color Doppler sonography.

 Colo-Doppler imaging is an extension of conventional gray-scale sonography and shows regions of blood flow or tissue motion in color.

Linear array presentation of color Doppler information is sometimes inadequate when the vessel runs parallel to the skin surface because the pulses (and scan lines) run perpendicular to the transducer surface (and therefore to the skin surface), resulting in a 90-degree Doppler angle where the pulses intersect the flow in the vessel. If the flow is parallel to the vessel walls, the 90-degree Doppler angle would yield no Doppler shift, and hence no color within the vessel. To solve this problem, phasing is used to steer each emitted pulse from the array in a given direction (e.g., 20 degrees away from perpendicular). All the color pulses and color scan lines are steered at the same angle, resulting in a parallelogram presentation of color Doppler information on the display (Figure 5-18).

Instruments

The color Doppler display is part of a sonographic instrument (see Figure 4-1, A). The beam former, signal

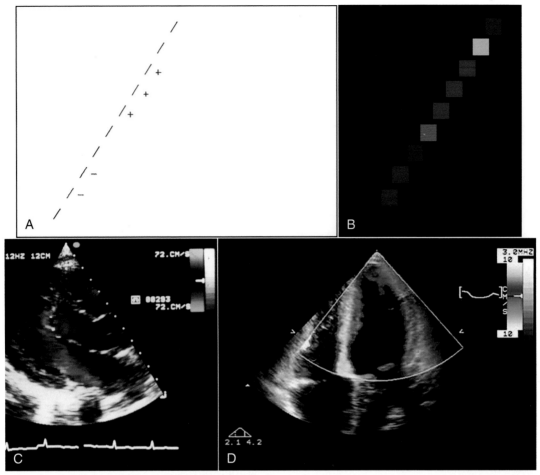

FIGURE 5-17 A, Ten echoes are received as a pulse travels through tissues. Three (red) have positive Doppler shifts, and two (blue) have negative shifts. **B,** These echoes are shown (in this example) as red and blue pixels, respectively, on the color Doppler display. As in gray-scale sonography, a two-dimensional cross-sectional image is made up of many scan lines. **C,** A parasternal long-axis image of normal mitral valve blood flow. **D,** A parasternal short-axis view of myocardial tissue motion (color kinesis).

processor, image processor, and display perform the same functions as they do in anatomic imaging. In addition, the signal processor has the ability to detect Doppler shifts, and the display is capable of presenting echoes in color.

 Color Doppler uses conventional sonographic instruments that have the ability to detect Doppler shifts and present them on the display in color.

Doppler Shift Detection

The signal processor receives the digitized voltages from the beam former that represent the echoes returning from the tissue. Non–Doppler-shifted echoes are processed conventionally, as in any sonographic instrument. Doppler-shifted echoes are commonly detected in the signal processor using a mathematical technique called **autocorrelation,** which rapidly determines the mean and **variance** of the Doppler shift signal (Figure 5-19) at each location along the scan line (at each selected echo arrival time during pulse travel). The autocorrelation technique is a mathematical process that yields Doppler shift information for each sample time (and corresponding depth down the scan line) following pulse emission. The sign, mean, and variance of the Doppler signal are stored at appropriate locations in the memory corresponding to anatomic sites where the Doppler shifts have been found. Typically 100 to 400 Doppler samples (locations) per scan line are shown on a **color Doppler display.** Depending on the depth and width of the color presentation, typically 5 to 50 frames per second can be shown. Recall that for gray-scale sonography, a single pulse produces one scan line. For multiple foci, multiple pulses per scan line are required. In color Doppler instruments, multiple pulses are involved in all images because they are required in the autocorrelation process. A three-pulse minimum is required for one speed estimate. More pulses are required for improved accuracy of the estimates, for variance determinations, or to improve detection of lower-frequency mean Doppler shifts (slower flows).

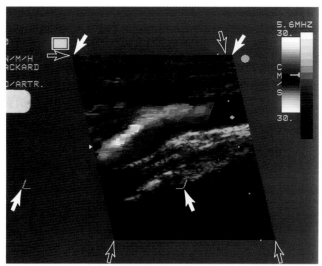

FIGURE 5-18 A perpendicular Doppler angle is avoided in this image by electronically steering the color-producing Doppler pulses to the left of vertical. The corners of the resulting parallelogram in which color can be displayed are shown by the solid arrows. Note that on this instrument, the gray-scale anatomic imaging pulses can also be steered (in this case, to the right of vertical). The corners of the resulting gray-scale parallelogram are shown by the open arrows. *(From Kremkau FW: Principles and pitfalls of real-time color-flow imaging. In Bernstein EF, editor: Vascular diagnosis, 4th ed, St. Louis, 1993, Mosby.)*

 Autocorrelation is the mathematical process commonly used to detect Doppler shifts in color Doppler instruments.

Color Controls

Color controls (Figure 5-20) include gain, color **window** location, width and depth, steering angle, color inversion, **wall filter, priority, baseline shift**, velocity range (pulse repetition frequency [PRF]), color map selection, variance, smoothing, and **ensemble length**. Steering angle control permits avoidance of 90-degree angles (Figure 5-21). Color inversion alternates the color assignments on either side of the zero-Doppler-shift baseline on the color map (Figure 5-21, *D–E*). The wall filter allows elimination of **clutter** caused by tissue and wall motion (Figure 5-22). However, one must take care not to set the wall filter too high, or slower blood flow signals will be removed (see Figure 5-22, *C*). The operator of a gray-scale sonographic instrument does not have direct control of pulse repetition frequency. But in Doppler operation, the operator does control pulse repetition frequency with the scale control. This control sets the pulse repetition frequency and the limit at the color bar extremes. Decreasing the value permits observation of slower flows (smaller Doppler shifts) (see Figure 5-22, *F*) but increases the probability of an artifact, called *aliasing*, for faster flows (aliasing is described in Chapter 6). Priority selects the gray-scale echo strength below which color, instead of gray level, will be shown at each

pixel location (Figure 5-23). Baseline control allows shifting the baseline up or down to correct aliasing. Smoothing (also called *persistence*) provides frame-to-frame averaging to reduce noise (Figure 5-24). Ensemble length is the number of pulses used for each color scan line. The minimum is 3, with 10 to 20 being common. Greater ensemble lengths provide more accurate estimates of mean Doppler shift, improved detection of slow flows, and complete representation of flow within a vessel (see Figure 5-24) but at the expense of longer time per frame and therefore lower frame rates. Wider color windows (viewing areas) also reduce frame rates because more scan lines are required for each frame (Figure 5-25).

Color-Doppler Limitations

Several aspects of color Doppler imaging are, by their nature, limiting. These aspects include angle dependence, lower frame rates, and lack of detailed spectral information. Spectral Doppler presents the entire range of Doppler shift frequencies received as they change over the cardiac cycle. Color Doppler displays present only a statistical representation of the complete spectrum at each pixel location on the display. The sign, mean value, and, if chosen, the power or the variance of the spectrum are color coded into combinations of **hue, saturation,** and **luminance** that are presented at each display pixel location. Some Doppler displays have the capability of reading the quantitative digital values for mean Doppler shifts (sometimes converted to angle-corrected equivalent flow speed) at chosen pixel locations (Figure 5-26). One must realize that these are mean values that must be compared carefully with the peak systolic values, which are used commonly to evaluate spectral displays. Because color Doppler techniques require several pulses per scan line (as opposed to one pulse per scan line for single-focus, gray-scale anatomic imaging), frame rates are lower than those for gray-scale anatomic imaging. Therefore multiple foci are not used in color Doppler imaging. The relationship between penetration (*pen*), line density, and frame rate is the same as that presented in Chapter 4, except that ensemble length (*n*) replaces number of foci. The maximum permissible frame rate (*FR$_m$*) is as follows:

$$FR_m\,(Hz) = \frac{77,000\,(cm/s)}{[pen\,(cm) \times LPF^* \times n]}$$

 If ensemble length increases, frame rate decreases.

Doppler Shift Displays

Where Doppler-shifted echoes have been stored, hue, saturation, and luminance appropriate to the shift infor-

---

*LPF, Lines per frame.

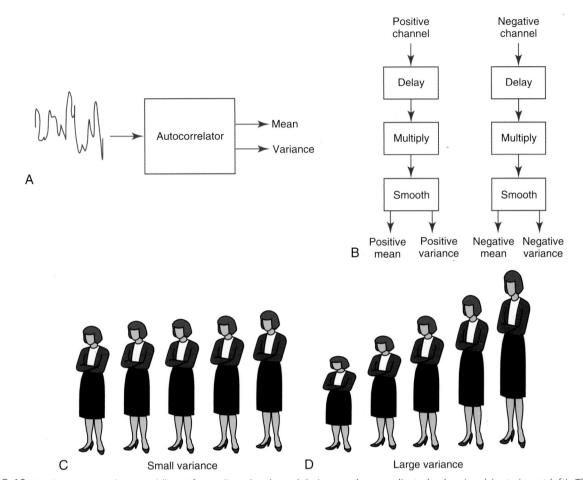

FIGURE 5-19 **A,** The autocorrelator rapidly performs Doppler demodulation on the complicated echo signal (entering at left). The outputs of the autocorrelator yield the magnitude of the mean and the variance of Doppler shifts at each location in the scanned cross-section. These items of information are stored in each pixel location in the memory. Color assignments are selected appropriately to indicate these items of information two-dimensionally on the display. **B,** After division of the Doppler signal into positive and negative Doppler shift channels, each signal is multiplied by a version of itself delayed by one pulse repetition period. High-frequency variations are filtered out (smoothed) to yield the mean and variance of Doppler shifts. Variance is a measure of data spread around a mean. Variance is equal to the standard deviation squared. **C–D,** Two groups of women with equal mean heights but unequal variances.

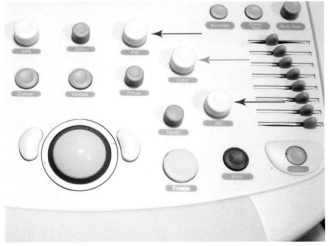

FIGURE 5-20 **Color-Doppler gain control** *(green arrow).* The gray-scale *(blue arrow)* and spectral Doppler *(red arrow)* gain controls also are indicated.

mation are presented according to a choice of schemes, the one selected being presented on the display as a color map (Figure 5-27). The map allows the observer to interpret what the hue, saturation, and luminance mean at each location in terms of the sign, magnitude, and variance of Doppler shifts. Hue indicates the sign of the Doppler shift. Changes in hue, saturation, or luminance up or down the map from the center indicate increasing Doppler shift magnitude. When selected, variance is shown as a change in hue from left to right across the map.

 The color map, always shown on the display, is the key to understanding how image colors are related to Doppler characteristics.

Text continued on p. 146

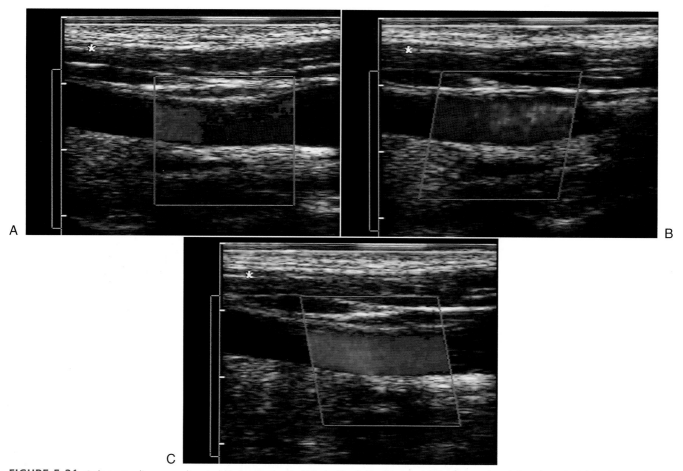

FIGURE 5-21 Color scan lines are directed down vertically **(A),** to the left of vertical **(B),** and to the right of vertical **(C).** Flow is from left to right, producing positive (red) or negative (blue) Doppler shifts, depending on the relationship between scan lines and flow.

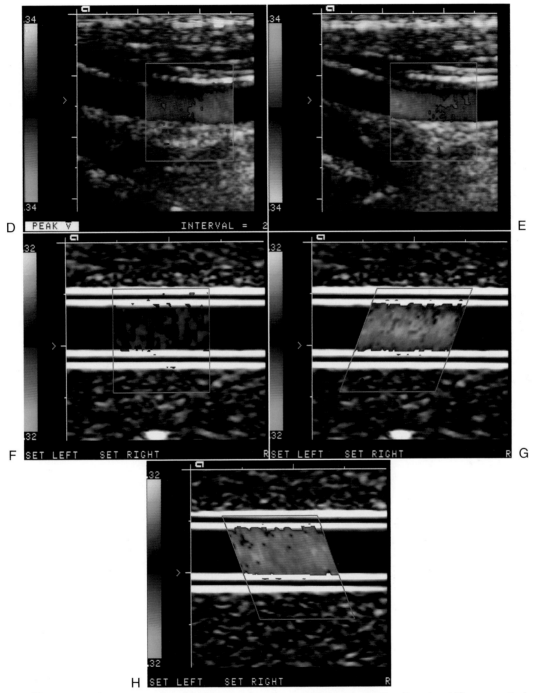

FIGURE 5-21, cont'd D, In this hue map, red and blue are assigned to positive and negative Doppler shifts, respectively, progressing to yellow and cyan (by the addition of green) at the map limits. **E,** In this map, the color assignments are reversed from those presented in *D* (i.e., blue and red are assigned to positive and negative Doppler shifts, respectively). Note the color change occurring within each color window. This is caused by vessel curvature. **F,** With flow in a straight tube, positive and negative Doppler shifts are distributed equally throughout the color window with a Doppler angle of 90 degrees. **G,** Uniform positive Doppler shifts are observed with the color window steered 20 degrees to the left (70-degree Doppler angle). **H,** Uniform negative Doppler shifts are observed with the color window steered to the right. (*A–C from Kremkau FW: Doppler principles, Semin Roentgenol 27:6–16, 1992; D–E from Kremkau FW: Principles and pitfalls of real-time color-flow imaging. In Bernstein EF, editor: Vascular diagnosis, 4th ed, St Louis, 1993, Mosby.*)

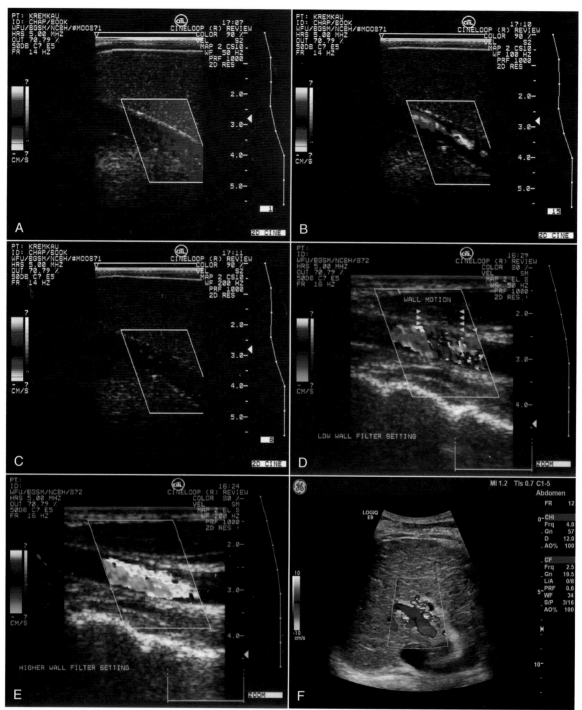

FIGURE 5-22 A, Tissue motion causes clutter, obscuring the flow in the vessel and clouding the gray-scale tissue with color Doppler information. **B,** Wall filter has been increased to 100 Hz, thereby eliminating the color clutter. **C,** Wall filter has been increased (too much) to 200 Hz, eliminating virtually all the color Doppler information derived from the vessel. **D,** With a low wall filter setting (50 Hz), wall motion appears in color on the image. **E,** With a higher wall filter setting (200 Hz), this motion no longer appears in color. **F,** Slow portal flow imaged with low PRF. (*A–C from Kremkau FW: Principles and pitfalls of real-time color-flow imaging. In Bernstein EF, editor: Vascular diagnosis, 4th ed, St Louis, 1993, Mosby; D–E from Kremkau FW: Principles and instrumentation. In Merritt CRB, editor: Doppler color imaging, New York, 1992, Churchill Livingstone.*)

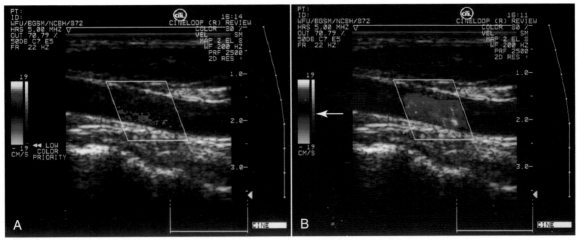

FIGURE 5-23 A, With the color priority set low *(at the bottom of the gray bar)*, weak, non–Doppler-shifted reverberation and off-axis echoes within the vessel take precedence over the Doppler-shifted echoes, and little color is displayed. **B,** With a higher color priority setting *(halfway up the gray bar [arrow])*, the Doppler-shifted echoes *(color)* take precedence over the weaker gray-scale echoes. *(From Kremkau FW: Principles and instrumentation. In Merritt CRB, editor:* Doppler color imaging, *New York, 1992, Churchill Livingstone.)*

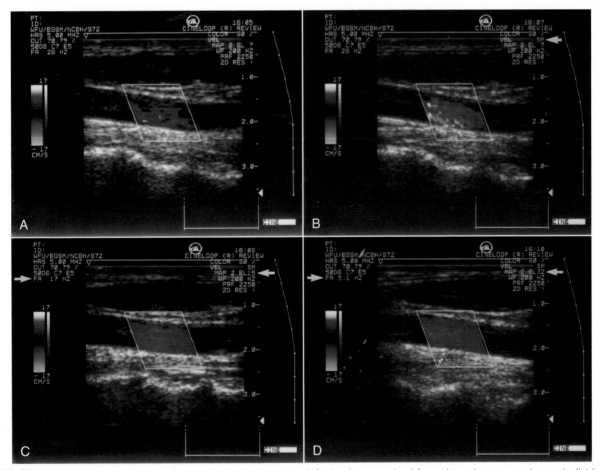

FIGURE 5-24 A, With no smoothing (persistence), only the Doppler-shifted echoes received from the pulses generating an individual frame are shown. **B,** With smoothing, consecutive frames are averaged, filling gaps in the presentation and presenting a smoother but less detailed representation of flow. **C–D,** More accurate and complete detection of flow information is obtained with increasing ensemble lengths. The ensemble lengths shown are 7 (see **B**), 15 (see **C**), and 32 (see **D**). Note the decrease in frame rate from 26 to 17 to 5.1 frames per second. *(From Kremkau FW: Principles and instrumentation. In Merritt CRB, editor:* Doppler color imaging, *New York, 1992, Churchill Livingstone.)*

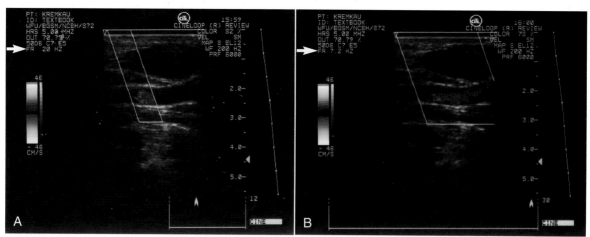

FIGURE 5-25 Tripling the color window width decreases the frame rate from 20 Hz **(A)** to 7.2 Hz **(B)**. *(From Kremkau FW: Principles and instrumentation. In Merritt CRB, editor:* Doppler color imaging, *New York, 1992, Churchill Livingstone.)*

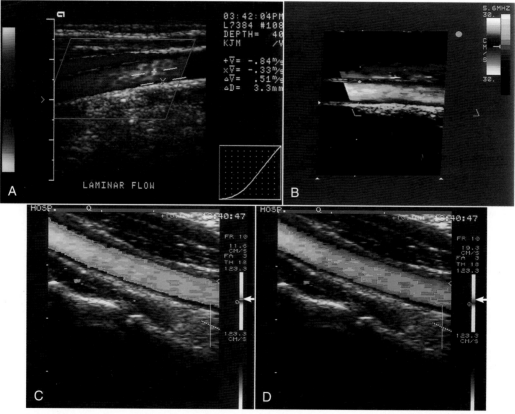

FIGURE 5-26 A, Digital readout of stored mean Doppler shift (converted to mean flow speed) at specific pixel locations. Conversion to speed requires angle correction. The value at the vessel center (84 cm/s) is greater than at the edge (33 cm/s), as expected for laminar flow. **B,** Laminar flow. The color bar used in this scan progresses from dark red and dark blue to bright white (indicating decreasing saturation and increasing luminance). The regions near the vessel wall are dark, with progressive brightening and decreasing saturation to white at the center left. This corresponds to the low flow speeds at the vessel wall and high flow speeds at the vessel center that are characteristic of laminar flow. **C,** The green tag is set at a specific level (11.6; *arrow*) on an angle-corrected, calibrated color bar. The green region on the display, therefore, indicates areas where that specific flow speed exists. **D,** The green tag is set at 19.3. As the set flow speed value increases, the indicated region *(green)* moves to the center, where higher speeds are expected. (**A** *from Kremkau FW: Doppler principles,* Semin Roentgenol *27:6–16, 1992;* **B–D** *from Kremkau FW: Principles and instrumentation. In Merritt CRB, editor:* Doppler color imaging, *New York, 1992, Churchill Livingstone.)*

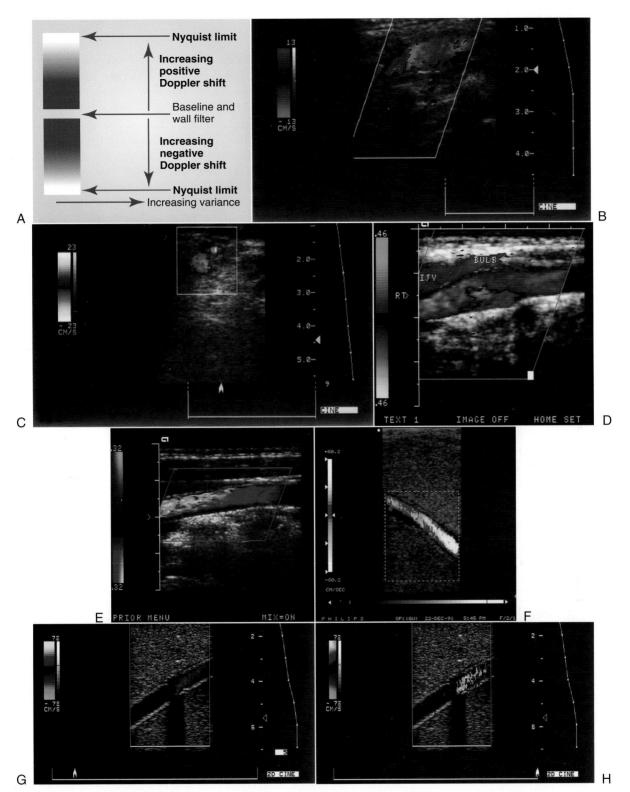

FIGURE 5-27 Color map information. A, Diagram describing the information contained in a color map or color bar. **B,** A luminance map. Increasing luminance of red or blue indicates, respectively, increasing positive or negative mean Doppler shifts. **C,** A saturation map is used to show flow transversely in two vessels. Flow in the upper vessel is toward the transducer, yielding positive Doppler shifts *(red)*. Flow in the lower vessel is away from the transducer, yielding negative Doppler shifts *(blue)*. On this color map, red and blue progress to white (decreasing saturation, increasing luminance) with increasing positive and negative Doppler shift means, respectively. **D,** A hue map showing flow in the carotid artery (with reversal in the bulb) and jugular vein. Increasingly positive Doppler shifts progress from dark blue to bright cyan *(blue plus green)*. Increasingly negative Doppler shifts progress from dark red to bright yellow *(red plus green)*. **E,** A luminance *(dark blue and red to bright blue and red)* map with variance included. Increasing variance adds green to red or blue *(producing yellow or cyan)*, progressing from left to right across the map. **F,** A saturation map. Red and blue progress toward white. **G,** A stenosis in a tube *(located at the shadow)* increases the flow speed. Proximal to (left of) the stenosis, flow speed is too slow to be detected, whereas distal to (right of) the stenosis, positive Doppler shifts are seen. **H,** The variance map shows spectral broadening *(green)* in the turbulent flow region distal to the stenosis. (**A** *from Kremkau FW: Principles and instrumentation. In Merritt CRB, editor:* Doppler color imaging, *New York, 1992, Churchill Livingstone;* **B–F** *from Kremkau FW:* Principles of color flow imaging, *J Vasc Technol 15:104–111, 1991.)*

Angle

As with any Doppler technique, angle is important. Figure 5-28 shows convex array and linear array views of vascular flow. Note that the images are similar in appearance, with red on the left and blue on the right. But note that the relative position of the color bars is inverted. How is this inconsistency explained? In fact, why does the color change at all, considering that there is no reason not to expect unidirectional flow in these vessels? The color changes in the vessel in Figure 5-28, *A* because, with the sector image format, pulses and scan lines travel in different directions away from the transducer. Thus they have different Doppler angles with the flow in a straight vessel. Some pulses view the flow upstream and some downstream. At the 90-degree Doppler angle point, the color changes because the situation changes from upstream to downstream. However, this is not the case in Figure 5-28, *C*. All the pulses travel in the same direction (straight down) from this linear-array transducer. If the color change is not due to changing scan line directions, then it must be due to changing flow direction. Careful inspection of Figure 5-28, *C* reveals that the vessel is not perfectly straight but curves up. Flow is from right to left in

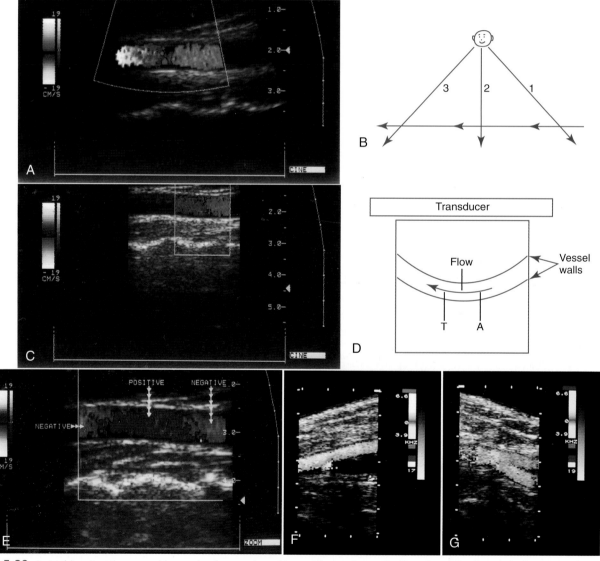

FIGURE 5-28 **A,** In this saturation map, blue and red are assigned to positive and negative Doppler shifts, respectively, progressing to white at the extremes. **B,** With flow moving from right to left, an observer looking to the right *(1)* is looking upstream; when looking to the left *(3)*, the observer has a downstream view. The perpendicular view *(2)* is neither upstream nor downstream. **C,** In this map, the color assignments are reversed from those in **A** (i.e., red and blue are assigned to positive and negative Doppler shifts, respectively). **D,** Exaggerated representation of the image in **C** in which point A represents flow away from the transducer and point T represents flow toward the transducer. **E,** Extension to the left of the color box in **C** reveals another color change caused by vessel curvature (concave-down). **F,** The profunda branch off the femoral artery appears to have no flow (no color within it). **G,** This view of the profunda shows color within it. The 90-degree Doppler angle in **F** causes no Doppler shift, and therefore color is lacking. (*A–C* from Kremkau FW: *Principles of color flow imaging, J Vasc Technol 15:104–111, 1991; E from Kremkau FW: Color flow color assignments, CJ Vasc Technol 15:265–266, 1991.*)

the vessel, so flow is away from the transducer on the right (negative Doppler shift is blue on this map) and toward the transducer on the left (positive Doppler shift is red; see Figure 5-28, *D*). A view further to the left reveals a second color change caused by the curve downward (see Figure 5-28, *E*). Figure 5-28, *F*, shows an example of lack of color in a vessel. This lack of Doppler shift could be caused by lack of flow or flow viewed with a 90-degree Doppler angle. With an acceptable angle (see Figure 5-28, *G*), flow is revealed.

 Changing Doppler angle in an image produces various colors in different locations.

Figure 5-29, *A*, shows various Doppler shifts as the Doppler angle changes across the display in the sector format. Yellow corresponds to a large positive shift, red to a small positive shift, black to a zero shift, blue to a small negative shift, and cyan to a large negative shift. Flow is from left to right. Figure 5-29, *B–F*, confirms all this by spectral displays, which are discussed later in this chapter.

In Figure 5-30, some interesting questions arise. First, in *A*, what is the blood flow direction? According to the color map in the upper left-hand corner of the figure, negative Doppler shifts are coded in red and yellow, whereas positive Doppler shifts are coded in blue and cyan. The color scan lines (and pulses) are steered to the left, and negative Doppler shifts (red and yellow) are

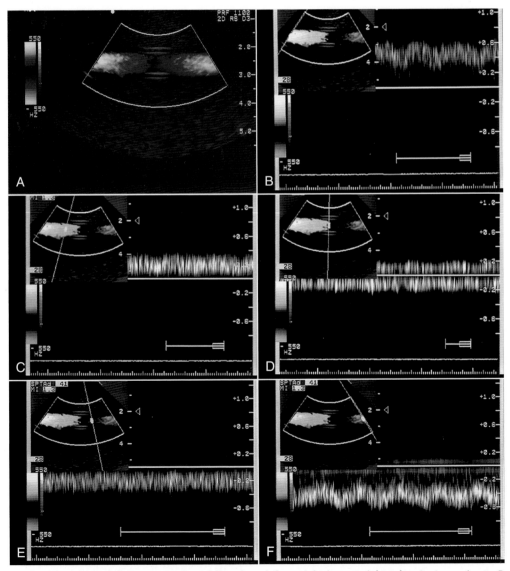

FIGURE 5-29 Sector format, color-Doppler presentation of flow from left to right in a straight tube. A, Approximate Doppler shifts (from the color map) are yellow (500 Hz), red (200 Hz), black (0 Hz), blue (−200 Hz), and cyan (−500 Hz). Spectra from these five regions (shown in **B–F)** confirm these estimates. Doppler shifts decrease as Doppler angles increase toward the center of the color window.

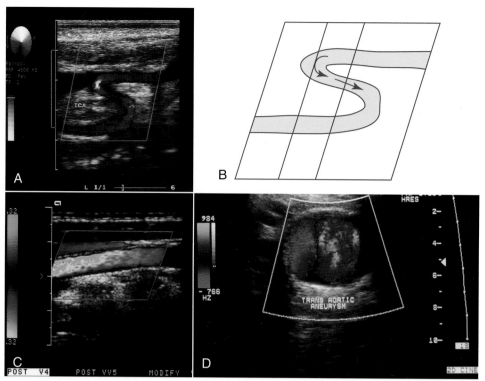

FIGURE 5-30 A, A tortuous artery. **B,** This drawing shows the angle relationships depicted in **A. C,** A (nearly) straight artery. **D,** Circular flow in an aneurysm. The black area between the red and blue areas indicates true flow reversal. (**A–C** *from Kremkau FW: Color interpretation, J Vasc Technol 16:215–216, 1992.*)

received from the blood flowing within the vessel in the upper and lower portions of the figure. If we are looking to the left and seeing blood flowing away from us (negative Doppler shifts), the blood must be flowing from right to left in the upper and lower horizontal portions of the vessel. What about the central portion of the vessel? Clearly, the blood would have to be flowing from left to right there, but why are negative Doppler shifts also seen in this portion? The answer is that this portion of the vessel is not horizontal but is angled down, so even though the blood is flowing from left to right, it is also flowing away from the transducer because of the downward direction (more precisely, it is flowing from upper left to lower right). Thus negative Doppler shifts are found throughout the vessel in this scan. In other words, the flow direction gets close to, but never crosses, the perpendicular to the scan lines (see Figure 5-30, *B*).

Another intriguing question arises with respect to Figure 5-30, *A:* Does the yellow region in the bend at the upper left indicate where the blood flows the fastest? According to the color map, this region is where the highest negative Doppler shifts are generated. Does that mean, however, that this is where the highest flow speeds are encountered? The answer in this case is no. The highest negative Doppler shifts are found in this region because the smallest Doppler angles are encountered there, and not because high flow speeds are found there. In this region, the flow is approximately parallel to the scan lines (see Figure 5-30, *B*), yielding Doppler angles

of around zero. No evidence of vessel narrowing is present to explain increased flow speed. The increased Doppler shift can be explained purely on grounds of angle.

In Figure 5-30, *C*, the region shown in cyan (aqua or blue-green) indicates positive Doppler shifts according to the color map, whereas the blood flow in the rest of the vessel is generating negative Doppler shifts (red and yellow). Again, the scan lines are steered to the left, so negative Doppler shifts indicate that we are looking downstream, seeing flow away from the transducer. Therefore blood flow is from right to left in this carotid artery, with the head oriented to the left as usual. How then can we explain the positive Doppler shifts found in the upper left-hand portion of the vessel? Possibilities include turbulent flow, flow reversal, and flow speed exceeding 32 cm/s in this region, which produce aliasing. Flow reversal and turbulent flow can be eliminated because the region between the negative (red and yellow) and positive (cyan) Doppler shift regions contains no dark or black region (baseline indicating flow reversal). One can easily distinguish between true flow reversal (which involves dark regions, as shown around the baseline of the color bar) (see Figure 5-30, *D*) and aliasing (which involves bright colors, as indicated at the bar extremes). Thus the aqua region is a region of flow away from the transducer that has exceeded the negative aliasing limit of 32 cm/s and has become an aliased positive Doppler shift (cyan).

Does this mean that the flow speed in the aliased aqua region exceeds 32 cm/s? In this case the answer is no. The aliasing limit, which is one half the pulse repetition frequency, has been exceeded. This aliasing limit has been converted, using the Doppler equation, to an equivalent flow speed of 32 cm/s, as indicated at the map extremes. However, because there is no angle correction in this scan, an angle of zero was assumed in the conversion from the Doppler shift to flow speed. Therefore aliased flow exceeds 32 cm/s only when it is parallel to the scan lines. Because the Doppler angle in this example is approximately 60 degrees, the Doppler shifts are only about one half what they would be at zero degrees. Therefore the flow in the aliased region has exceeded approximately 64 cm/s. One must exercise care in estimating flow speeds with tagging (see Figure 5-26, C–D) or aliasing limits that are converted to flow speed units without correcting for angle.

 Proper understanding of the effects of angle on the Doppler shift and of how color is related to the Doppler shift is necessary to interpret complex images properly.

Doppler Power Displays

Doppler shift displays encode mean Doppler shifts in a two-dimensional matrix according to the color map selected. **Doppler power displays** (also called power-Doppler) present two-dimensional Doppler information by color-encoding the *strength* of Doppler shifts. This approach is free of aliasing and angle dependence and is more sensitive to slow flow as well as flow in small or deep vessels. Names applied to this technique include *color power Doppler*, *ultrasound angio*, *color Doppler energy*, and *color power angio*. Rather than assigning various hue, saturation, and luminance values to mean Doppler shift frequency values, as in Doppler shift displays, this technique assigns these values to Doppler shift *power* values. The power of Doppler shifts is determined by the *concentration* of moving scatterers producing Doppler shifts and is independent of Doppler shift frequency (and thus independent of the Doppler angle). In addition to the colors already encountered, magenta (a combination of red and blue) is used on some Doppler power maps.

 Doppler-power-displays color-encode Doppler shift power values on the display.

Advantages and Disadvantages

The Doppler detector in color Doppler imaging instruments yields the sign, mean, variance, and amplitude and power of the **Doppler spectrum** (Figure 5-31, A) at each of the hundreds of **sample volume** locations in an anatomic cross-section. Traditionally, in color Doppler imaging, sign and mean Doppler shift, and sometimes variance (usually in cardiac applications), are color encoded and displayed. These parameters depend on the Doppler angle and are subject to aliasing (Figure 5-32, A). Power Doppler integrates the area under the spectrum (see Figure 5-31, B). This area is independent of angle and aliasing, displaying the effects of neither (see Figure 5-32, B). Thus an advantage of **Doppler power display** is the uniform (angle-independent and alias-free) presentation of flow information, although this is accomplished with a loss in direction, speed, and flow character information. This extends even through regions of 90-degree Doppler angle (see Figure 5-32, B–C) because the Doppler shift spectrum there has a nonzero area (see Figure 5-31, B), even though its mean is zero, yielding a black region in color Doppler imaging displays (see Figure 5-32, A, C). Power Doppler is also essentially free of variations in flow speed (as in the cardiac cycle) and thus can be frame averaged to improve the signal-to-noise ratio and sensitivity substantially (Figure 5-33). Because aliasing is not a problem in power Doppler, lower pulse repetition frequencies can be used to detect slow flows. Box 5-3 lists the advantages and disadvantages of Doppler power displays. In general, Doppler ultrasound can determine (1) the presence or absence of flow, (2) the direction and (3) speed of flow, and (4) the character of flow. Power Doppler is superior in terms of the first, but at the expense of the other three. Table 5-6 compares color Doppler displays.

 Doppler power displays do not have direction, speed, or flow character information included and are insensitive to angle effects and aliasing. They are more sensitive than Doppler shift displays in that they can present slower flows as well as flows in deeper or tinier vessels.

BOX 5-3	Advantages and Disadvantages of Doppler-Power Displays With Respect to Doppler Shift Displays

Advantages
- Angle independence
- No aliasing
- Improved sensitivity (deeper penetration, smaller vessels, slower flows)

Disadvantages
- No directional information
- No flow speed information
- No flow character information

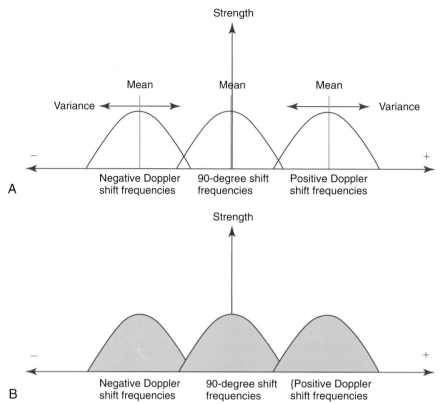

FIGURE 5-31 A. Spectra for flow toward (positive) and away from (negative) the transducer and perpendicular (90 degrees) to the sound beam. Conventional color Doppler imaging determines and displays, in color-coded form, the sign and mean (and sometimes the variance) of the Doppler shift frequency spectrum. **B.** Doppler power determines and displays, in color-coded form, the size of the area under the spectral curve. The axes of the spectral graph represent strength (amplitude, power, energy, or intensity) versus frequency.

TABLE 5-6	Comparison of Doppler Shift Display and Doppler Power Display	
	Doppler Shift Display	**Doppler Power Display**
Quantitative	No	No
Global	Yes	Yes
Perfusion	No	Yes

SPECTRAL-DOPPLER DISPLAYS

In addition to color Doppler operation, two types of spectral-Doppler operation—continuous-wave (CW) and pulsed-wave (PW)—are used for Doppler detection of flow in the heart and in blood vessels. All three are combined into one multipurpose instrument (Figure 5-34). CW operation detects Doppler-shifted echoes in the region of overlap between the beams of the transmitting and receiving transducer elements. Differences between other transducers and those designed exclusively for CW Doppler use are that the latter are not damped and that they have separate sending and receiving elements. PW operation emits ultrasound pulses and receives echoes using a single element transducer or an array. Because of the required Doppler frequency shift detection, the pulses are longer than those used in imaging. Through **range gating**, PW Doppler has the ability to select information from a particular depth along the beam. To use PW Doppler effectively, it commonly is combined with gray-scale sonography. Such instruments are called *duplex scanners* because of their dual functions (anatomic imaging and flow measurement). CW and PW operations present Doppler shift information in an audible form and as a visual display.

Continuous-Wave Operation

Spectral Doppler operation provides continuous or pulsed voltages to the transducer and converts echo voltages received from the transducer to audible and visual information corresponding to scatterer motion. If an instrument distinguishes between positive and negative Doppler shifts, it is called **bidirectional**. **Continuous wave Doppler** instruments include a CW oscillator and a Doppler detector that detects the changes in frequency (Doppler shifts) resulting from scatterer motion and presents them as audible sounds and as a visual display corresponding to the motion.

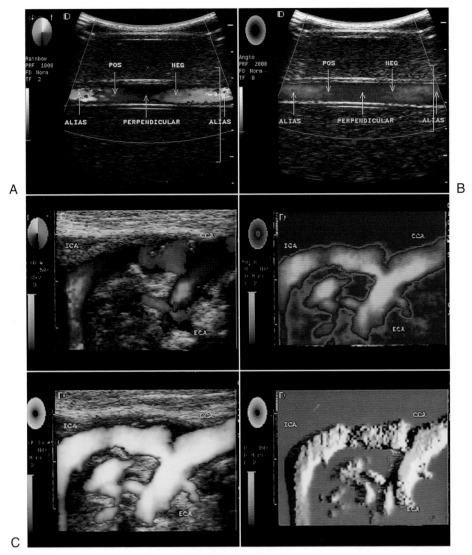

FIGURE 5-32 A, A color Doppler shift image of flow in a straight tube, acquired in sector format. The varying Doppler angle from left to right yields aliasing and positive, negative, and zero Doppler-shift regions. **B,** A Doppler power presentation of the situation shown in **A** yields a uniform image, free of angle dependence and aliasing. However, it contains no directional, speed, or dynamic information. **C,** Angle independence is seen in the Doppler power images of the carotid artery; compare them with the Doppler shift display *(upper left)*. Doppler power imaging is shown in color, topographic, and gray-scale forms *(clockwise from upper right)*. (See also Figure 1-13, *B–C.*)

Components of a Continuous-Wave Doppler System

A diagram of the components of a CW Doppler system is presented in Figure 5-35, *A*. The oscillator produces a continuously alternating voltage with a 2- to 10-MHz frequency, which is applied to the source transducer element. The ultrasound frequency is determined by the oscillator and is set to equal the operating frequency of the transducer. In the transducer assembly is a separate receiving transducer element that produces voltages with frequencies equal to the frequencies of the returning echoes. If there is scatterer motion, the reflected ultrasound and the ultrasound produced by the source transducer will have different frequencies. The Doppler detector detects the difference between these two fre-

quencies, which is the Doppler shift, and drives a loudspeaker at this frequency. Doppler shifts are typically one thousandth of the operating frequency, which puts them in the audible range. Doppler shifts also are commonly sent through a **spectrum analyzer** to a **spectral-Doppler display** for visual observation and evaluation.

The detector (see Figure 5-35, *B*) amplifies the echo voltages it receives from the receiving element, detects the Doppler shift information in the returning echoes, and determines the motion direction from the sign of the Doppler shift. Doppler shifts are determined by mixing the returning voltages with the CW voltage from the oscillator. This produces the sum and difference of the oscillator and echo frequencies (see Figure 5-35, *B*). The difference is the desired Doppler shift. The sum is a much higher frequency (approximately double the

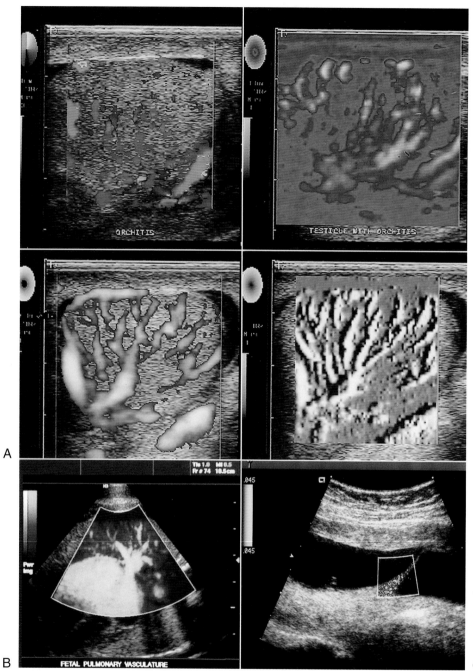

FIGURE 5-33 A, Improved sensitivity to testicular flow compared with Doppler shift imaging *(upper left).* Small vessel flow is imaged in fetal pulmonary vasculature **(B)** and within the membrane separating a twin gestation **(C).**

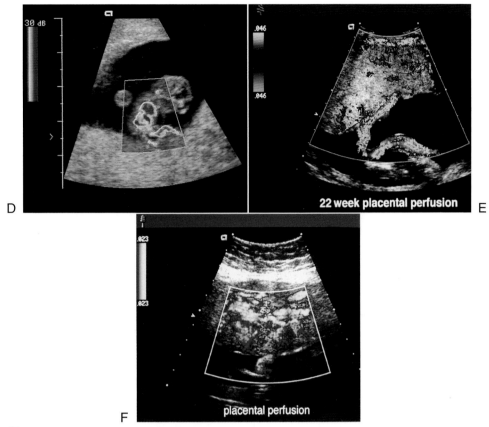

FIGURE 5-33, cont'd D, First-trimester fetal circulation. A comparison of placental Doppler shift imaging **(E)** and Doppler power imaging **(F)** reveals improved flow detection with the latter.

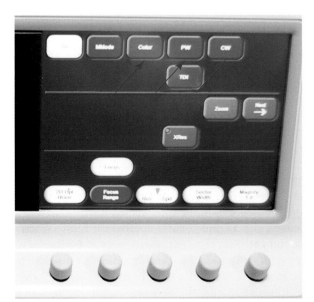

FIGURE 5-34 Continuous-wave (CW), pulsed-wave (PW), and color Doppler modes are available in one instrument, with each mode selectable from the control panel *(arrows)*.

operating frequency) and is filtered out. The difference is zero for echoes returning from stationary structures. In the case of echoes from moving structures or flowing blood, this difference is the Doppler shift, which provides information about motion and flow (positive or negative).

> The Doppler detector detects Doppler shifts and determines their sign (positive or negative).

Positive and negative shifts indicate motion toward and away from the transducer, respectively. The detector shown in Figure 5-35, *B*, does not provide this directional information. Determining direction and separating Doppler shift voltages into separate forward and reverse channels is accomplished by the **phase quadrature** detector (Figure 5-36).

The forward and reverse channel signals are sent to separate loudspeakers so that forward and reverse Doppler shifts can be heard separately. The signals also are sent to a visual display to show positive and negative Doppler shifts above and below the display baseline, which represents zero Doppler shift (Figure 5-37).

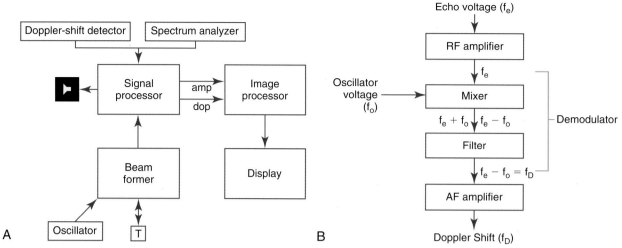

FIGURE 5-35 A, Block diagram of a sonographic instrument functioning in continuous-wave Doppler mode. The oscillator (part of the beam former) produces a continuously alternating voltage that drives the source transducer element *(T)*. The receiving transducer element *(T)* produces a continuous voltage in response to echoes it is continuously receiving. The signal processor includes a Doppler shift detector that detects differences in frequency between the voltages produced by the oscillator and by the receiving element. The Doppler shifts produce voltages that drive the loudspeakers and a visual display. The frequency of the audible sound is equal to the Doppler shift and is proportional to the reflector speed and to the cosine of the angle between the sound propagation direction and the boundary motion. **B,** Block diagram of a continuous-wave Doppler detector. The radio frequency *(RF)* amplifier increases the echo voltage amplitude. The frequency of the echo voltage is f_e. In the mixer, this frequency is combined with the oscillator voltage, the frequency of which is f_o. The mixer yields the sum and difference of these two frequency inputs ($f_e + f_o$ and $f_e - f_o$). The low-pass (high-frequency rejection) filter removes $f_e + f_o$, leaving $f_e - f_o$, which is the Doppler shift frequency (f_D). This frequency then is strengthened in the audio frequency *(AF)* amplifier. The mixer and filter together constitute the Doppler demodulator.

Continuous-Wave Sample Volume

CW operation detects flow that occurs anywhere within the intersection of the transmitting and receiving beams of the dual-transducer assembly (Figure 5-38). The **sample volume** is the region from which Doppler-shifted echoes return and are presented audibly or visually. In this case, the sample volume is the overlapping region of the transmitting and receiving beams. Because the sample volume is large, CW Doppler systems can give complex and confusing presentations if two or more different motions or flows are included in the sample volume (e.g., two blood vessels being viewed simultaneously). **Pulsed Doppler** systems solve this problem by detecting motion or flow at a selected depth with a relatively small sample volume. However, the large sample volume of a CW system is helpful when searching for a Doppler maximum associated with a vascular or valvular stenosis.

Because a distribution of flow velocities is encountered by the beam as it traverses a vessel, a distribution of many Doppler-shifted frequencies returns to the transducer and the instrument. In arterial circulation or in the heart, these Doppler shifts are changing continually over the cardiac cycle and are displayed as a function of time with appropriate real-time frequency-spectrum processing (Figure 5-39). These displays provide quantitative data for evaluating Doppler-shifted echoes. The display device is, again, the flat-panel display. The displayed Doppler information is stored in the digital memory before it is displayed so that it can be frozen and backed up over the last few seconds of preceding information.

Angle Incorporation or Correction

To convert a display correctly from the Doppler shift versus time to flow speed versus time, the Doppler angle must be incorporated accurately into the calculation process (Figure 5-40). This incorporation is commonly called "angle correction." Either term is appropriate because lack of angle incorporation leaves the instrument to assume that the Doppler angle is zero, which is incorrect unless the angle is, in fact, zero. Figure 5-40, *B–C*, illustrates the importance of accurate angle correction. Figure 5-40, *C–F*, shows errors encountered when the Doppler angle is handled incorrectly. Recall that as angle increases, the Doppler shift decreases. Thus, when the angle indicator on the instrument is set at 60 degrees, the instrument responds by doubling the calculated flow speed from what it would have been at a Doppler angle of zero. In other words, the Doppler equation, arranged to have the calculated flow speed alone on one side of the equal sign, has the cosine Doppler angle in the denominator on the other side. As the angle indicator is increased, the cosine decreases, increasing the calculated speed value. This compensates for the reduction in the Doppler shift caused by the Doppler angle actually involved in the ultrasound beam and flow intersection. For example, if the

Text continued on p. 157

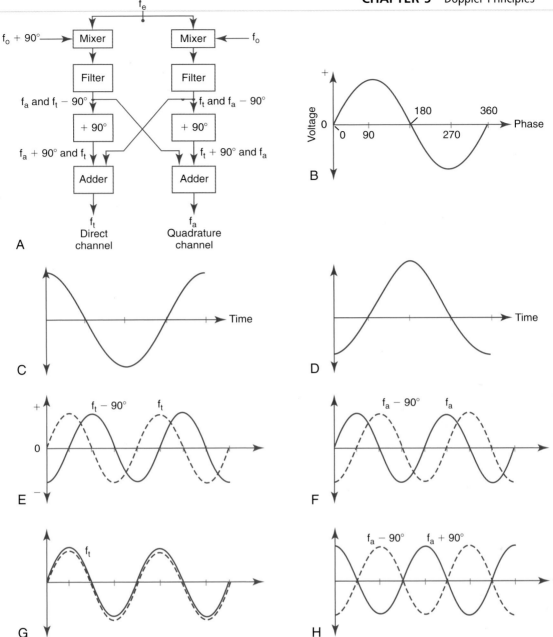

FIGURE 5-36 A, The phase quadrature detector detects the positive f_t and negative f_a Doppler shifts contained in the incoming echo voltage (f_e) and separates them into separate channels for delivery to the loudspeakers and the visual display. These channels are designated as direct and quadrature *(on the left and right, respectively).* Detection proceeds as described in the following. The echo voltage is mixed with the oscillator voltage (f_o) in two mixers. The oscillator voltage in the direct channel leads that in the quadrature channel by one-quarter cycle (90 degrees). This is illustrated in **C,** which leads **B** by 90 degrees (one-quarter cycle). **B,** One complete variation (cycle) of alternating voltage that may be thought of as traveling around a 360-degree circle. One quarter of a cycle is 90 degrees of phase angle. Phase is a description of progression through a cycle (analogous to the phase of the moon). One quarter of a cycle is 90 degrees, and one half of a cycle is 180 degrees. The completion of a cycle occurs at 360 degrees, but this is also the zero-degree phase of the next cycle. **D** lags **B** by 90 degrees. **C–D,** If the voltages in **C** and **D** are added together, a zero voltage results. (The two voltages are equal and opposite, so they cancel each other when summed.) Returning to **A,** the frequency sum ($f_e + f_o$) is filtered out, as in Figure 5-35, *B,* yielding the Doppler shift f_D, which is $f_e - f_o$. The Doppler shift may be positive (f_t, for flow toward the transducer) or negative (f_a, for flow away from the transducer). Because of the oscillator-voltage phase difference ($f_o + 90$ degrees versus f_o), the two filter outputs are different. Positive shifts in the direct channel lag those in the quadrature channel by 90 degrees. This is illustrated in **E.** In **E–H,** the solid curves refer to the direct channel, whereas the dashed curves refer to quadrature. The vertical and horizontal axes represent voltage and time, respectively. **E,** Positive Doppler shifts (f_t) at the output of the direct channel filter lag those in the quadrature channel by 90 degrees. **F,** Negative Doppler shifts (f_a) at the output of the quadrature channel lag those in the direct channel by 90 degrees. **G,** Positive Doppler shifts at the input to the direct channel adder are in phase (zero-degree phase difference), yielding an f_t output. **H,** Negative Doppler shifts at the input to the direct channel adder are 180 degrees out of phase, yielding a zero f_a output. Returning to **A,** negative shifts in the quadrature channel lag those in the direct channel by 90 degrees **(F).** Next, another 90-degree phase shift results in the separation of the positive and negative shifts into separate channels—direct and quadrature, respectively—as follows. The phase-shifted positive Doppler shifts in the direct channel are now in phase with the unshifted ones in the quadrature channel **(G),** whereas the negative shifts are 180 degrees out of phase **(H).** When added together, the negative shifts will cancel **(C–D),** yielding positive shifts as the output voltage in the direct channel. A similar process in the quadrature channel yields negative shifts as output.

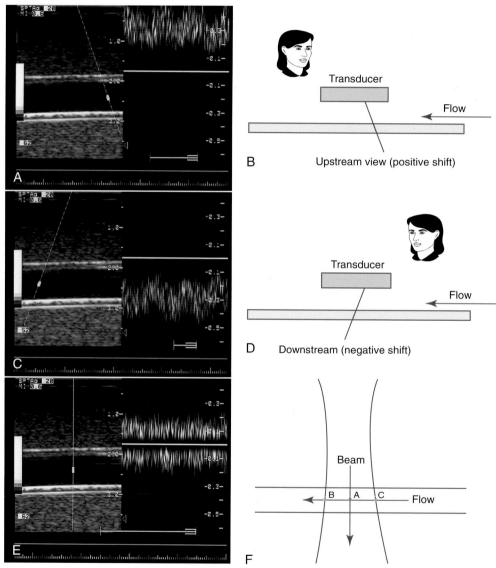

FIGURE 5-37 The beam is steered to the right and positive Doppler shifts are received **(A).** Thus this is an upstream view **(B),** and flow is from right to left. Therefore steering the beam to the left **(C)** would provide a downstream view **(D)** with negative Doppler shifts. With the beam perpendicular to the flow **(E),** Doppler shifts are received, both positive and negative, because of beam spreading **(F);** that is, a portion of the beam views upstream while a portion views downstream. The beam axis portion (90-degree angle) yields a zero Doppler shift.

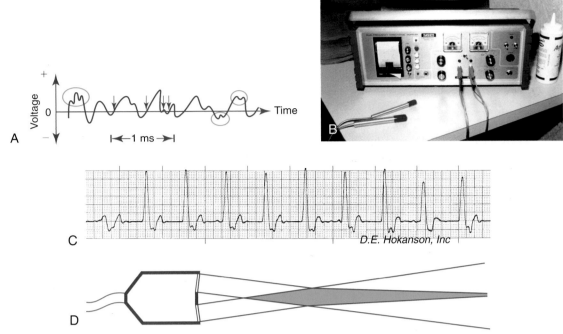

FIGURE 5-38 **A,** A zero-crossing detector counts the number of zero crossings per second in the positive or negative direction. In the 1-ms period shown, four zero crossings (negative to positive) occurred *(arrows)*, corresponding to a mean frequency of 4 kHz. Higher frequencies that are missed by the zero-crossing technique are circled. **B,** A zero-crossing continuous-wave Doppler instrument. **C,** Chart output from a zero-crossing instrument shows a time-varying average Doppler shift. **D,** Continuous-wave Doppler systems have dual-element transducer assemblies, one for transmitting and one for receiving. The region over which Doppler information can be acquired (Doppler sample volume) is the region of overlap between the transmitting and receiving beams *(green region)*.

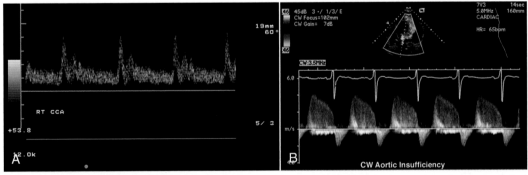

FIGURE 5-39 **A,** A display of Doppler shift frequencies as a function of time. This is a pulsed-wave Doppler spectral display. **B,** A cardiac continuous-wave Doppler spectral display.

actual Doppler angle is 60 degrees, the Doppler shift is half what it would have been at zero degrees. If the angle is set properly on the instrument at 60, the cosine in the denominator of the Doppler equation is set at 0.5. This doubles the calculated flow speed to the correct value.

 The Doppler sample volume of a continuous-wave Doppler instrument is relatively large, being the overlapping region of the transmission and reception beams.

Wall Filter

In Doppler studies, a wall filter that rejects frequencies below an adjustable value is used to eliminate the high-intensity, low-frequency Doppler shift echoes, called *clutter*, caused by heart or vessel wall or cardiac valve motion with pulsatile flow (Figure 5-41). Sometimes called *wall-thump filter*, the **filter** rejects these strong echoes that otherwise would overwhelm the weaker echoes from blood. These strong echoes have low

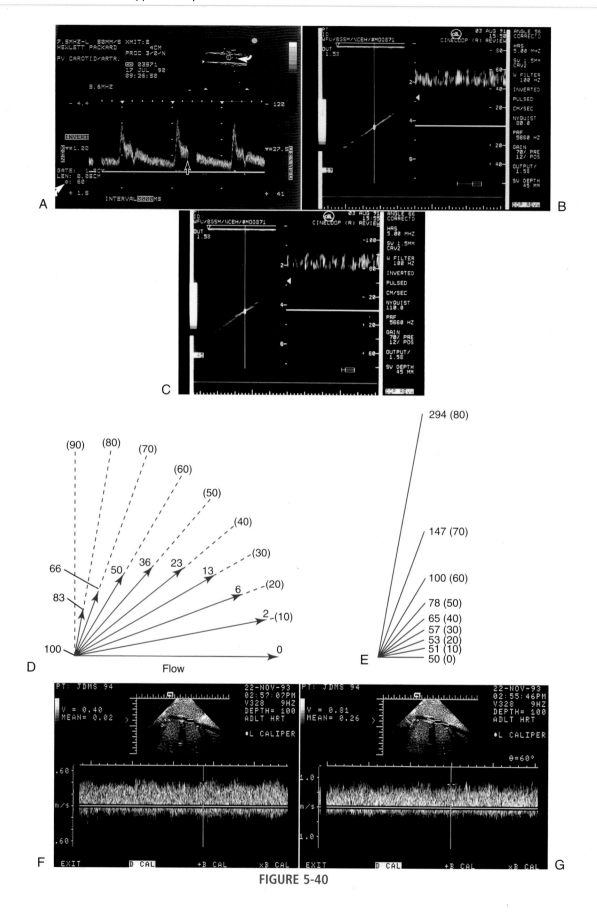

FIGURE 5-40

FIGURE 5-40 A, A spectral display with Doppler-shift (kilohertz) calibration of the vertical axis on the left and flow speed (cm/s, centimeters per second) calibration on the right. Conversion from the former to the latter requires angle incorporation *(curved arrows).* The Doppler angle in this example is 60 degrees. The gap in Doppler information *(open arrow)* occurs when the instrument takes time to generate a frame of the anatomic image *(upper right).* **B–C,** A moving-string test object is imaged, resulting in the Doppler spectral display shown. With proper angle incorporation (56 degrees) the 50 cm/s string speed is shown correctly **(B).** With improper angle incorporation (66 degrees), an incorrect string speed of 70 cm/s is shown **(C).** This is a 40% error. **D,** If a zero Doppler angle is assumed correctly, there is zero error in the calculated flow speed. However, if the angle is actually nonzero, error results. The error in flow speed increases as the angle error (in parentheses) increases. For example, if the Doppler angle is 10 degrees but is assumed to be zero, the calculated flow speed will be 2% less than the correct value. At 60 and 80 degrees, the errors are 50% and 83%, respectively. At 90 degrees, there is zero Doppler shift. The calculated flow speed is zero (100% error). **E,** If the Doppler angle is zero but is assumed to be some other value, the calculated flow speeds are too large. Here, the correct value is 50 cm/s. The error increases with angle *(in parentheses).* For example, at 60 and 80 degrees, the calculated values are 100 and 294 cm/s, respectively. **F,** No angle correction is used in this display. The instrument assumes a Doppler angle of zero and calculates flow speed *(v)* at 40 cm/s. However, the Doppler angle is actually 60 degrees, yielding half the Doppler shift that a zero-degree angle would. **G,** When the cosine of 60 degrees (0.5) is incorporated into the Doppler equation, the result is 81 cm/s. *(B–C from Kremkau FW: Doppler principles, Semin Roentgenol 27:6–16, 1992; F–G from Kremkau FW: Doppler, J Diagn Med Sonogr 10:337–338, 1994. Reprinted by permission of Sage Publications, Inc.)*

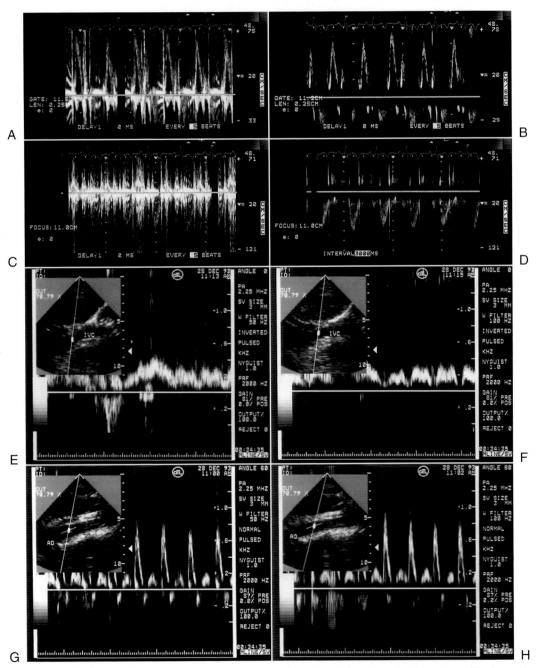

FIGURE 5-41 A, Clutter in the spectrum of inflow at the mitral valve is shown. **B,** The clutter in **A** is removed by increasing the wall filter setting. **C,** Clutter in the spectrum of the left ventricular outflow tract. **D,** The clutter in **C** is removed with an increase in the wall filter setting. **E,** Clutter in the display of inferior vena caval flow. **F,** The clutter shown in **E** is removed by adjusting the wall filter from 50 to 100 Hz. **G,** Clutter in the display of aortic flow. **H,** The clutter shown in **G** is removed by adjusting the wall filter.

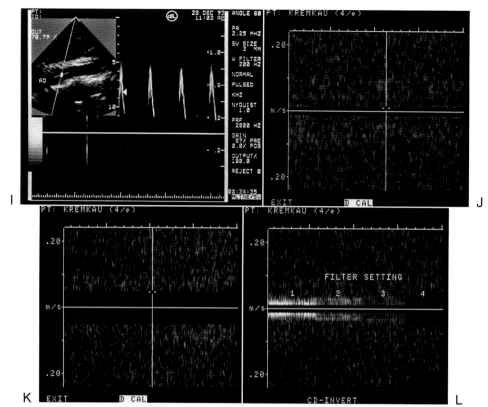

FIGURE 5-41, cont'd I, The wall filter is set too high (200 Hz), eliminating all but the peak systolic portion of the spectrum. **J,** Using electronic noise on the spectrum (with high Doppler gain), a low wall filter setting eliminates Doppler shifts corresponding to flow speeds of less than 1 cm/s. **K,** A higher setting eliminates speeds of less than 5 cm/s. **L,** Four wall filter settings reduce or eliminate frequencies as shown.

Doppler shift frequencies because the tissue structures do not move as fast as blood does. The upper limit of the filter is adjustable over a range of about 25 to 3200 Hz. However, the filter, if not properly used, can erroneously alter conclusions with regard to diastolic flow and distal flow resistance.

 Wall filters remove clutter (low-frequency Doppler shifts from moving tissue).

Pulsed-Wave Operation

A diagram of the components of pulsed-wave Doppler operation is given in Figure 5-42, *A*. The pulser (in the beam former) functions as in sonographic imaging, except that it generates pulses of several cycles of voltage that drive the transducer where ultrasound pulses are produced. Recall that imaging pulses are two or three cycles long. Pulses used in Doppler instruments, however, have pulse lengths of about 5 to 30 cycles. This is necessary to determine the Doppler shifts of returning echoes accurately. Echo voltages from the transducer are processed in the detector. In the detector, echo voltages are amplified, their frequency is compared with the pulser frequency, and Doppler shifts are determined. Doppler shifts are sent to loudspeakers for audible output and to

the display for visual observation. Based on their arrival time (recall the 13 μs/cm rule), echoes coming from reflectors at a given depth may be selected by the amplifier **gate**. Thus motion information may be obtained from a specific depth. This is called *range gating*. The operator controls the gate length and location.

 Range gating enables depth selectivity and a small Doppler sample volume.

A PW Doppler instrument does not detect the complete Doppler shift as a CW instrument does but, rather, obtains samples of it because the PW instrument is a sampling system, with each pulse yielding a sample of the Doppler shift signal. The Doppler shifts are determined as described previously, except that the mixer does not receive a continuous input echo voltage but, rather, a sampled one. Echoes arrive from the sample volume depth in pulsed form at a rate equal to pulse repetition frequency. Each of these returning echoes yields a sample of the Doppler shift from the Doppler detector. These samples are connected and smoothed (filtered) to yield the sampled waveform (see Figure 5-42, *B-E*).

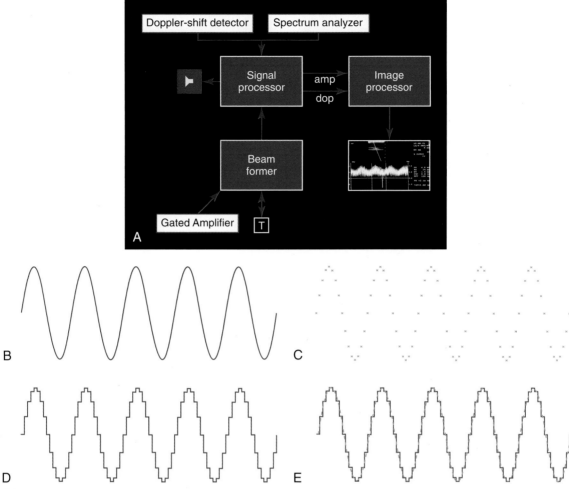

FIGURE 5-42 A, Block diagram of a sonographic instrument functioning in pulsed-wave Doppler mode. The beam former produces voltage pulses of several cycles each, which drive the transducer (*T*). The signal processor includes a Doppler shift detector, where shift frequencies are compared with the frequency of the outgoing pulses. The difference (the Doppler shift) is sent to the loudspeakers and, through the spectrum analyzer and image processor, to the display. The beam former also contains a gate that selects echoes from a given depth according to arrival time and thus gives motion information from a selected depth. **B,** Five cycles of a 500-Hz Doppler shift frequency occurring in 10 ms of time. **C,** In a pulsed-wave Doppler instrument, each pulse yields echoes from the sample volume. These echoes, after Doppler detection, yield samples (*x*) of the Doppler shift from the sample volume. In this example, 80 samples are determined in a 10-ms time period. Therefore, the pulse repetition frequency of the instrument is 8 kHz (with each pulse yielding one sample of the Doppler shift). **D,** The pulsed-wave Doppler gate is also called a *sample-and-hold amplifier*. It samples the returning stream of echoes (resulting from one emitted pulse of ultrasound) at the appropriate time for the desired depth (see Table 5-7) and holds the value until the next pulse and sample are accomplished. **E,** Low-pass filtering (which removes higher frequencies) smooths the sampled result *(solid line)*, yielding the desired Doppler shift waveform *(dashed line))* comparable with that shown in *B*.

 A pulsed wave Doppler system is a sampling system.

Range Gate

The gate selects the sample volume location from which returning Doppler-shifted echoes are accepted (Table 5-7 and Figures 5-43 to 5-45). The width of the sample volume is equal to the beam width. The gate has some length over which it permits reception (Table 5-8). For example (applying the 13 μs/cm rule), a gate that passes echoes arriving from 13 to 15 μs after pulse generation is listening over a depth range of 10.0 to 11.5 mm. In

this case, the gate is located at a depth of 10.8 mm with a length (depth range) of ±0.8 mm. Longer gate lengths are used when searching for the desired vessel and flow location, and shorter gate lengths are used for spectral analysis and evaluation. The shorter gate length improves the quality of the spectral display.

The Doppler sample volume is determined by beam width, gate length, and emitted pulse length. One half the pulse length (the same as axial resolution in sonography) is added to gate length to yield effective sample volume length (Table 5-9). Thus pulse length must shorten as gate length is reduced. The sample volume width is equal to the beam width at the sample volume depth.

TABLE 5-7	Echo Arrival Time for Various Reflector Depths (Gate Locations)
Depth (mm)	Time (μs)
10	13
20	26
30	39
40	52
50	65
60	78
70	91
80	104
90	117
100	130
150	195
200	260

TABLE 5-8	Spatial Gate Length for Various Temporal Gate Lengths
Length (mm)	Time (μs)
1	1.3
2	2.6
3	3.9
4	5.2
5	6.5
10	13.0
15	19.5
20	26.0

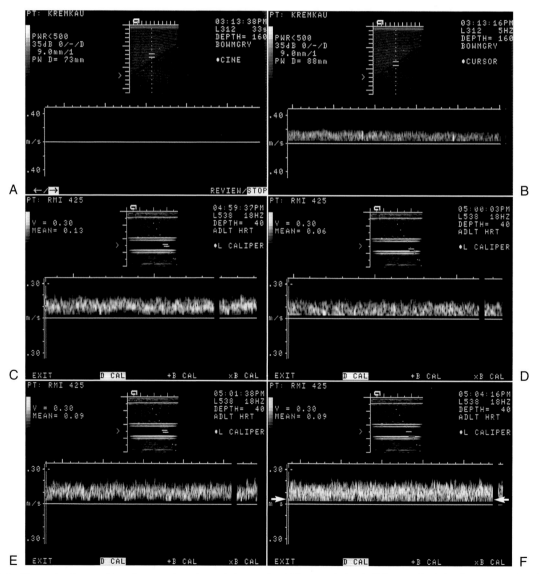

FIGURE 5-43 A, The pulsed-wave Doppler sample volume is located at 73 mm of depth (95 μs arrival time). No Doppler shift is seen on the lower display because Doppler shifted echoes from within the tube arrive at about 114 μs. **B,** When the gate is open later (corresponding to a depth of 88 mm), Doppler shifts are received and displayed (indicating a constant flow rate in the tube). **C,** The gate is located in the center of the tube. **D,** The gate is located near the tube wall. Mean flow speed is 6 cm/s compared with 13 cm/s in C. This is the expected result with laminar flow. **E,** The gate is again located at the center of the tube. **F,** The gate length is extended to include the flow from the center, out to the tube wall. Note the strengthening of the lower flow speeds (Doppler shifts) *(arrows)* compared with **E,** where the slower flow is not included in the sample volume.

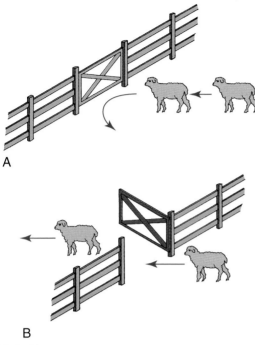

TABLE 5-9	The Amount Added to Effective Gate Length by Pulse Length for Various Cycles per Pulse and Frequencies	
Amount Added (mm)	**Cycles**	**f (MHz)**
1.9	5	2
3.8	10	2
7.7	20	2
0.8	5	5
1.5	10	5
3.1	20	5
0.4	5	10
0.8	10	10
1.5	20	10

FIGURE 5-44 A, Two sheep arrive at a closed gate and are not received into the pen. **B,** Two sheep arrive later at the gate, when it is open, and are received into the pen. In a Doppler detector the gate accepts and rejects echoes in a similar manner.

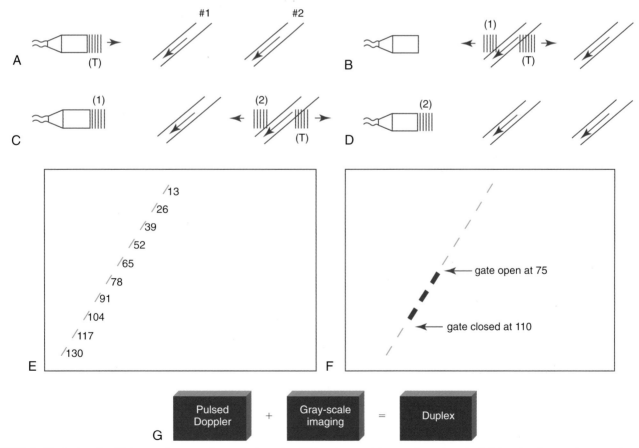

FIGURE 5-45 A, A pulse (T) leaves the transducer. **B,** An echo (1) is generated in vessel number 1. **C,** Echo 1 arrives at the transducer. At the same time, another echo (2) is generated at vessel number 2. **D,** Echo 2 arrives at the transducer after echo 1. These echoes will be processed by the instrument if the gate is open when they arrive. **E,** Echoes from 1-, 2-, 3-, 4-, 5-, 6-, 7-, 8-, 9-, and 10-cm depths arrive at the times (microseconds) indicated. **F,** If the gate is open from 75 to 110 μs after pulse emission, only the echoes in **E,** arriving at 78, 91, and 104 μs, will be accepted. The others will be rejected. **G,** A duplex instrument is a sonographic instrument with pulsed-wave Doppler capability incorporated.

Duplex Instrument

Including PW Doppler capability in a gray-scale sonographic instrument yields what is commonly called a **duplex instrument** (see Figure 5-45, *G*). The duplex instrument has the capacity to image anatomic structures and to analyze motion and flow at a known point in the anatomic field. Imaging allows intelligent positioning of the gate and angle correction in a PW Doppler system.

Duplex systems must be time shared; that is, imaging and Doppler flow measurements cannot be done simultaneously. Electronic scanning with arrays permits rapid switching between imaging and Doppler functions (several times per second), allowing what can appear to be simultaneous acquisition of real-time image and Doppler flow information. Imaging frame rates are slowed to allow for the acquisition of Doppler information between frames. Likewise, a time-out from the spectral display is taken to present a sonographic frame (see Figure 5-40, *A, open arrow*).

 Duplex instruments enable intelligent use of the Doppler sample volume by showing its location in the gray-scale anatomic display.

Spectral Analysis

The Doppler shift voltage from the detector does not go directly to the display but undergoes further processing,

otherwise it would look like Figure 5-46, *A*. This is the visual picture of what a listener hears from the loudspeaker. **Spectral analysis** (see Figure 5-46, *B*) provides a more meaningful and useful way to present the Doppler information visually. The presentation is in the form of a Doppler **frequency spectrum.**

Frequency Spectrum

The term *spectral* means "relating to a spectrum." A spectrum is an array of the components of a wave, separated and arranged in order of increasing frequency. The term *analysis* comes from the Greek word meaning "to break up" or "to take apart." Thus spectral analysis is the breaking up of the frequency components of a complex wave or signal and spreading them out in order of increasing frequency.

 Spectral analysis presents Doppler shift frequencies in frequency order.

The human auditory system analyzes sound. The ear and brain break down the complex sounds we receive into the component frequencies contained in the sounds. Thus we can listen to a Doppler signal and recognize normal and abnormal flow sounds. Visual presentation of these sounds provides additional capability for recognition of flow characteristics and for diagnosis of disease.

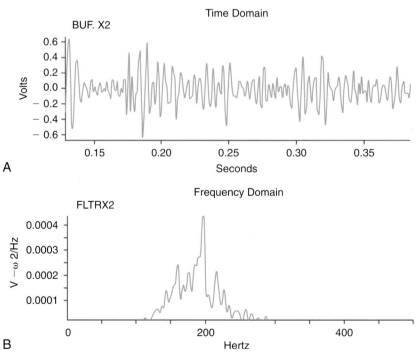

FIGURE 5-46 A, Demodulated Doppler shift signal for microspheres flowing at nearly uniform speed. When applied to a loudspeaker, a mix of many frequencies is heard. Approximately 10 cycles occur over a period of 0.20 to 0.25 second. Thus the fundamental period of this signal is about 50 ms, yielding a fundamental frequency of 200 Hz. **B,** After the Fourier transform is applied, a frequency spectrum is obtained. The center frequency is approximately 200 Hz. This is what was predicted in **A.** *(From Burns PN: The physical principles of Doppler and spectral analysis,* J Clin Ultrasound *15:567–590, 1987. Reprinted by permission of John Wiley & Sons, Inc.)*

Various kinds of flow occur in blood vessels. Changes in vessel size, turns, and abnormalities such as the presence of plaque or stenoses can alter the flow character. We have seen that flow can be characterized as *plug, laminar, parabolic, disturbed,* and *turbulent.* Portions of the blood flowing within a vessel are moving at different speeds (even for normal flow) and sometimes in different directions. Thus as the ultrasound beam intersects this flow and produces echoes, many different Doppler shifts are received from the vessel by the system, even from a small sample volume. These Doppler shifts are called the *Doppler frequency spectrum.* The extent of the range of generated Doppler shift frequencies depends on the character of the flow. For near-plug flow, a narrow range of Doppler shift frequencies is received. In disturbed and turbulent flows, broader and much broader ranges of Doppler shift frequencies, respectively, can be received.

 Different flow conditions produce various spectral presentations.

Fast Fourier Transform

The **fast Fourier transform** is the mathematical technique the instrument uses to derive the Doppler spectrum from the returning echoes of various frequencies (Figure 5-47). Fast Fourier transform displays can show **spectral broadening,** which is widening of the Doppler shift spectrum (i.e., an increase in the range of Doppler shift frequencies present) caused by a broader range of flow speeds and directions encountered by the sound beam with disturbed or turbulent flow.

 The fast Fourier transform is used to generate Doppler shift spectral displays.

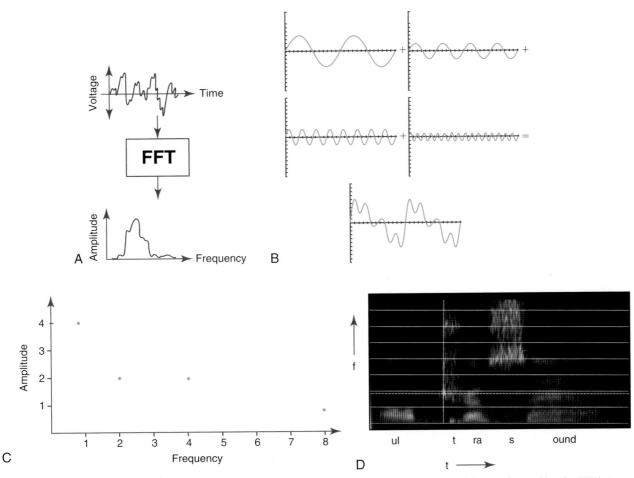

FIGURE 5-47 Fast fourier transform (FFT). A, The Doppler shift signal (containing many frequencies) is transformed by the FFT into a spectrum. (See Figure 5-46 for an example of the Doppler signal before **[A]** and after **[B]** FFT processing.) **B,** Four voltages of different frequencies are combined to give the complex result. **C,** The FFT analysis of this combined voltage yields this spectrum of four frequency components (a frequency of 1 with amplitude 4, two frequencies [2 and 4] with amplitude 2, and one frequency of 8 with amplitude of 1). **D,** Spectral analysis of the word *ultrasound.* Time progresses to the right as the word is uttered, and about 100 FFTs are performed. The vertical axis represents frequency. The low frequencies of the *ul, ra,* and *ound* syllables are seen, along with the high frequencies of the *t* and *s* sounds.

Spectral Displays

The received Doppler signal is a combination of many Doppler shift frequencies, yielding a complex waveform (see Figures 5-46, *A*, and 5-47, *B*). Using the fast Fourier transform, these frequencies are separated into a spectrum that is presented on a two-dimensional display as Doppler shift frequency on the horizontal axis and power or amplitude of each frequency component on the vertical axis (see Figures 5-46, *B*, and 5-47, *A*, *C*). Depending on the speed of the processor, about 100 to 1000 spectra can be generated per second. In the case of venous flow, such a spectral display usually would be rather constant. However, in the case of the pulsatile flow in arterial circulation, such a presentation changes continually, shifting to the right in systole as the blood accelerates and Doppler shifts increase, shifting to the left in dias-

tole, and changing in amplitude distribution over the cardiac cycle. Interpretation of this changing presentation is difficult; indeed, the character of the changes over the cardiac cycle could be important. Therefore, presentation of this changing spectrum as a function of time is valuable and useful. Such a trace is shown in Figures 5-47, *D*, 5-48, and 5-49. In these presentations the vertical axis represents Doppler shift frequency and the horizontal represents time (Figure 5-50). The amplitude or power of each Doppler shift frequency component at any instant is now presented as brightness (gray scale; see Figure 5-39, *A*) or color (see Figure 1-14). Doppler signal power is proportional to blood cell concentration (number of cells per unit volume). A bright spot on a spectral display means that a strong Doppler shift frequency component was received at that instant of time (see Figure 5-39). A dark spot means that a Doppler-shift

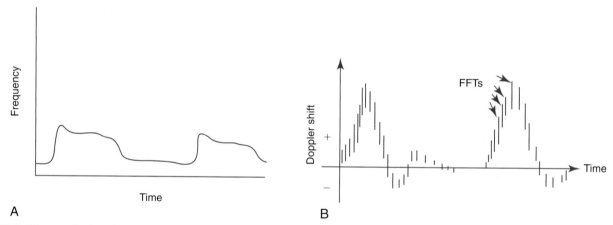

A

B

FIGURE 5-48 **A,** A display of Doppler shift as a function of time for pure plug flow. The Doppler shift frequency is represented on the vertical axis. The amplitude of the Doppler shift frequency at each instant of time is represented by gray level or color. In this example, there is only a single shift frequency at each instant of time (i.e., no spectrum). **B,** A spectral display for nonplug flow is composed of several (about 100–1000 per second) fast Fourier transform (FFT) spectra arranged vertically next to each other across the time (horizontal) axis.

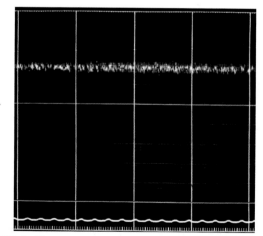

FIGURE 5-49 A spectral display of the signal shown in Figure 5-46. The flow is constant, yielding Doppler shift frequencies of approximately 200 Hz. (The horizontal markers represent 100 Hz.) *(From Burns PN: The physical principles of Doppler and spectral analysis,* J Clin Ultrasound *15:567–590, 1987. Reprinted by permission of John Wiley & Sons, Inc.)*

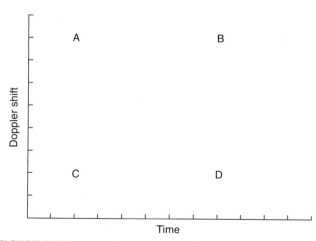

FIGURE 5-50 **Four points on a spectral display.** Points *A* and *C* occur at an earlier time, compared with points *B* and *D*, which occur later. Points *A* and *B* represent higher Doppler shift frequencies than points *C* and *D*.

frequency component was weak or nonexistent at that point in time. Intermediate values of gray shade or brightness indicate intermediate amplitudes or powers of frequency components at the given times. A strong signal at a particular frequency and time means that many scattering blood cells are moving at speeds and directions corresponding to that Doppler shift. A weak frequency means that few cells are traveling at speeds and directions corresponding to that Doppler shift at that point in time.

 The spectral display is a presentation of Doppler spectra versus time.

Spectral Broadening

Spectral trace presentations provide information about flow that can be used to discern conditions at the site of measurement and at sites proximal or distal to it. Peak flow speeds and spectral broadening are indicative of the degree of stenosis. Spectral broadening is a vertical thickening of the spectral trace (Figure 5-51). If all the cells were moving at the same speed, the spectral trace would be a thin line (see Figure 5-48, *A*). As stated previously, though, this is not the case in practice. However, narrow spectra can be observed, particularly in large vessels (Figure 5-52, *A*). The apparent narrowing of the spectrum as the blood accelerates in systole can

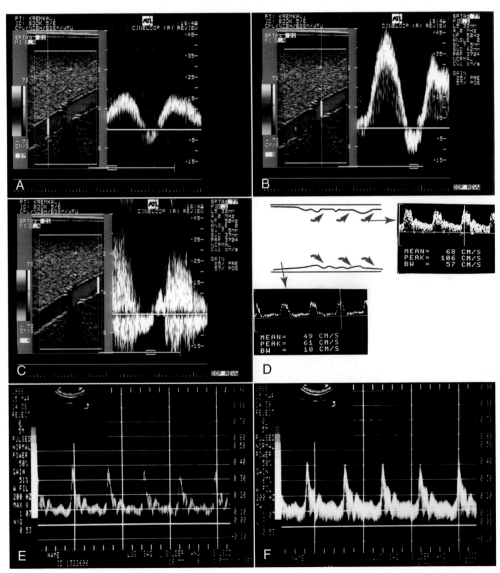

FIGURE 5-51 Flow *(lower left to upper right)* **in a tube with a stenosis in tissue-equivalent material. A,** Proximal to the stenosis, a narrow spectrum is observed (indicating approximately plug [i.e., blunted] flow). **B,** At the stenosis, a reasonably narrow spectrum still is seen, but the Doppler shifts have tripled because of the high flow speed through the stenosis. **C,** Distal to the stenosis, a broad spectrum is observed, along with negative Doppler shifts, both of which are caused by turbulent flow. Compare these observations with the flow conditions in and beyond a narrow gorge (see Figure 5-7). **D,** Spectral broadening produced by atheroma. **E,** Display produced at a correct Doppler gain setting. **F,** Artifactual spectral broadening caused by excessive gain. (**D–F** *from Taylor KJW, Holland S: Doppler US. Part I. Basic principles, instrumentation, and pitfalls,* Radiology *174:297–307, 1990.*)

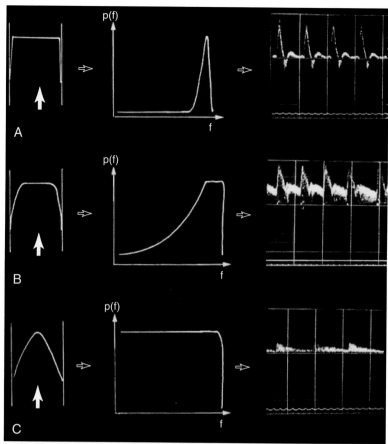

FIGURE 5-52 Flow speed profiles *(left)*, Doppler spectra (power versus frequency; *center*), and spectral displays *(right)* are shown for nearly plug flow in the aorta **(A)**, blunted parabolic flow in the celiac trunk **(B)**, and parabolic flow in the ovarian artery **(C)**. *(From Burns PN: The physical principles of Doppler and spectral analysis, J Clin Ultrasound 15:567–590, 1987. Reprinted by permission of John Wiley & Sons, Inc.)*

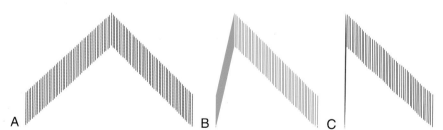

FIGURE 5-53 **Apparent spectral narrowing in rapidly accelerating flow. A,** Slowly accelerating and decelerating flow shows that the spectral widths (bandwidths) are all equal. **B–C,** As the acceleration phase becomes steeper, the bandwidths appear to narrow. However, the vertical lines representing bandwidth in all cases are the same.

be misinterpreted. A spectrum of consistent width appears to be thinner in a steep-rise portion of a curve (Figure 5-53). As flow is disturbed or becomes turbulent, greater variation in velocities of various portions of the flowing blood produce a greater range of Doppler shift frequencies. This results in a broadened spectrum presented on the spectral display (see Figure 5-51, *C, D*). Thus spectral broadening is indicative of disturbed or turbulent flow and can be related to a pathologic condition. However, spectral broadening can also be produced artificially by excessive Doppler gain (see Figure 5-51, *E–F*), and some broadening is produced by beam spreading (see Figure 5-37, *F*), particularly with wide-aperture arrays.

 Disturbed or turbulent flow conditions produce spectral broadening

Downstream (Distal) and Upstream (Proximal) Conditions

Doppler flow measurements can yield information about downstream (distal) conditions. Flow reversal in early diastole and lack of flow in late diastole (see Figures 5-8 and 5-52, *A*) indicate high resistance to flow downstream (e.g., because of vasoconstriction of arterioles). If flow resistance is reduced because of vasodilation, significant differences in the spectral display are observed (Figure 5-54). A comparison between low-resistance and high-resistance flow spectra is given in Figure 5-55. Stenoses upstream (proximal) produce spectral displays that have the so-called *tardus-parvus* character (see Figure 5-55, *C*).

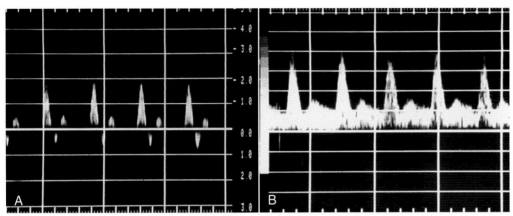

FIGURE 5-54 A, High distal resistance flow in the popliteal artery with the patient's leg at rest. **B,** Low distal resistance flow is observed after exercise. *(From Taylor KJW, Holland S: Doppler US. Part I. Basic principles, instrumentation, and pitfalls, Radiology 174:297–307, 1990.)*

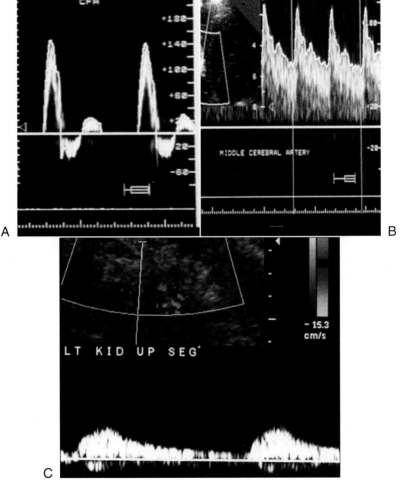

FIGURE 5-55 A, High distal resistance flow is seen in the common femoral artery of the resting lower limb. **B,** Low distal resistance flow is seen in the middle cerebral artery. Although these spectral displays are very different, they are both normal for the locations and conditions given. **C,** *Tardus-parvus* waveform typical of flow with proximal stenosis.

TABLE 5-10	Comparison of Doppler Shift Display, Doppler Power Display, and Spectral Display		
	Color Doppler Shift Display	Color Doppler Power Display	Spectral Display
Quantitative	No	No	Yes
Global	Yes	Yes	No
Perfusion	No	Yes	No

Normal vessels can be occluded in diastole when pressure drops below the critical value for flow. When this happens, no diastolic Doppler shift is detected.

 High- and low-impedance conditions upstream and downstream give rise to various spectral displays.

Table 5-10 compares the three types of Doppler displays: (1) color Doppler shift, (2) color Doppler power, and (3) spectral displays.

REVIEW

The key points presented in this chapter are the following:

- The heart provides the pulsatile pressure necessary to produce blood flow.
- Volumetric flow rate is proportional to the pressure difference at the ends of a tube.
- Volumetric flow rate is inversely proportional to flow resistance.
- Flow resistance increases with viscosity and tube length and decreases strongly with increasing tube diameter.
- Flow classifications include steady, pulsatile, plug, laminar, parabolic, disturbed, and turbulent.
- In a stenosis, flow speeds up, pressure drops (Bernoulli effect), and flow is disturbed or turbulent.
- Pulsatile flow is common in arterial circulation.
- Diastolic flow and/or flow reversal occur in some locations within the arterial system.
- The Doppler effect is a change in frequency resulting from motion.
- In medical ultrasound applications, blood flow and tissue motion are the sources of the Doppler effect.
- The change in frequency of the returning echoes with respect to the emitted frequency is called the *Doppler shift*.
- For flow toward the transducer, the Doppler shift is positive.

- For flow away from the transducer, the Doppler shift is negative.
- The Doppler shift depends on the speed of the scatterers of sound, the Doppler angle, and the operating frequency of the Doppler system.
- Greater flow speeds and smaller Doppler angles produce larger Doppler shifts but not stronger Doppler-shifted echoes.
- Higher operating frequencies produce larger Doppler shifts.
- Typical ranges of flow speeds (10 to 100 cm/s), Doppler angles (30 to 60 degrees), and operating frequencies (2 to 10 MHz) yield Doppler shifts in the range of 100 Hz to 11 kHz for vascular studies.
- In Doppler echocardiography, in which zero angle and speeds of a few meters per second can be encountered, Doppler shifts can be as high as 30 kHz.
- Color Doppler imaging acquires Doppler-shifted echoes from a two-dimensional cross-section of tissue scanned by an ultrasound beam.
- Doppler-shifted echoes are presented in color and superimposed on the gray-scale anatomic image of nonshifted echoes that were received during the scan.
- Flow echoes are assigned colors according to the color map chosen.
- Several pulses (the number is called *ensemble length*) are needed to generate a color scan line.
- Color controls include gain, map selection, variance on/off, persistence, ensemble length, color/gray priority, scale (pulse repetition frequency), baseline shift, wall filter, and color window angle, location, and size.
- Doppler shift displays are subject to Doppler angle dependence and aliasing.
- Doppler power displays color-coded Doppler-shift strengths into angle-independent, aliasing-independent, more sensitive presentations of flow information.
- Continuous-wave Doppler systems provide motion and flow information without depth selection capability.
- Pulsed-wave Doppler systems provide the ability to select the depth from which Doppler information is received.
- Spectral analysis provides visual information on the distribution of Doppler shift frequencies resulting from the distribution of the scatterer speeds and directions encountered.
- The Doppler spectrum is generated by the range of scatterer velocities encountered by the ultrasound beam.
- The spectrum is derived electronically using the fast Fourier transform and is presented on the display as Doppler shift versus time, with brightness indicating power.
- Flow conditions at the site of measurement are indicated by the width (vertical thickness) of the

spectrum, with spectral broadening being indicative of disturbed and turbulent flows.
- Flow conditions downstream, especially distal flow impedance, are indicated by the relationship between peak systolic and end diastolic flow speeds.

EXERCISES

1. Which of the following are parts of the circulatory system? (more than one correct answer)
   a. Heart
   b. Cerebral ventricle
   c. Artery
   d. Arteriole
   e. Capillary
   f. Bile duct
   g. Venule
   h. Vein
2. The _____ are the tiniest vessels in the circulatory system.
3. In which of the following can Doppler ultrasound detect flow? (more than one correct answer)
   a. The heart
   b. Arteries
   c. Arterioles
   d. Capillaries
   e. Venules
   f. Veins
4. To flow is to move in a _____.
5. The characteristic of a fluid that offers resistance to flow is called _____.
   a. resistance
   b. viscosity
   c. inertia
   d. impedance
   e. density
6. Poise is a unit of _____.
7. Pressure is _____ per unit area.
8. Pressure is _____.
   a. nondirectional
   b. unidirectional
   c. omnidirectional
   d. all of the above
   e. none of the above
9. Flow is a response to pressure _____ or _____.
10. If the pressure is greater at one end of a liquid-filled tube or vessel than it is at the other, the liquid will flow from the _____-pressure end to the _____-pressure end.
    a. higher, lower
    b. lower, higher
    c. depends on the liquid
    d. all of the above
    e. none of the above

11. The volumetric flow rate in a tube is determined by _____ difference and _____.
12. Flow increases if _____ increase(s).
    a. pressure difference
    b. pressure gradient
    c. resistance
    d. a and b
    e. all of the above
13. As flow resistance increases, volumetric flow rate _____.
14. If pressure difference is doubled, volumetric flow rate is _____.
    a. unchanged
    b. quartered
    c. halved
    d. doubled
    e. quadrupled
15. If flow resistance is doubled, volumetric flow rate is _____.
    a. unchanged
    b. quartered
    c. halved
    d. doubled
    e. quadrupled
16. Flow resistance in a vessel depends on _____.
    a. vessel length
    b. vessel radius
    c. blood viscosity
    d. all of the above
    e. none of the above
17. Flow resistance decreases with an increase in _____.
    a. vessel length
    b. vessel radius
    c. blood viscosity
    d. all of the above
    e. none of the above
18. Flow resistance depends most strongly on _____.
    a. vessel length
    b. vessel radius
    c. blood viscosity
    d. all of the above
    e. none of the above
19. Volumetric flow rate decreases with an increase in _____.
    a. pressure difference
    b. vessel radius
    c. vessel length
    d. blood viscosity
    e. c and d
20. When the speed of a fluid is constant across a vessel, the flow is called _____ flow.
    a. volume
    b. parabolic
    c. laminar
    d. viscous
    e. plug

21. The type of flow (approximately) seen in Figure 5-56, *A*, is _____.
    a. volume
    b. steady
    c. parabolic
    d. viscous
    e. plug

22. The type of flow seen in Figure 5-56, *B*, is _____.
    a. volume
    b. steady
    c. parabolic
    d. viscous
    e. plug

23. _____ flow occurs when straight parallel streamlines describing the flow are altered.

24. _____ flow involves random and chaotic flow patterns, with particles flowing in all directions.

25. Turbulent flow is more likely proximal or distal to a stenosis. _____

26. A narrowing of the lumen of a tube is called a _____.

27. Proximal to, at, and distal to a stenosis, _____ must be constant.
    a. laminar flow
    b. disturbed flow
    c. turbulent flow
    d. volumetric flow rate
    e. none of the above

28. For the answer to Exercise 27 to be true, flow speed at the stenosis must be _____ that proximal and distal to it.
    a. greater than
    b. less than
    c. less turbulent than
    d. less disturbed than
    e. none of the above

29. Poiseuille's equation predicts a(n) _____ in flow speed with a decrease in vessel radius.

30. The continuity rule predicts a(n) _____ in flow speed with a localized decrease (stenosis) in vessel diameter.

31. In a stenosis, the pressure is _____ the proximal and distal values.
    a. less than
    b. equal to
    c. greater than
    d. depends on the fluid
    e. none of the above

32. Added forward flow and flow reversal in diastole can occur with _____ flow.
    a. volume
    b. turbulent
    c. laminar
    d. disturbed
    e. pulsatile

33. As stenosis diameter decreases, _____ pass(es) through a maximum.
    a. flow speed at the stenosis
    b. flow speed proximal to the stenosis
    c. volumetric flow rate
    d. the Doppler shift at the stenosis
    e. a and d

34. In Figure 5-57, at which point is pressure the lowest?
    a. P
    b. S
    c. D
    d. P and D
    e. None of the above

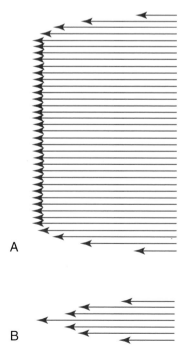

A

B

FIGURE 5-56 Two types of flow patterns. Illustration to accompany Exercises 21 and 22.

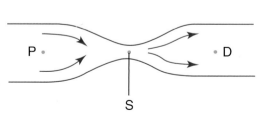

S

FIGURE 5-57 Proximal to *(P)*, at *(S)*, and distal to *(D)* a stenosis. Illustration to accompany Exercises 34 to 37. *(From Kremkau FW: Fluid flow, J Vasc Technol 17:153–154, 1993. Reproduced with permission.)*

35. In Figure 5-57, at which point is flow speed the lowest?
    a. P
    b. S
    c. D
    d. P and D
    e. None of the above
36. In Figure 5-57, at which point is volumetric flow rate the lowest?
    a. P
    b. S
    c. D
    d. P and D
    e. None of the above
37. In Figure 5-57, at which point is pressure energy the greatest?
    a. P
    b. S
    c. D
    d. P and D
    e. None of the above
38. The _____ effect is used to detect and measure _____ in vessels.
39. Motion of an echo-generating structure causes an echo to have a different _____ from that of the emitted pulse.
40. If the incident frequency is 1 MHz, the propagation speed is 1600 m/s, and the reflector speed is 16 m/s toward the source, the Doppler shift is _____ MHz, and the reflected frequency is _____ MHz.
41. If 2-MHz ultrasound is reflected from a soft tissue boundary moving at 10 m/s toward the source, the Doppler shift is _____ MHz.
42. If 2-MHz ultrasound is reflected from a soft tissue boundary moving at 10 m/s away from the source, the Doppler shift is _____ MHz.
43. The Doppler shift is the difference between _____ and _____ frequencies.
44. When incident sound direction and reflector motion are not parallel, calculation of the reflected frequency involves the _____ of the angle between these directions.
45. If the angle between incident sound direction and reflector motion is 60 degrees, the Doppler shift and reflected frequency in Exercise 40 are _____ MHz and _____ MHz.
46. If the angle between incident sound direction and reflector motion is 90 degrees, the cosine of the angle is _____, and the reflected frequency in Exercise 40 is _____ MHz.
47. For an operating frequency of 2 MHz, a flow speed of 10 cm/s, and a Doppler angle of 0 degrees, calculate the Doppler shift.
48. For an operating frequency of 6 MHz, a flow speed of 50 cm/s, and a Doppler angle of 60 degrees, calculate the Doppler shift.

49. For blood flowing in a vessel with a plug flow profile, the Doppler shift is _____ across the vessel.
50. Which Doppler angle yields the greatest Doppler shift?
    a. −90
    b. −45
    c. 0
    d. 45
    e. 90
51. To proceed from a measurement of Doppler shift frequency to a calculation of flow speed, _____ _____ must be known or assumed.
52. If operating frequency is doubled, the Doppler shift is _____.
53. If flow speed is doubled, the Doppler shift is _____.
54. If Doppler angle is doubled, the Doppler shift is _____.
55. Color Doppler instruments present two-dimensional, color-coded images representing _____ that are superimposed on gray-scale images representing _____.
56. Which of the following on a color Doppler display is (are) presented in real time?
    a. Gray-scale anatomy
    b. Flow direction
    c. Doppler spectrum
    d. a and b
    e. All of the above
57. Color Doppler instruments use an _____ technique to yield Doppler information in real time.
58. The information in Exercise 57 includes _____ Doppler shift, _____, _____, and _____.
59. The angle dependencies of Doppler shift displays and Doppler power displays are different. True or false?
60. Do the different colors appearing in Figure 5-28, A and C indicate that flow is going in two different directions in the vessel?
61. In color Doppler instruments, color is used only to represent flow direction. True or false?
62. In practice, approximately _____ pulses are required to obtain one line of color Doppler information.
    a. 1
    b. 10
    c. 100
    d. 1000
    e. 1,000,000
63. About _____ frames per second are produced by a color Doppler instrument.
    a. 10   d. 80
    b. 20   e. More than one of the above
    c. 40

64. Doppler shift displays are not dependent on Doppler angle. True or false?

65. If a color Doppler instrument shows two colors in the same vessel , it always means flow is occurring in opposite directions in the vessel. True or false?

66. A region of bright color on a Doppler shift display always indicates the highest flow speeds. True or false?

67. Increasing the ensemble length _____ the frame rate.

68. The _____ technique is commonly used to detect echo Doppler shifts in color Doppler instruments.

69. Which of the following reduce the frame rate of a color Doppler image? (more than one correct answer)
    a. Wider color window
    b. Longer color window
    c. Increased ensemble length
    d. Higher transducer frequency
    e. Higher priority setting

70. Lack of color in a vessel containing blood flow may be attributable to _____. (more than one correct answer)
    a. low color gain
    b. a high wall filter setting
    c. a low priority setting
    d. baseline shift
    e. aliasing

71. Increasing ensemble length _____ color sensitivity and accuracy and _____ frame rate.
    a. improves, increases
    b. degrades, increases
    c. degrades, decreases
    d. improves, decreases
    e. none of the above

72. Which control can be used to help with clutter?
    a. Wall filter
    b. Gain
    c. Baseline shift
    d. Pulse repetition frequency
    e. Smoothing

73. Color map baselines are always represented by _____.
    a. white
    b. black
    c. red
    d. blue
    e. cyan

74. Doubling the width of a color window produces a(n) _____ frame rate.
    a. doubled
    b. quadrupled
    c. unchanged
    d. halved
    e. quartered

75. Steering the color window to the right or left produces a(n) _____ frame rate.
    a. doubled
    b. quadrupled
    c. unchanged
    d. halved
    e. quartered

76. Autocorrelation produces _____. (more than one correct answer)
    a. the color of the Doppler shift
    b. the mean value of the Doppler shift
    c. variance
    d. spectrum
    e. peak Doppler shift

77. Steering the color window to the right or left changes _____.
    a. frame rate
    b. pulse repetition frequency
    c. the Doppler angle
    d. the Doppler shift
    e. more than one of the above

78. Color Doppler frame rates are _____ gray-scale rates.
    a. equal to
    b. less than
    c. more than
    d. depends on color map
    e. depends on priority

79. In a single frame, color can change in a vessel because of _____.
    a. vessel curvature
    b. sector format
    c. helical flow
    d. diastolic flow reversal
    e. all of the above

80. Angle is not important in transverse color Doppler views through vessels. True or false?

81. Compared with Doppler-shift imaging, Doppler-power imaging is _____.
    a. more sensitive
    b. angle independent
    c. aliasing independent
    d. speed independent
    e. all of the above

82. Doppler-power imaging indicates (with color) the _____ of flow.
    a. presence
    b. direction
    c. speed
    d. character
    e. more than one of the above

83. Doppler-shift imaging indicates (with color) the _____ of flow.
    a. presence
    b. direction
    c. speed
    d. character
    e. more than one of the above

84. The functions of a Doppler detector include _____.
    a. amplification
    b. phase quadrature detection
    c. Doppler shift detection
    d. sign determination
    e. all of the above

85. An earlier gate time means _____ sample volume depth.
    a. a later
    b. a shallower
    c. a deeper
    d. a stronger
    e. none of the above

86. Doppler signal power is proportional to _____.
    a. volume flow rate
    b. flow speed
    c. the Doppler angle
    d. cell concentration
    e. more than one of the above

87. Doppler ultrasound provides information about flow conditions only at the site of measurement. True or false?

88. Stenosis affects _____.
    a. peak systolic flow speed
    b. end diastolic flow speed
    c. spectral broadening
    d. window
    e. all of the above

89. Spectral broadening is a _____ of the spectral trace.
    a. vertical thickening
    b. horizontal thickening
    c. brightening
    d. darkening
    e. horizontal shift

90. If all the cells in a vessel were moving at the same constant speed, the spectral trace would be a _____ line.
    a. thin horizontal
    b. thin vertical
    c. thick horizontal
    d. thick vertical
    e. none of the above

91. Disturbed flow produces a narrower spectrum. True or false?

92. Turbulent flow produces a narrower spectrum. True or false?

93. As stenosis progresses, which of the following increase(s)?
    a. Lumen diameter
    b. Systolic Doppler shift
    c. Diastolic Doppler shift
    d. Spectral broadening
    e. More than one of the above

94. Higher flow speed always produces a higher Doppler shift on a spectral display. True or false?

95. Flow reversal in diastole indicates _____.
    a. a stenosis
    b. an aneurysm
    c. high distal resistance
    d. low distal resistance
    e. more than one of the above

96. Decreased distal resistance normally causes end diastolic flow to _____.
    a. increase
    b. decrease
    c. be disturbed
    d. become turbulent
    e. more than one of the above

97. If angle correction is set at 60 degrees but should be zero degrees, the display indicates a flow speed of 100 cm/s. The correct flow speed is _____ cm/s.
    a. 25
    b. 50
    c. 100
    d. 200
    e. 400

98. If angle correction is set at zero degrees but should be 60 degrees, the display indicates a flow speed of 100 cm/s. The correct flow speed is _____ cm/s.
    a. 25
    b. 50
    c. 100
    d. 200
    e. 400

99. If a 5-kHz Doppler shift corresponds to 100 cm/s, then a 2.5-kHz shift corresponds to _____ cm/s.

100. Which of the following is increased if Doppler angle is increased?
    a. Aliasing
    b. Doppler shift
    c. Effect of angle error
    d. b and c
    e. None of the above

Artifacts

Revised by Flemming Forsberg and Frederick W. Kremkau

LEARNING OBJECTIVES

After reading this chapter, the student should be able to do the following:

- List reasons for incorrect presentation of anatomic structures by sonographic gray-scale images
- List reasons for incorrect presentation of motion and flow information by spectral and color Doppler displays
- Describe how specific artifacts can be recognized
- Explain how to deal with artifacts in order to avoid the pitfalls and misdiagnoses that they can cause

OUTLINE

Propagation
  Slice Thickness
  Speckle
  Reverberation
  Mirror Image
  Refraction
  Grating Lobes
  Speed Error

Range Ambiguity
Attenuation
  Shadowing
  Enhancement
Spectral Doppler
  Aliasing
  Nyquist Limit
  Range Ambiguity

Mirror Image
Color Doppler
  Aliasing
  Mirror Image, Shadowing,
    Refraction, Clutter, and Noise
Review
Exercises

KEY TERMS

Aliasing
Anechoic
Comet tail
Cross-talk
Enhancement
Hypoechoic

Mirror image
Multiple
Multiple angle artifact
Nyquist limit
Range ambiguity
Reverberation

Slice thickness
Shadowing
Speckle
Speed error

In imaging, an artifact is anything that does not correctly display the structures or functions (such as blood flow and motion) imaged. An artifact is caused by some problematic aspect of the imaging technique. In addition to helpful artifacts, there are several that hinder correct interpretation and diagnosis. One must avoid these artifacts or handle them properly when encountered.

Artifacts are incorrect representations of anatomy or function.

Artifacts in sonography occur as apparent structures that are one of the following:

1. Not real
2. Missing
3. Misplaced
4. Of incorrect brightness, shape, or size

Some artifacts are produced by improper equipment operation or settings (e.g., incorrect gain and compensation settings). Other artifacts are inherent in the sonographic and Doppler methods of today's scanners

BOX 6-1 | Sonographic Artifacts

Propagation Group
- Comet tail
- Grating lobe
- Mirror image
- Range ambiguity
- Refraction
- Reverberation
- Ring-down
- Slice (section) thickness
- Speckle
- Speed error

Attenuation Group
- Enhancement
- Focal enhancement
- Refraction (edge) shadowing
- Shadowing

and can occur even with proper equipment and technique. Artifacts that occur in sonography are listed in Box 6-1, where they are grouped as they are considered in the following sections.

The assumptions inherent in the design of sonographic instruments include the following:

- Sound travels in straight lines
- Echoes originate only from objects located on the beam axis
- The amplitude of returning echoes is related directly to the reflecting or scattering properties of distant objects
- That the distance to reflecting or scattering objects is proportional to the round-trip travel time (13 μs/cm of depth).

If any of these assumptions are violated, an artifact occurs.

Several artifacts are encountered in Doppler ultrasound, including incorrect display of Doppler flow information, either in color Doppler or in spectral format. The most common of these is **aliasing**. Others include **range ambiguity** and spectrum mirror image.

PROPAGATION

Slice Thickness

Limited detail resolution can introduce artifacts, because a failure to resolve means a loss of detail, and two adjacent structures may be visualized as one. The beam width perpendicular to the scan plane (the third dimension; Figure 6-1, A) results in slice-thickness artifacts; for example, the appearance of false debris in a simple echo-free cyst (Figure 6-1, B). These artifacts occur because of the finite thickness of the interrogating beam used to scan the patient. Echoes originate not only from the

center of the main beam, but also from off-center (the slice thickness). These echoes are all collapsed into a zero-thickness, two-dimensional image that is composed of echoes that have come from a not-so-thin tissue volume scanned by the beam. The slice-thickness artifact is also called the section-thickness or partial-volume artifact. It may be possible to resolve this artifact by using tissue harmonic imaging, as the sound beam in this mode is narrower than in regular gray-scale mode (Figure 6-1, C).

 Beam width perpendicular to the scan plane causes section slice thickness artifact.

Speckle

Apparent detail resolution can be deceiving. The detailed echo pattern often is not related directly to the scattering properties of tissue (called tissue texture) but is a result of the interference effects of the scattered sound from the distribution of all the scatterers within the tissue. There are many small scatterers (smaller than the wavelength) included in the ultrasound pulse at any instant as it travels through the tissue. Their echoes can combine constructively or destructively, which produces the familiar pattern of bright and dark spots in a gray-scale image. This phenomenon is called acoustic **speckle** (Figure 6-2) and may obstruct the detection of low-contrast objects in an otherwise homogenous background (for example liver lesions). Strictly speaking, speckle is not an artifact as it results from the underlying distribution of scatterers. Given how difficult it is to predict speckle patterns in practice, most modern instruments have implemented some form of speckle reduction techniques (see Figure 6-2).

 Speckle is the granular appearance of images that is caused by the interference of echoes from the distribution of scatterers in tissue.

Reverberation

Multiple reflections (reverberations) can occur between two strong reflectors or between the transducer and a strong reflector (Figure 6-3, A). When these multiple echoes are received by the scanner, they may be sufficiently strong to be detected by the instrument and then displayed. This may cause confusion in the interpretation of the displayed image. The process by which they are produced is shown in Figure 6-3, B. Reverberations are shown in the sonographic image as additional reflectors that don't represent real structures (Figure 6-4). The multiple reflections are displayed beneath the real reflector at intervals equal to the distance between the transducer and the real reflector. Each subsequent reflection is weaker than prior ones, but this drop in echo strength is counteracted (at least partially) by the attenuation

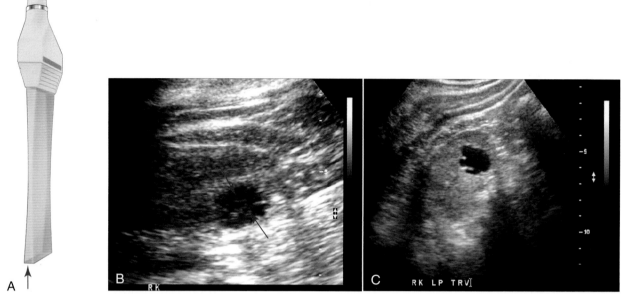

FIGURE 6-1 A, The scan "plane" through the tissue is really a three-dimensional volume. Two dimensions (axial and lateral) are in the scan plane, but there is a third dimension (called *slice thickness* or *section thickness*). The third dimension *(arrow)* is collapsed to zero thickness when the image is displayed in two-dimensional format. **B,** A simple renal cyst that should be echo-free is filled with echoes *(arrows)*, which could lead to concern that this might be a solid renal lesion. These off-axis echoes are a result of scan-plane slice thickness. **C,** When tissue harmonic imaging is activated (resulting in a narrower beam-profile), the slice-thickness artifact disappears.

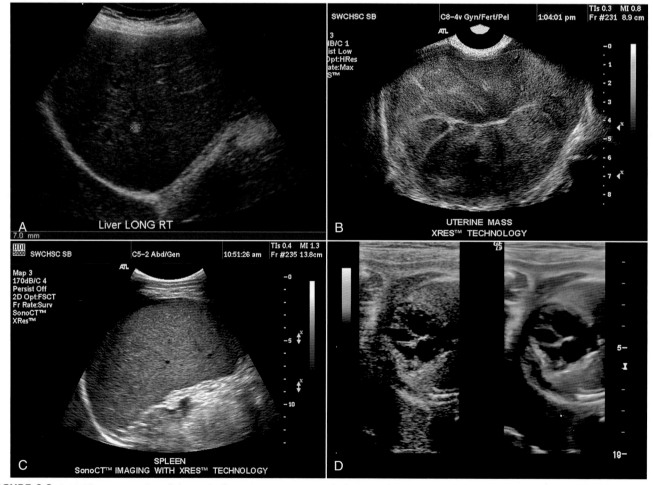

FIGURE 6-2 A–C, Three examples of the typically grainy appearance of ultrasound images that is not primarily the result of detail resolution limitations but rather of speckle. Speckle is the interference pattern resulting from constructive and destructive interference of echoes returning simultaneously from many scatterers within the propagating ultrasound pulse at any instant. **D,** Approaches to speckle reduction (right image compared with the left) are implemented in modern instruments.

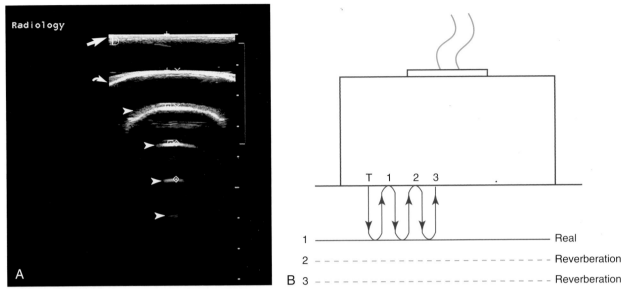

FIGURE 6-3 A, Reverberation *(arrowheads)* resulting from multiple reflection through a water path between a linear array transducer *(straight arrow)* and the surface of an apple *(curved arrow).* **B,** The behavior in **A** is explained as follows: A pulse *(T)* is transmitted from the transducer. A strong echo is generated at the real reflector and is received (1) at the transducer, allowing correct imaging of the reflector. However, the echo is reflected partially at the transducer so that a second echo (2) is received, as well as a third (3). Because these echoes arrive later, they appear deeper on the display, where there are no reflectors. The lateral displacement of the reverberating sound path is for figure clarity. In fact, the sound travels down and back the same path repeatedly.

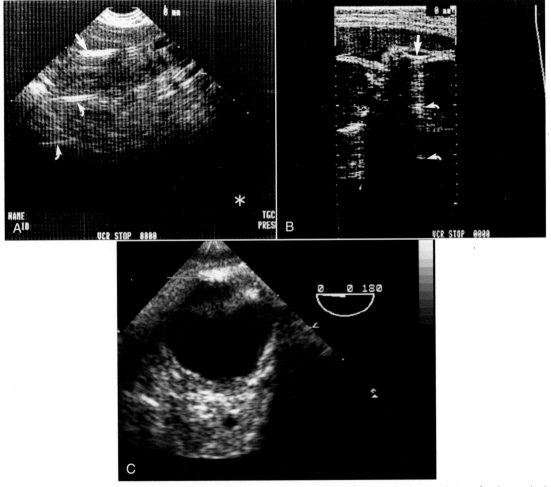

FIGURE 6-4 A, A chorionic villi sampling catheter *(straight arrow)* and two reverberations *(curved arrows).* **B,** A fetal scapula *(straight arrow)* and two reverberations *(curved arrows).* **C,** Reverberation *(red arrow)* from hyperechoic region *(green arrow)* in transesophageal scan of the ascending aorta.

compensation (TGC) function. The **comet tail** artifact is a particular case of reverberation, where two closely spaced surfaces generate a series of closely spaced, discrete echoes (Figure 6-5). Moreover, if these two surfaces are the front and back of the transducer crystal then the artifact is often referred to as the (transducer) ringdown artifact. It is relatively rare to observe a significant ringdown artifact on a modern scanner.

 Reverberations are multiple reflections between a structure and the transducer or between structures or within a structure.

Mirror Image

The mirror-image artifact, also a form of reverberation, shows structures that exist on one side of a strong reflector as being present on the other side as well. Figure 6-6 explains how this happens and shows examples. Mirror-image artifacts are common around the diaphragm and pleura because of the total reflection from air-filled lung. They occasionally occur in other locations. Sometimes the mirrored structure is not in the unmirrored scan plane (Figure 6-6, C).

 Mirror-image artifact duplicates a structure on the opposite side of a strong reflector.

Refraction

Refraction of light enables lenses to focus and distorts the presentation of objects, as shown in Figure 6-7. Refraction can cause a reflector to be positioned improperly (laterally) on a sonographic display (Figure 6-8). This is likely to occur, for example, when the transducer is placed on the abdominal midline (Figures 6-8, C, and 6-9), producing doubling of single objects. Beneath are the rectus abdominis muscles, which are surrounded by fat. These tissues present refracting boundaries because of their different propagation speeds.

 Refraction displaces structures laterally from their correct locations.

Grating Lobes

Side lobes are beams that propagate from a single element in directions different from the primary or main beam. Grating lobes are additional beams emitted from an array transducer that are stronger than the side lobes of individual elements (Figure 6-10). Side and grating lobes are weaker than the primary beam and normally do not produce echoes that are displayed in the image, particularly if they fall on a normally echogenic region of the scan. However, if grating lobes encounter a strong reflector (e.g., bone or gas), their echoes may well be displayed, particularly if they fall within an **anechoic** region.

If so, they appear in incorrect locations as in these obstetrical examples (Figure 6-11). Note that the grating lobe artifact is normally weaker than the correct presentation of the structure. However, that may not always be the case with very strong reflectors, such as metallic needles (Figure 6-12).

 Grating lobes duplicate structures laterally to the true ones.

Speed Error

Propagation **speed error** occurs when the assumed value for the speed of sound in soft tissues (1.54 mm/µs, leading to the 13 µs/cm rule) is incorrect. If the propagation speed that exists over a path traveled is greater than 1.54 mm/µs, the calculated distance to the reflector is too small, and the display will place the reflector too close to the transducer (Figure 6-13). This occurs because the increased speed causes the echoes to arrive sooner. If the actual speed is less than 1.54 mm/µs, the reflector will be displayed too far from the transducer (Figure 6-14) because the echoes arrive later. Refraction and propagation speed error can also cause a structure to be displayed with an incorrect shape.

 Propagation speed error displaces structures axially.

Range Ambiguity

In sonographic imaging, it is assumed that for each pulse all echoes are received before the next pulse is emitted. If this were not the case, error could result (Figures 6-15 and 6-16). The maximum depth imaged correctly by an instrument is determined by its pulse repetition frequency (PRF). To avoid range ambiguity, PRF automatically is reduced in deeper imaging situations. This also causes a reduction in frame rate.

 The range-ambiguity artifact places structures much closer to the surface than they should be.

Sometimes two artifacts combine to present even more challenging cases. An example involving range ambiguity is shown in Figure 6-17.

ATTENUATION

Shadowing

Shadowing is the reduction in echo amplitude from reflectors that lie behind a strongly reflecting or attenuating structure (Figure 6-18). A strongly attenuating or reflecting structure weakens the sound distal to it, causing echoes from the distal region to be weak and thus to appear darker, like a shadow. Of course, the returning

Text continued on p. 187

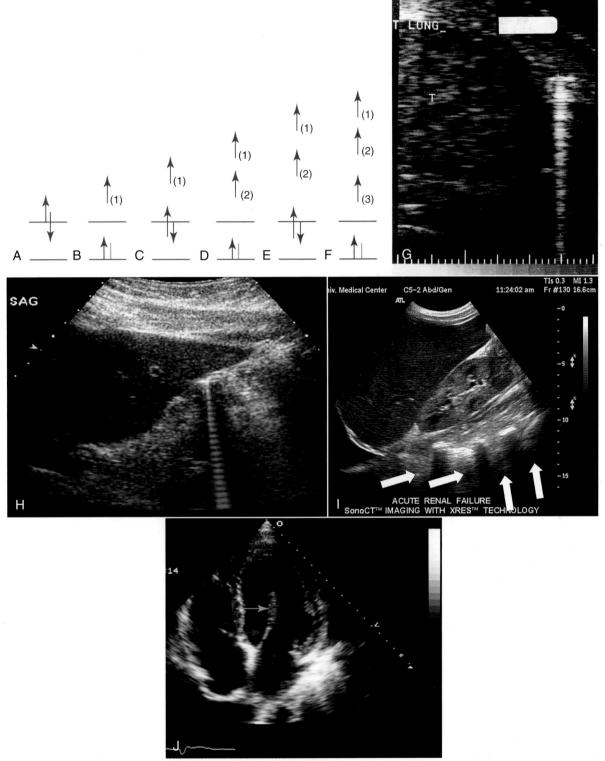

FIGURE 6-5 **Generation of comet-tail artifact (closely spaced reverberations).** Action progresses in time from left to right. **A,** An ultrasound pulse encounters the first reflector, is reflected partially and transmitted partially. **B,** Reflection and transmission at the first reflector are complete. Reflection at the second reflector is occurring. **C,** Reflection at the second reflector is complete. Partial transmission and partial reflection are again occurring at the first reflector as the second echo passes through. **D,** The echoes from the first *(1)* and second *(2)* reflectors are traveling toward the transducer. A second reflection (repeat of **B**) is occurring at the second reflector. **E,** Partial transmission and reflection are again occurring at the first reflector. **F,** Three echoes are now returning—the echo from the first reflector *(1)*, the echo from the second reflector *(2)*, and the echo from the second reflector *(3)*—that originated from the back side of the first reflector **(C)** and reflected again from the second reflector **(D).** A fourth echo is being generated at the second reflector **(F). G,** Comet-tail artifact from an air rifle BB shot pellet *(B)* adjacent to the testicle *(T).* The front and rear surface of the BB shot are the two reflecting surfaces involved in this example. **H,** Comet-tail artifact from gas bubbles in the duodenum. **I,** Comet tail *(arrows)* from diaphragm. **J,** Apical four-chamber view of comet tail artifact *(green arrow)* in the left ventricle. Artifact is connected to anterior mitral leaflet *(red arrow)*. *(G from Kremkau FW, Taylor KJW: Artifacts in ultrasound imaging,* J Ultrasound Med 5:227, 1986.)

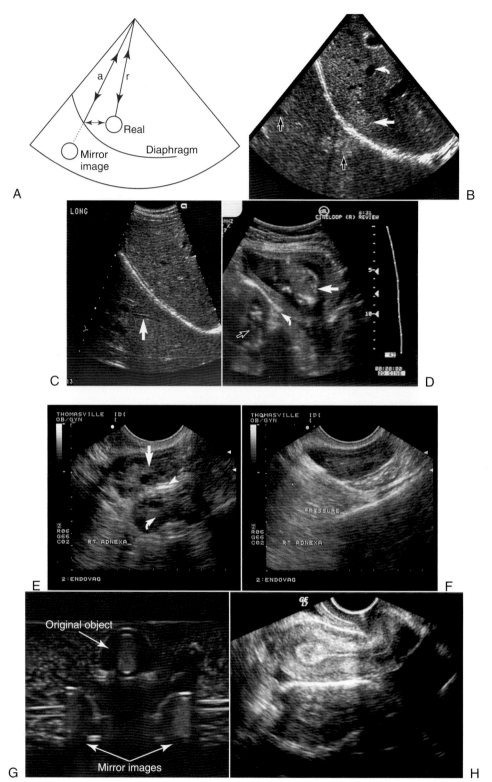

FIGURE 6-6 A, When pulses encounter a real hepatic structure directly *(scan line r),* the structure is imaged correctly. If the pulse first reflects off the diaphragm *(scan line a)* and returns along the same path, the structure is displayed on the other side of the diaphragm. **B,** A hemangioma *(straight arrow)* and vessel *(curved arrow)* with their mirror images *(open arrows).* **C,** A vessel is mirror-imaged *(arrow)* superior to the diaphragm but does not appear inferior because it is outside the unmirrored scan plane. **D,** A fetus *(straight arrow)* also appears as a mirror image *(open arrow).* The mirror *(curved arrow)* is probably echogenic muscle. **E,** Ovary *(arrow)* with mirror image *(curved arrow)* that could be mistaken for an adnexal mass or ectopic pregnancy. Bowel gas *(arrowhead)* is apparently the mirror in this case. **F,** Applying external abdominal pressure displaces the gas, eliminating the mirror image. **G,** Mirror image of a thick-walled vessel in a tissue-equivalent phantom. The echoes are being reflected from the echogenic scatterers used in the circulating fluid and the vessel wall resulting in two (2) mirror images split on either side of the center line *(arrows).* **H,** Uterus with its mirror image below it.

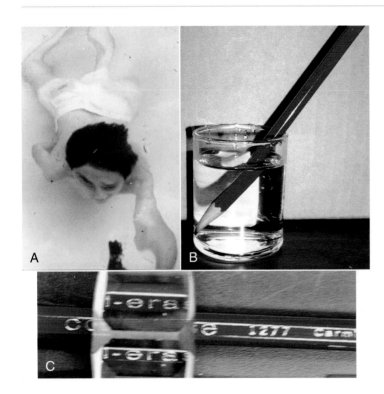

FIGURE 6-7 A, Refracted light from a child in a swimming pool distorts his appearance. We see a thin arm and a thick one, a large eye and a small one, a thin leg, a thick one, and even a third lower limb emerging. **B,** A pencil in water appears to be broken. **C,** A pencil beneath a prism appears to be split in two.

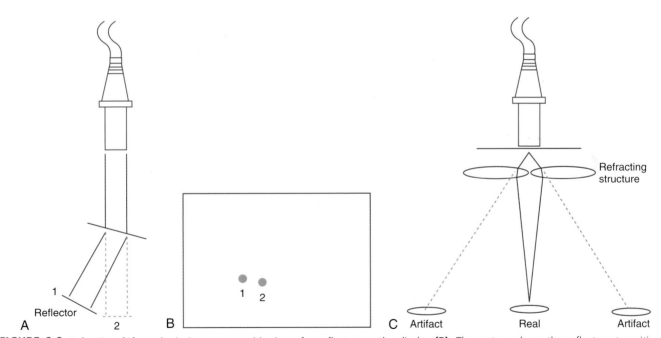

FIGURE 6-8 Refraction **(A)** results in improper positioning of a reflector on the display **(B).** The system places the reflector at position 2 (because that is the direction from which the echo was received), when in fact the reflector is actually at position 1. **C,** One real structure is imaged as two artifactual objects because of the refracting structure close to the transducer. If unrefracted pulses can propagate to the real structure, a triple presentation (one correct, two artifactual) will result.

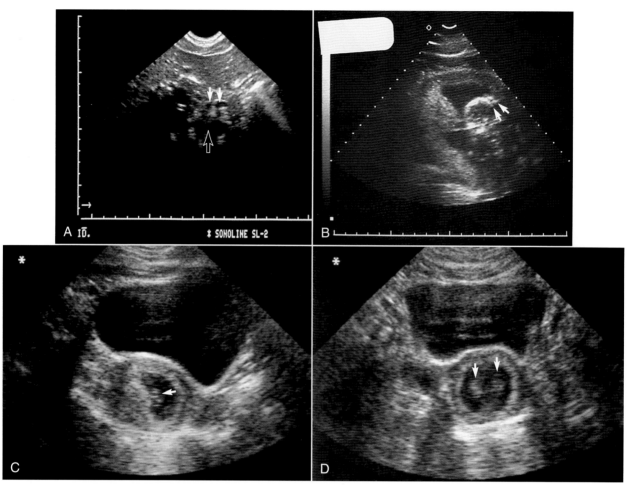

FIGURE 6-9 **A,** Refraction (probably through the rectus abdominis muscle) has widened the aorta *(open arrow)* and produced a double image of the celiac trunk *(arrows)*. **B,** Refraction has produced a double image of a fetal skull *(arrows)*. Refraction also may cause a single gestation **(C)** to appear as a double gestation **(D).**

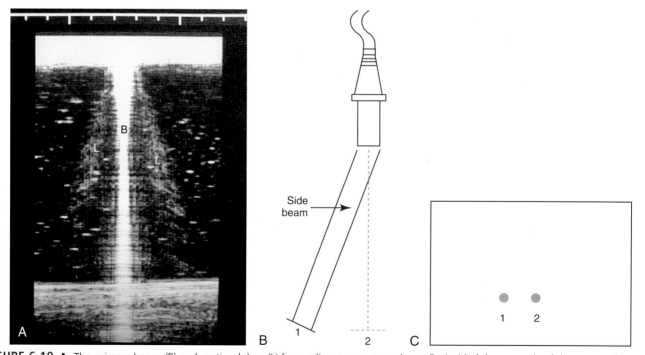

FIGURE 6-10 **A,** The primary beam *(B)* and grating lobes *(L)* from a linear array transducer. **B,** A side lobe or grating lobe can produce and receive a reflection from a "side view." **C,** This will be placed on the display at the proper distance from the transducer but in the wrong location (direction) because the instrument assumes that echoes originate from points along the main beam axis. The instrument shows the reflector at position 2 because that is the direction in which the main beam travels. The reflector is actually in position 1.

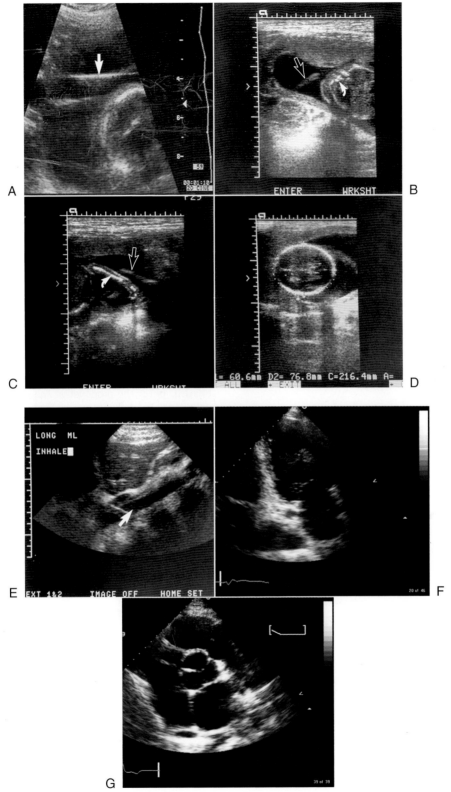

FIGURE 6-11 Grating lobes in obstetric scans can produce the appearance of amniotic sheets or bands. A, A real amniotic sheet *(arrow).* **B–C,** Grating lobe duplication *(open arrows)* of fetal bones *(curved arrows)* resembles amniotic bands or sheets. **D,** Grating lobe duplication of a fetal skull. **E,** Artifactual grating lobe echoes *(arrow)* cross the aorta. In these examples, we observe that the grating lobe artifact is always weaker than the correct presentation of the structure. **F,** Apical two-chamber view of grating-lobe artifact *(arrow)* in left ventricle. **G,** Short-axis view of aortic and tricuspid valves with grating lobe artifact *(arrow).*

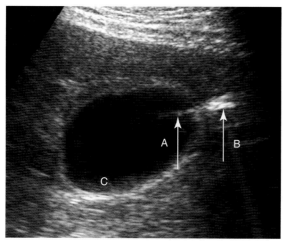

FIGURE 6-12 Needle tip *(A arrow)* is correctly seen in a cyst for aspiration, while grating lobes show the out-of-plane body of the needle *(B arrow)*. In this example, there is also a slice thickness artifact depicting non-existent sludge in the cyst *(labeled C)*.

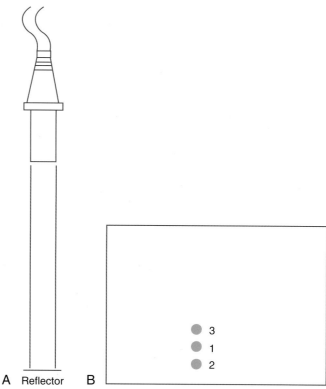

FIGURE 6-13 The propagation speed over the traveled path **(A)** determines the reflector position on the display **(B).** The reflector is actually in position 1. If the actual propagation speed is less than that assumed, the reflector will appear in position 2. If the actual speed is more than that assumed, the reflector will appear in position 3.

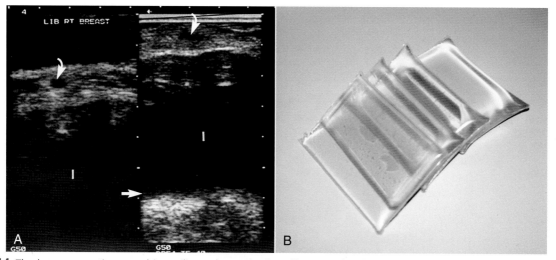

FIGURE 6-14 The low propagation speed in a silicone breast implant *(I)* causes the chest wall *(straight arrow)* to appear deeper than it should **(A).** Note that a cyst *(curved arrow)* is shown more clearly on the left image than on the right because a gel standoff pad **(B)** has been placed between the transducer and the breast, moving the beam focus closer to the cyst.

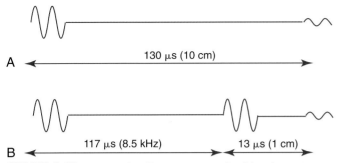

FIGURE 6-15 A, An echo (from a 10-cm depth) arrives 130 µs after pulse emission. **B,** If the pulse repetition period were 117 µs (corresponding to a pulse repetition frequency of 8.5 kHz), the echo in **A** would arrive 13 µs after the next pulse was emitted. The instrument would place this echo at a 1-cm depth rather than the correct value. This range location error is known as the *range-ambiguity artifact.*

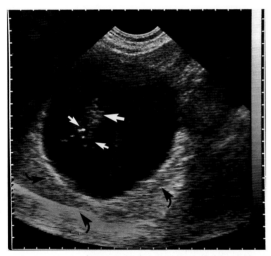

FIGURE 6-16 A large renal cyst (diameter about 10 cm) has artifactual range-ambiguity echoes within it *(white arrows).* They are generated from structure(s) below the display. These deep echoes arrive after the next pulse is emitted. Because the time from the emission of the last pulse to echo arrival is short, the echoes are placed closer to the transducer than they should be. Echoes arrive from much deeper (later) than usual in this case because the sound passes through the long, low-attenuation paths in the cyst. These echoes may have come from bone or a far body wall. Low attenuation in the cyst is indicated by the enhancement below it *(curved black arrows).*

echoes also must pass through the attenuating structure, adding to the shadowing effect. Examples of shadowing structures include calcified plaques (Figure 6-18, *A*), stiff breast lesions (Figure 6-18, *B*), and stones (Figure 6-19, *A*). Shadowing also can occur behind the edges of objects that are not necessarily strong attenuators (Figure 6-20). In this case the cause may be the defocusing action of a refracting curved surface. Alternatively, it may be attributable to destructive interference caused by portions of an ultrasound pulse passing through tissues with different propagation speeds and subsequently getting out of

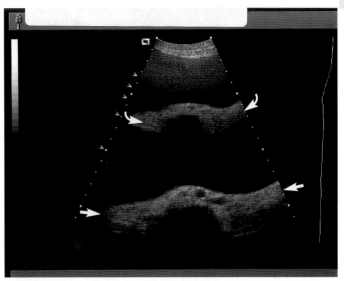

FIGURE 6-17 Abdominal ascites produces a large echo-free region in this scan. A structure is located at a depth of about 13 cm *(straight arrows).* Located in the anechoic region at a depth of about 6 cm is a structure *(curved arrows)* shaped like that at 13 cm. How could this artifact appear closer than the actual structure, implying that these echoes arrived earlier than those from the correct location? It turns out that the artifact is actually a combination of two: reverberation and range ambiguity. The artifact seen is a reverberation from the deep structure and the transducer. But a reverberation should appear at twice the depth of the actual structure, that is, at about 26 cm. However, the arrival of the reverberation echoes occurs about 78 µs after the next pulse is emitted so that they are placed at a 6-cm depth. Single artifacts are difficult enough. Fortunately, combinations like this occur infrequently.

phase. In either case the intensity of the beam decreases beyond the edge of the structure, causing echoes to be weakened.

> Shadowing is the weakening of echoes distal to a strongly attenuating or reflecting structure or from the edges of a refracting structure.

Enhancement

Enhancement is the strengthening of echoes from reflectors that lie behind a weakly attenuating structure (see Figures 6-16 and 6-19). Shadowing and enhancement result in reflectors being displayed on the image with amplitudes that are too low and too high, respectively. Brightening of echoes also can be caused by the increased intensity in the focal region of a beam because the beam is narrow there. This is called focal enhancement or focal banding (Figure 6-21). Shadowing and enhancement artifacts are often useful for determining the nature of masses and structures. Shadowing and enhancement are reduced with spatial compounding (and other speckle reduction techniques), because several directional approaches to each

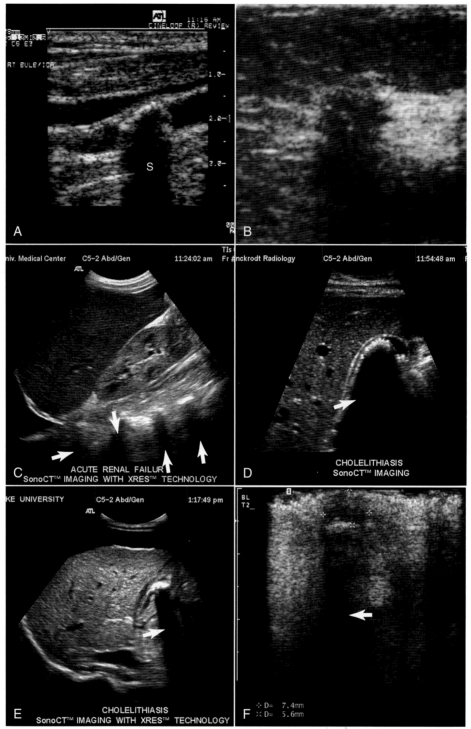

FIGURE 6-18 A, Shadowing *(S)* from a high-attenuation calcified plaque in the common carotid artery. **B,** Shadowing from a stiff breast lesion. **C–F,** Examples of shadowing *(arrows)*.

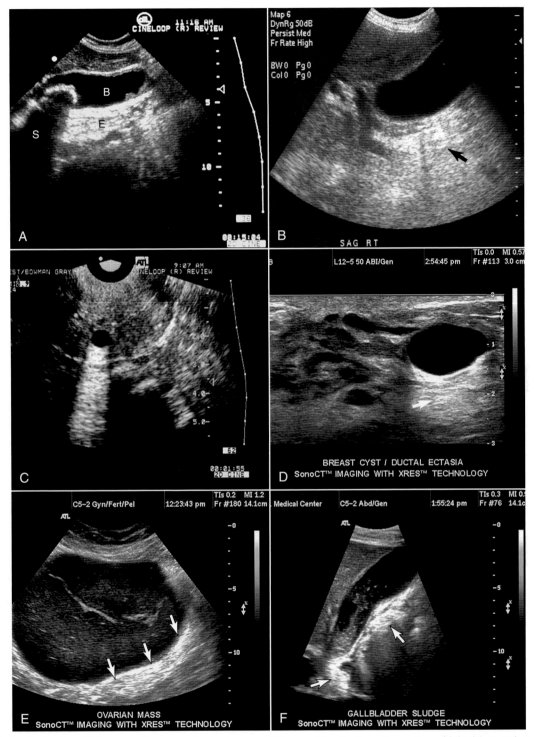

FIGURE 6-19 A, Shadowing *(S)* from a gallstone and enhancement *(E)* caused by the low attenuation of bile *(B)*. **B,** Enhancement *(arrow)* from the low attenuation of bile in the gallbladder. **C,** Enhancement beyond a cervical cyst. **D–F,** Examples of enhancement *(arrows)*.

anatomic site are used to form the final image, allowing the beam to "get around" the attenuating or enhancing structure. This may be useful with shadowing because it can uncover structures (especially pathologic ones) that were not imaged because they were located in the shadow.

 Enhancement is the strengthening of echoes distal to a weakly attenuating structure.

External influences also can produce artifacts. As an example, interference from electronic equipment adds unwanted noise to the image (Figure 6-22).

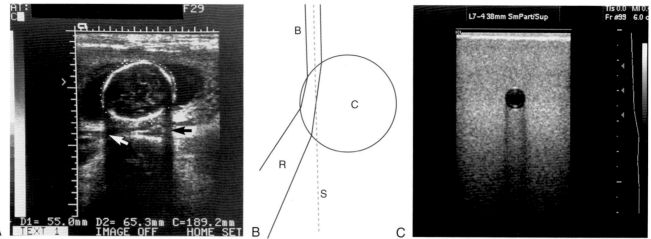

FIGURE 6-20 A, Edge shadows *(arrows)* from a fetal skull. **B,** As a sound beam *(B)* enters a circular region *(C)* of higher propagation speed, it is refracted, and refraction occurs again as it leaves. This causes spreading of the beam with decreased intensity. The echoes from region *R* are presented deep to the circular region in the neighborhood of the dashed line. Because of beam spreading, these echoes are weak and thus cast a shadow *(S).* **C,** Edge shadows from a tube (shown in transverse view) embedded in tissue-equivalent material in a flow phantom.

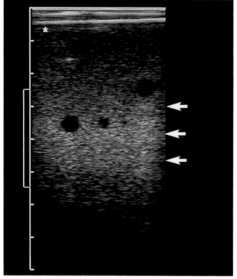

FIGURE 6-21 Focal banding *(arrows)* is the brightening of echoes around the focus, where intensity is increased by the narrowing of the beam.

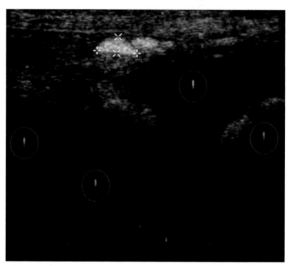

FIGURE 6-22 Interference *(circled random white specks)* from nearby electronic equipment seen below a small lymph node.

SPECTRAL DOPPLER

Aliasing

Aliasing is the most common artifact encountered in Doppler ultrasound. The word *alias* comes from Middle English *elles,* Latin *alius,* and Greek *allos,* which mean "other" or "otherwise." Contemporary meanings for the word include (as an adverb) "otherwise called" or "otherwise known as" and (as a noun) "an assumed or additional name." Aliasing in its technical use indicates improper representation of information that has been sampled insufficiently. The sampling can be spatial or temporal. Inadequate spatial sampling can result in

improper conclusions about the object or population sampled. For example, we could assemble 10 families, each consisting of a father, a mother, and a child, and line them up in that order—father, mother, child, father, mother, child—for all the families. If we wanted to sample the contents of these families by taking 10 photographs, we could choose to photograph one out of every three persons (e.g., the first, fourth, and seventh persons in the line). However, if we did this, we would conclude that all families are made up of three adult males, no women, and no children. In this example, spatial undersampling of one third of the population would result in an incorrect conclusion regarding the total population.

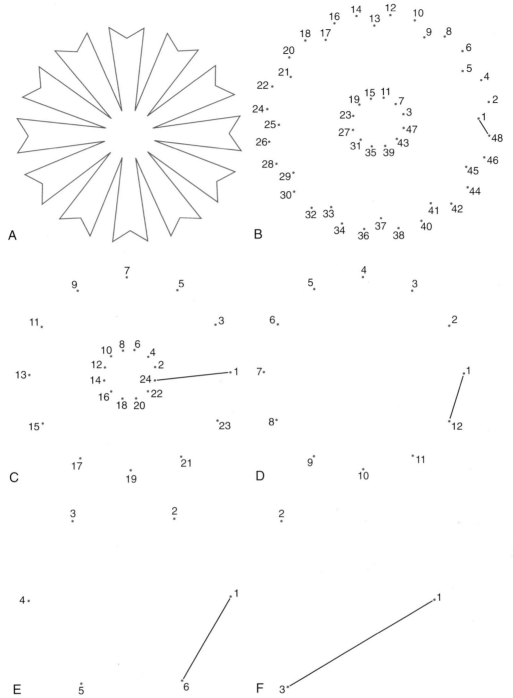

FIGURE 6-23 A, A "Doppler flower." **B,** Forty-eight samples. **C,** Twenty-four samples. **D,** Twelve samples. **E,** Six samples. **F,** Three samples. *(From Kremkau FW: Doppler artifacts, J Vasc Technol 14:41–42, 1990.)*

Another example of inadequate spatial sampling is shown in Figure 6-23. In *A* we see what we might call a "Doppler flower," containing 12 double-pointed petals. Each petal is made up of four lines. If we sample at the intersections of these lines, we get a 46-point dot-to-dot child's puzzle, as shown in Figure 6-23, *B*. Connecting the dots properly will yield the flower shown in Figure 6-23, *A*. In Figure 6-23, *C*, the even-numbered dots from Figure 6-23, *B* have been eliminated so that there are now 24 dots (samples). When these dots are connected,

a reasonable representation of the original flower results, but it is not as good as the representation in Figure 6-23, *B*. The higher-frequency information delineating the double pointing of the petals has been lost. In Figure 6-23, *D* the even-numbered dots from Figure 6-23, *C* have been eliminated. This representation of the flower, containing 12 samples, yields a 12-sided polygon that approximates a circle and is a poor representation of the original flower. The lower-frequency information about the 12 petals has been lost. In Figure 6-23, *E* and *F*, each eliminates half of the previous samples, yielding a hexagon and a triangle, respectively. Figure 16-23, *F* yields virtually no information regarding the round, double-pointed, 12-petaled flower.

In these examples, we see that inadequate spatial sampling yields an incorrect representation of the object sampled. This is similar to a disguise (false appearance or assumed identity) or alias. As the sampling was reduced, we first lost the double-pointed character of each petal, then the presence of the 12 petals, and finally the circular nature of the flower. In each case, we were experiencing spatial aliasing.

An optical form of temporal aliasing occurs in motion pictures when wagon wheels appear to rotate at various speeds and in reverse direction. Similar behavior is observed when a fan is lighted with a strobe light. Depending on the flashing rate of the strobe light, the fan may appear stationary or rotating clockwise or counterclockwise at various speeds.

Nyquist Limit

Pulsed wave Doppler instruments are sampling instruments. Each emitted pulse yields a sample of the desired Doppler shift. The upper limit to Doppler shift that can be detected properly by pulsed instruments is called the **Nyquist limit** (NL). If the Doppler-shift frequency exceeds one half the PRF (which is typically in the 5- to 30-kHz range for pulsed Doppler instruments), temporal aliasing occurs.

$$NL\,(kHz) = \frac{1}{2} \times PRF\,(kHz)$$

Improper Doppler shift information (improper direction and improper value) results. Higher PRFs (Table 6-1) permit higher Doppler shifts to be detected, but also increase the chance of the range-ambiguity artifact occurring. Continuous wave Doppler instruments do not experience aliasing. However, recall that neither do they provide depth localization (localized sample volume).

TABLE 6-1	Aliasing and Range-Ambiguity Artifact Values	
Pulse Repetition Frequency (kHz)	**Doppler Shift Above Which Aliasing Occurs (kHz)**	**Range Beyond Which Ambiguity Occurs (cm)**
5.0	2.5	15
7.5	3.7	10
10.0	5.0	7
12.5	6.2	6
15.0	7.5	5
17.5	8.7	4
20.0	10.0	3
25.0	12.5	3
30.0	15.0	2

 Aliasing is the appearance of Doppler spectral information on the wrong side of the baseline.

Figures 6-24 and 6-25 illustrate aliasing in the carotid artery and in the aorta of a normal subject. Also illustrated is how aliasing can be reduced or eliminated (Box 6-2) by increasing PRF, increasing Doppler angle (which decreases the Doppler shift for a given flow), or by shifting the baseline. The latter is an electronic cut-and-paste technique that moves the misplaced aliasing peaks over to their proper location. The technique is successful as long as there are no legitimate Doppler shifts in the region of the aliasing. If there are legitimate Doppler shifts, they will get moved over to an inappropriate location along with the aliasing peaks. Baseline shifting is not helpful if the desired information (e.g., peak systolic Doppler shift) is buried in another portion of the spectral display (see Figure 6-24, *G*). Other approaches to eliminating aliasing include changing to a lower-frequency (see Figure 6-25) or switching to continuous wave operation. The common and convenient solutions to aliasing are shifting the baseline, increasing PRF, or doing both in extreme cases.

 Aliasing is caused by undersampling of the Doppler shifts.

Aliasing occurs with a pulsed Doppler system because it is a sampling system; that is, a pulsed Doppler system acquires samples of the desired Doppler shift frequency from which it must be synthesized (see Figure 5-42). If samples are taken often enough, the correct result is achieved. Figure 6-26 shows temporal sampling of a signal. Sufficient sampling yields the correct result. Insufficient sampling yields an incorrect result.

The Nyquist limit, or Nyquist frequency, describes the minimum number of samples required to avoid aliasing. At least two samples per cycle of the desired Doppler shift must be made for the image to be obtained correctly. For a complicated signal, such as a Doppler signal containing many frequencies, the sampling rate must be such that at least two samples occur for each cycle of the highest frequency present. To restate this rule, if the highest Doppler-shift frequency present in a signal exceeds one half the PRF, aliasing will occur (Figure 6-27).

BOX 6-2	Methods of Reducing or Eliminating Aliasing

1. Shift the baseline.
2. Increase the pulse repetition frequency.
3. Increase the Doppler angle.
4. Use a lower operating frequency.
5. Use a continuous wave device.

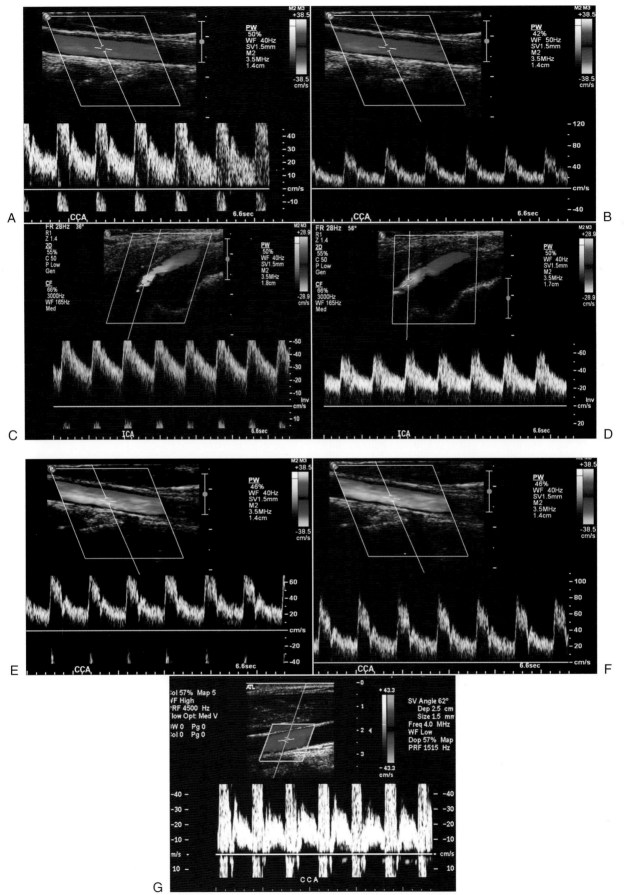

FIGURE 6-24 A, Aliasing in the common carotid artery (CCA). **B,** Pulse repetition frequency (PRF) is increased to eliminate the aliasing. **C,** Aliasing in the internal carotid artery at a 36° Doppler angle. **D,** When the Doppler angle is increased to 56° the aliasing is resolved. **E–F,** Baseline is shifted down to correct for aliasing in the CCA. **G,** An example where baseline shifting would not be helpful.

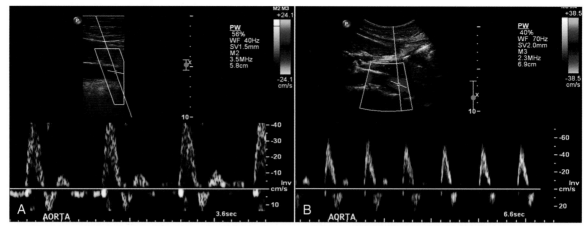

FIGURE 6-25 Aliasing in the aorta when imaged at 3.5 MHz **(A)** can be eliminated by imaging at a lower frequency of 2.3 MHz **(B)** in which the Doppler shifts are reduced to less than the Nyquist limit.

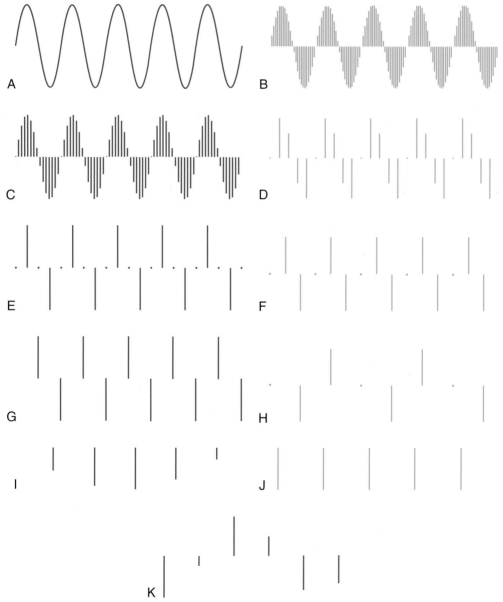

FIGURE 6-26 Decreasing sampling rate leads to aliasing. Sampling of a five-cycle voltage **(A)** is progressively decreased from 25 samples per cycle **(B)**, to 15 samples per cycle **(C)**, to 5 samples per cycle **(D)**, to 4 samples per cycle **(E)**, to 3 samples per cycle **(F)**, to 2 samples per cycle **(G)**, and finally to successive sampling of 1 sample per cycle **(H–K)**. In the last four cases, aliasing occurs.

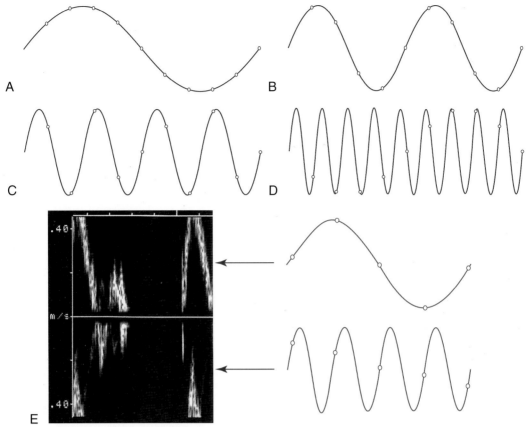

FIGURE 6-27 Increasing frequency leads to aliasing. Signal voltages are sampled at 10 points (o): **(A)** one cycle, **(B)** two cycles, **(C)** four cycles, and **(D)** nine cycles. As signal frequency is increased, aliasing occurs when the Nyquist limit is exceeded (in this case, beyond five cycles). Thus **D** is an example of aliasing. It can be seen that connecting the circles would yield a one-cycle representation of what is actually a nine-cycle signal voltage. **E,** In this spectral display the presentation above the baseline is correct (unaliased, five samples per cycle), whereas the systolic peaks appear incorrectly below the baseline (aliased, one sample per cycle).

 Aliasing is corrected by shifting the baseline, increasing the pulse repetition frequency, or both.

Two correction methods used less often are reduction of the operating frequency and switching to continuous wave mode. Operating frequency reduction reduces the Doppler shift. Continuous wave operation, because it is not pulsed, is not a sampling mode and is thus not subject to aliasing. However, it does not provide range discrimination.

Range Ambiguity

In attempting to solve the aliasing problem by increasing the PRF, one can encounter the range-ambiguity artifact, described previously. This artifact occurs when a pulse is emitted before all the echoes from the previous pulse have been received. When this happens, early echoes from the last pulse are received simultaneously with late echoes from the previous pulse. The system is unable to determine whether an echo is an early one (superficial) from the last pulse or a late one (deep) from the previous pulse (Figure 6-28). To deal with this problem, the instrument simply assumes that all echoes are derived

from the last pulse and that these echoes have originated from depths determined by the 13 µs/cm rule. As long as all echoes are received before the next pulse is sent out, this is true. However, with high PRFs, this may not be the case. Therefore Doppler flow information may come from locations other than the assumed one (the gate location). In effect, multiple gates or sample volumes are operating at different depths. Table 6-1 lists, for various PRFs, the ranges beyond which ambiguity occurs. Table 6-2 lists, for various depths, the maximum Doppler-shift frequency (Nyquist limit) that avoids aliasing and the range-ambiguity artifact. Maximum flow speeds that avoid aliasing for given angles also are listed. Instruments sometimes increase PRF (to avoid aliasing) into a range where range ambiguity occurs. Multiple sample gates are shown on the display to indicate this situation.

 High pulse repetition frequency causes Doppler range ambiguity. Multiple sample volumes appear as a result.

Mirror Image

The mirror-image artifact described previously can also occur with Doppler systems. This means that an image of a vessel and a source of Doppler-shifted echoes can

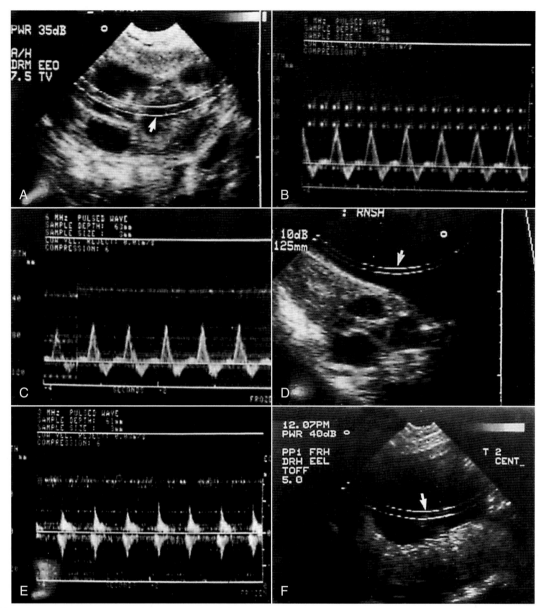

FIGURE 6-28 **Ambiguity is caused by sending out a pulse before all echoes from the previous pulse are received. A,** This transvaginal image shows the pulsed Doppler range gate *(arrow)* set at 33 mm within an ovary. **B,** The resulting Doppler spectrum shows a waveform typical of the external iliac artery. **C,** A signal identical to that shown in **B** was obtained when the range was increased to 63 mm, proving that the signal actually originated from the external iliac artery at this depth. **D,** A strong arterial Doppler signal was obtained when the range gate *(arrow)* was placed within the urinary bladder at a depth of 31 mm. **E,** A signal identical to that obtained in **D** was detected when the range gate depth was increased to 61 mm, indicating that the signal actually arose from an artery at this depth. **F,** The range gate *(arrow)* placed at a depth of 50 mm in the uterus of a pregnant woman (16 weeks' gestation).

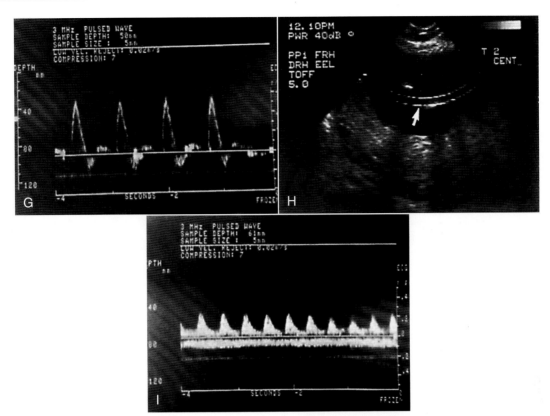

FIGURE 6-28, cont'd Range gate *(arrow)* from **F** produces signals typical of the external iliac artery **(G)**. **H,** In the same patient, a slight adjustment of the range gate *(arrow)* produced the desired umbilical artery signal **(I),** eliminating the artifactual iliac artery signal caused by range ambiguity. *(From Gill RW et al: New class of pulsed Doppler US ambiguity at short ranges, Radiology 173:272, 1989.)*

TABLE 6-2 | Aliasing and Range-Ambiguity Limits*

Maximum Flow Speed (cm/s) Depth (cm)	PRF (kHz)	Nyquist Limit (kHz)	0	30	60
1	77.0	38.5	593	685	1186
2	38.5	19.2	296	342	593
4	19.2	9.6	148	171	296
8	9.6	4.8	74	86	148
16	4.8	2.4	37	43	74

*For various depths the maximum pulse repetition frequency (PRF) that avoids range ambiguity and the corresponding maximum Doppler shift frequency (Nyquist limit) that avoids aliasing are listed. Maximum flow speeds corresponding to the maximum Doppler shift also are listed for three Doppler angles (0, 30, and 60 degrees), assuming a 5-MHz operating frequency.

be duplicated on the opposite side of a strong reflector. The duplicated vessel containing flow could be misinterpreted as an additional vessel that has a spectrum identical to that of the real vessel. Figure 6-29 shows an example of image and spectrum duplication of the subclavian artery. The strong reflector in this case is the air at the pleural boundary.

A **mirror image** of a Doppler spectrum can appear on the opposite side of the baseline when, indeed, flow is unidirectional and should appear only on one side of the baseline. This is an electronic duplication of the spectral information. The duplication can occur when Doppler gain is set too high (causing overloading in the amplifier and leakage, called **cross-talk**, of the signal from the

proper channel into the other channel; Figure 6-30). Duplication can also occur when the Doppler angle is near 90 degrees (Figure 6-31). In this situation the duplication is usually legitimate because beams are focused and not cylindrical. Thus while the beam axis is perpendicular to the flow direction, one edge of the beam is angled upstream and the other edge downstream.

 Spectral mirror image is the appearance of spectral information on both sides of the baseline. It occurs at high Doppler gains.

Doppler spectra have a speckle quality to them that is similar to that observed in gray-scale sonography,

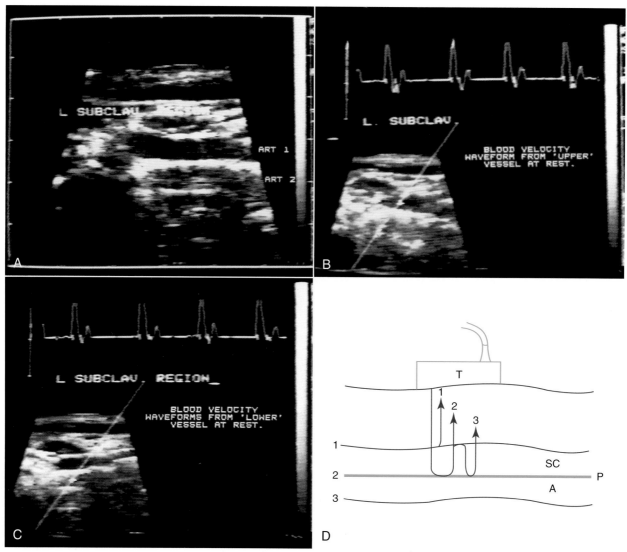

FIGURE 6-29 A, The subclavian artery *(ART 1)* and its mirror image *(ART 2).* **B,** Flow signal from artery. **C,** Flow signal from the mirror image of the artery. **D,** Multiple reflections produce a mirror image. Paths *1* and *2* are legitimate, but path 3 arrives late, producing the artifactual deep arterial wall. *T,* Transducer; *SC,* subclavian artery; *P,* pleura; *A,* artifactual artery; *(D from Kremkau FW: Principles and pitfalls of real-time color-flow imaging. In Bernstein EF, editor: Vascular diagnosis, ed 4, St Louis, 1993, Mosby.)*

discussed previously. Electromagnetic interference from nearby equipment can cloud the spectral display with lines or "snow" (Figure 6-32).

COLOR DOPPLER

Artifacts observed with color Doppler imaging are two-dimensional color presentations of artifacts that are seen in gray-scale sonography or Doppler spectral displays. They are incorrect presentations of two-dimensional motion information, the most common of which is aliasing. However, others occur, including anatomic mirror image, Doppler angle-effects, shadowing, and clutter.

Aliasing

Aliasing occurs when the Doppler shift exceeds the Nyquist limit (Figure 6-33), which happens more often

in color Doppler than in spectral Doppler due to the reduced PRFs employed in the former relative to the latter. The result is incorrect flow direction being displayed on the color Doppler image (Figure 6-34). Increasing the flow speed range (which is actually an increase in PRF) can solve the problem (Figures 6-34, *E–F* and 6-35). However, too high a range can cause loss of flow information, particularly if the wall filter is set high. This artifact can also be eliminated (or at least reduced) by angling the color-box (Figure 6-34, *C–D*). Baseline shifting can decrease or eliminate the effect of aliasing (Figure 6-34, *G–H*), as in spectral displays.

 Aliasing in color Doppler imaging appears as an incorrect color from the opposite side of the baseline on the color map.

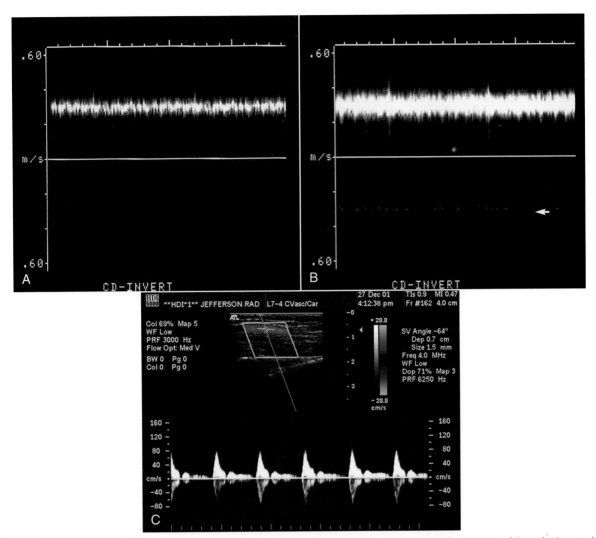

FIGURE 6-30 A, Spectrum produced by a string moving at 30 cm/s. **B,** An increase in gain produces spectral broadening and a mirror image *(arrow)*. **C,** High gain produces a mirror image of the carotid artery spectrum below the baseline.

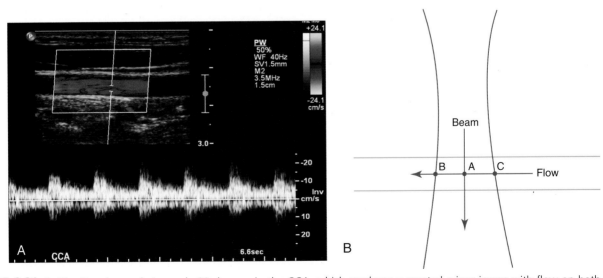

FIGURE 6-31 A, The Doppler angle is nearly 90 degrees in the CCA, which produces a spectral mirror image with flow on both sides of the baseline. **B,** Because beams are focused and not cylindrical, portions of the beam **(C)** can experience flow toward the transducer, whereas other portions **(B)** can experience flow away when the beam axis intersects **(A)** the flow at 90 degrees.

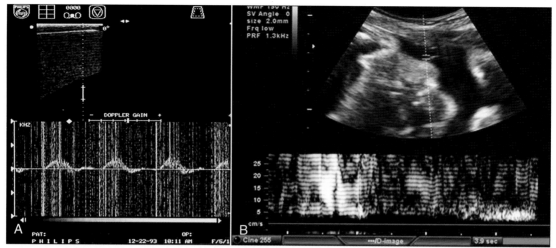

FIGURE 6-32 A, Interference from nearby electrical equipment clouds the spectral display with electric noise (the vertical "snow" lines). **B,** External interference produces bands of frequency that are fairly constant with time.

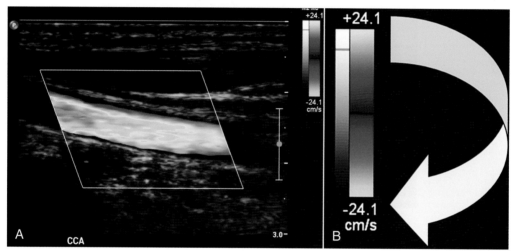

FIGURE 6-33 A, Negative *(blue)* Doppler shifts are shown in the arterial flow in this image. These are actually positive Doppler shifts that have exceeded the higher Nyquist limit (converted here to the equivalent flow speed: +24.1 cm/s) and are wrapped around to the negative portion of the color bar **(B).** (Likewise, negative shifts that exceed the -24.1 cm/s limit would alias to the positive side).

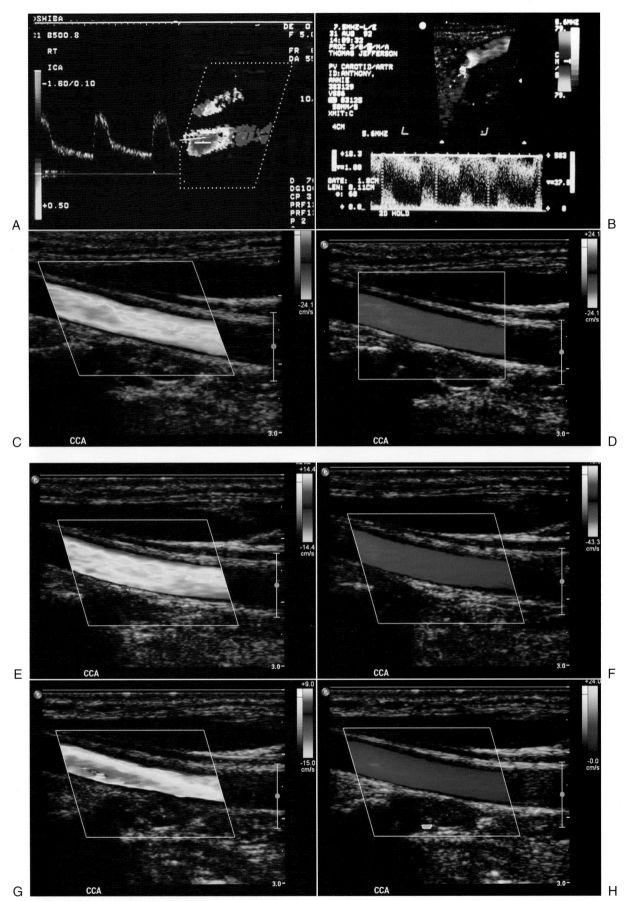

FIGURE 6-34 A, A color Doppler image with aliasing. The blue colors demonstrate aliasing, whereas the higher PRF associated with the spectral Doppler ensures that the spectral display is not aliased. **B,** An example in which both the color and spectral displays of the carotid are aliasing. **C,** Aliasing in the CCA with a color box angled incorrectly. **D,** Adjusting the angle of the color box eliminates the aliasing. **E–F,** Increasing the color PRF from 14.4 cm/s to 43.3 cm/s resolves the aliasing. **G–H,** The same result can be achieved by changing the baseline from covering -15 to 9.0 cm/s to covering the 0–24 cm/s range.

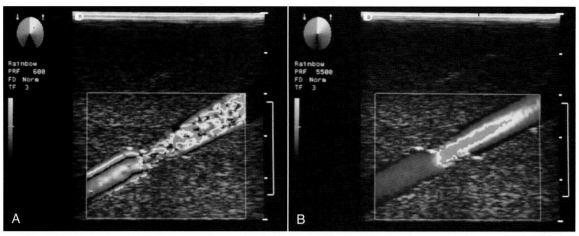

FIGURE 6-35 A, Flow in this phantom with an 80% stenosis is toward the upper right, producing positive Doppler shifts. The pulse repetition frequency (600 Hz) and Nyquist limit (300 Hz) are too low, resulting in aliasing (negative Doppler shifts) at the edge of the vessel as well as at the center of the flow in the vessel (positive Doppler shifts). **B,** With the pulse repetition frequency increased to 5500 Hz, the aliasing has been eliminated except for right in the stenosis, where the aliasing outlines the stenotic jet.

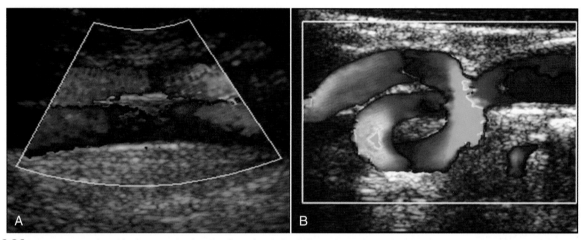

FIGURE 6-36. A, Two vessels with the anterior having flow from the left to the right and vice versa in the posterior vessel. Thus the flow in the anterior vessel is upstream from the transducer in the left half of the image (thus coded *red*) and down stream in the right half of the image (color coded *blue*). The posterior vessel has flow in the opposite direction and, hence, is color coded blue followed by red. **B,** The same effect can be observed in a tortuous carotid artery.

A related artifact is the **multiple angle artifact** - the Doppler angle in color Doppler displays is assumed (unrealistically) to be zero. Hence the color overlay is coded relative to the location of the transducer, which can lead to somewhat confusing displays (Figure 6-36).

Mirror Image, Shadowing, Refraction, Clutter, and Noise

In the mirror (or ghost) artifact (Figure 6-37), an image of a vessel and source of Doppler-shifted echoes can be duplicated on the opposite side of a strong reflector (e.g., pleura or diaphragm). This is a color Doppler extension of the gray-scale artifact of Figure 6-29. Shadowing is the weakening or elimination of Doppler-shifted echoes

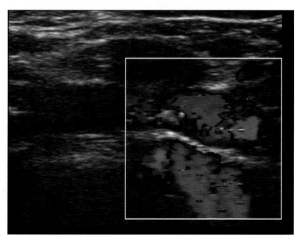

FIGURE 6-37 Longitudinal color doppler image of the subclavian vein. The pleura causes the mirror image. The diagram in Figure 6-29, *D* shows how this artifact occurs.

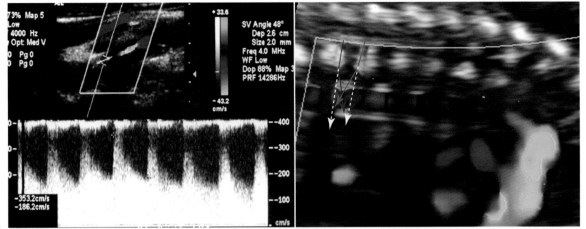

FIGURE 6-38 A, Shadowing from calcified plaque follows the gray-scale scan lines straight down. Notice how the color aliases. **B,** Refraction from ribs produces alternating positive and negative Doppler-shift regions in this fetal aorta. Positive Doppler shift is red. Flow is from right to left. The red sound path is refracted to an upstream view and presented red on the dashed scan line. The blue path is refracted to a downstream view and presented blue on its dashed scan line.

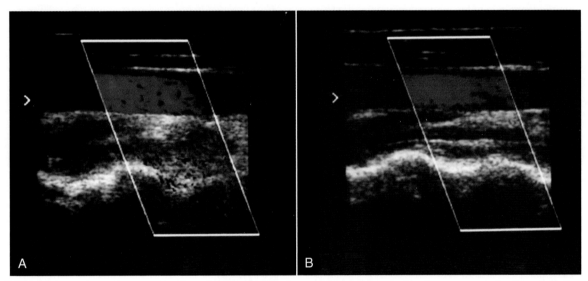

FIGURE 6-39 A, Clutter from tissue motion (i.e., flash artifact) in the neck (caused by speaking) appears as color Doppler below the CCA. **B,** When the speaking stops the clutter is gone, revealing the underlying tissue.

beyond a shadowing object, just as occurs with non–Doppler-shifted (gray-scale) echoes (Figure 6-38, *A*). Refraction can confuse the interpretation of color-Doppler presentations (Figure 6-38, *B*). Clutter, also known as the **flash artifact,** results from tissue, heart wall or valve, or vessel wall motion (Figure 6-39). Such clutter is eliminated by wall filters. Doppler angle effects include zero Doppler shift when the Doppler angle is 90 degrees (see Figure 5-28, *F*), as well as the change of color in a straight vessel viewed with a sector transducer (see Figure 5-28, *A*). Noise in the color Doppler electronics can mimic flow, particularly in **hypoechoic** or anechoic regions with gain settings too high (Figure 6-40).

This chapter has discussed several ultrasound imaging and flow artifacts, all of which are listed in Table 6-3, along with their causes. In some cases the names of the artifacts are identical to their causes. Shadowing and enhancement are useful in interpretation and diagnosis. Other artifacts can cause confusion and error. Artifacts seen in two-dimensional imaging are evidenced in three-dimensional imaging also, sometimes in unusual ways.[5] All of these artifacts can hinder proper interpretation and diagnosis and so must be avoided or handled properly when encountered. A proper understanding of artifacts and how to deal with them when they are encountered enables sonographers and sonologists to use them to advantage while avoiding the pitfalls that they can cause.

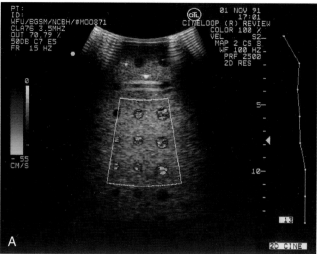

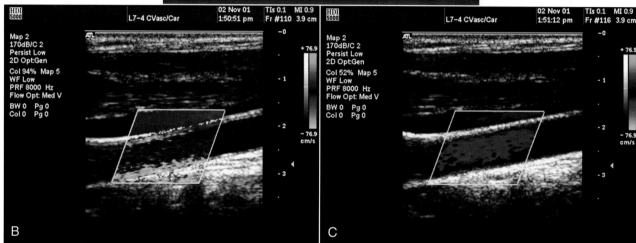

FIGURE 6-40 A, Color appears in echo-free (cystic) regions of a tissue-equivalent phantom. The color gain has been increased sufficiently to produce this effect. The instrument tends to write color noise preferentially in areas where non–Doppler-shifted echoes are weak or absent. **B–C,** a tissue can also be overwritten when the color gain is too high and reducing it (here from 94% to 52%) eliminates the artifact. (**A** *From Kremkau FW: Principles and pitfalls of real-time color-flow imaging. In Bernstein EF, editor: Vascular diagnosis, ed 4, St Louis, 1993, Mosby.*)

TABLE 6-3	Artifacts and Their Causes
Artifact	**Cause**
Axial resolution	Pulse length
Comet tail	Reverberation
Grating lobe	Grating lobe
Lateral resolution	Pulse width
Mirror image	Multiple reflection
Refraction	Refraction
Reverberation	Multiple reflection
Slice thickness	Pulse width
Speckle	Interference
Speed error	Speed error
Range ambiguity	Finite speed of sound in tissue
Shadowing	High attenuation
Edge shadowing	Refraction or interference
Enhancement	Low attenuation
Focal enhancement	Focusing
Aliasing	Exceeding the Nyquist Limit
Spectrum mirror	High Doppler gain

REVIEW

- The beam width perpendicular to the scan plane causes slice thickness artifacts.
- Apparent image details are not related directly to tissue texture but are a result of interference effects from a distribution of scatterers in the tissue (speckle).
- Reverberation produces a set of equally spaced artifactual echoes distal to the real reflector.
- In the mirror-image artifact, objects that are present on one side of a strong reflector are displayed on the other side as well.
- Refraction displaces echoes laterally.
- Propagation speed error and refraction can cause objects to be displayed in improper locations or incorrect sizes or both.
- Shadowing is caused by high-attenuation objects in the sound path.

- Refraction also can cause edge shadowing.
- Enhancement results from low-attenuation objects in the sound path.
- Aliasing occurs when the Doppler shift frequency exceeds one half the PRF.
- Aliasing can be reduced or eliminated by using baseline shift, increasing the PRF or Doppler angle, reducing operating frequency, or using continuous-wave operation.

EXERCISES

1. The pulser of an instrument automatically reduces the pulse repetition frequency for deeper imaging to avoid the _____ _____ artifact.

2. If an echo arrives 143 µs after the pulse that produced it was emitted, it should be located at a depth of _____ cm. If a second pulse was emitted 13 µs before the arrival of this echo, it will be placed incorrectly at a depth of _____ cm.

3. If the propagation speed in a soft tissue path is 1.60 mm/µs, a diagnostic instrument assumes a propagation speed too _____ and will show reflectors too _____ the transducer.
   a. High, close to
   b. High, far from
   c. Low, close to
   d. Low, far from

4. Mirror image can occur with only one reflector. True or false?

5. The most common artifact encountered in Doppler ultrasound is
   a. aliasing.
   b. range ambiguity.
   c. spectrum mirror image.
   d. location mirror image.
   e. electromagnetic interference.

6. Which of the following can reduce or eliminate aliasing?
   a. Increased pulse repetition frequency
   b. Increased Doppler angle
   c. Increased operating frequency
   d. Use of continuous wave mode
   e. More than one of the above

7. The fine texture in soft tissue indicates the excellent resolution that actually exists there. True or false?

8. The fact that a beam, as it scans through tissue, has some nonzero width perpendicular to the scan plane results in the _____ _____ artifact.

9. Which of the following can cause improper location of objects on a display? (more than one correct answer)
   a. Shadowing
   b. Enhancement
   c. Speed error
   d. Mirror image
   e. Refraction
   f. Grating lobe

10. Refraction can cause shadowing. True or false?

11. The transducer face is one of the reflectors involved in reverberations in which illustration, Figure 6-41, *A* or *B*?

12. Match these artifact causes with their result:
    a. Reverberation:
    b. Shadowing:
    c. Enhancement:
    d. Propagation speed error:
    e. Refraction:

    1. Unreal structure displayed
    2. Structure missing on the display
    3. Structure displayed with improper brightness
    4. Structure improperly positioned
    5. Structure improperly shaped

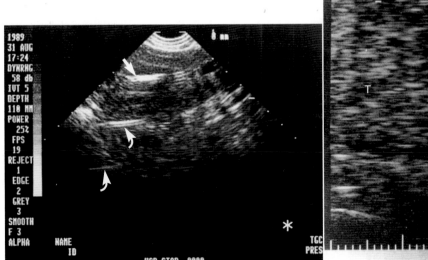
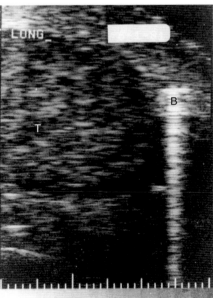

FIGURE 6-41 A–B, Illustrations to accompany Exercise 11.

13. Reverberation results in added reflectors being imaged with equal _____.
14. In reverberation, subsequent reflections are _____ than previous ones.
15. Enhancement is caused by a
    a. strongly reflecting structure.
    b. weakly attenuating structure.
    c. strongly attenuating structure.
    d. refracting boundary.
    e. propagation speed error.
16. Which of the following can decrease or eliminate aliasing?
    a. Decreased pulse repetition frequency
    b. Decreased Doppler angle
    c. Increased operating frequency
    d. Baseline shifting
    e. More than one of the above
17. Shadowing results in decreased echo amplitudes. True or false?
18. Propagation speed error results in improper _____ position of a reflector on the display.
    a. Lateral
    b. Axial
19. To avoid aliasing, a signal voltage must be sampled at least _____ time(s) per cycle.
    a. 1
    b. 2
    c. 3
    d. 4
    e. 5
20. If the highest Doppler-shift frequency present in a signal exceeds _____ the pulse repetition frequency, aliasing will occur.
    a. One tenth
    b. One half
    c. 2 times
    d. 5 times
    e. 10 times
21. When Doppler gain is set too high, which artifact is likely to occur?
    a. Aliasing
    b. Range ambiguity
    c. Spectrum mirror image
    d. Location mirror image
    e. Speckle
22. Which artifact should be suspected if one observes twin gestational sacs when scanning through the rectus abdominis muscle?
23. Range ambiguity can occur in which of the following?
    a. Imaging instruments
    b. Duplex instruments
    c. Pulsed wave Doppler instruments
    d. Color flow instruments
    e. All of the above

24. If the pulse repetition frequency is 4 kHz, which of the following Doppler shifts will cause aliasing?
    a. 1 kHz
    b. 2 kHz
    c. 3 kHz
    d. 4 kHz
    e. More than one of the above
25. If the pulse repetition frequency is 10 kHz, which of the following Doppler shifts will cause aliasing?
    a. 1 kHz
    b. 2 kHz
    c. 3 kHz
    d. 4 kHz
    e. None of the above
26. There is no problem with aliasing as long as the Doppler shifts are _____ half the pulse repetition frequency.
    a. Less than
    b. Approximately equal to
    c. Greater than
    d. All of the above
    e. None of the above
27. If Doppler shift is 2.6 kHz, no aliasing would result with a pulse repetition frequency of 10 kHz. True or false?
28. If there were a problem in Exercise 27, _____ Doppler ultrasound could be used to avoid it.
29. If red represents a positive Doppler shift and blue represents a negative one, what color is seen for normal flow toward the transducer? What color is seen for aliasing flow toward the transducer? What colors are seen for normal flow away and for aliasing flow away from the transducer?
30. When a pulse is emitted before all the echoes from the previous pulse have been received, which artifact occurs?
31. When a strong reflector is located in the scan plane, which of the following artifacts is likely to occur?
    a. Aliasing
    b. Range ambiguity
    c. Spectrum mirror image
    d. Location mirror image
    e. Speckle
32. Increasing pulse repetition frequency to avoid aliasing can cause the following:
    a. Baseline shift
    b. Range ambiguity
    c. Spectrum mirror image
    d. Location mirror image
    e. Speckle
33. Which of the following decreases the likelihood of range-ambiguity artifact?
    a. Decreasing operating frequency
    b. Decreasing pulse repetition frequency
    c. Decreasing Doppler angle
    d. Baseline shift
    e. Increasing pulser output

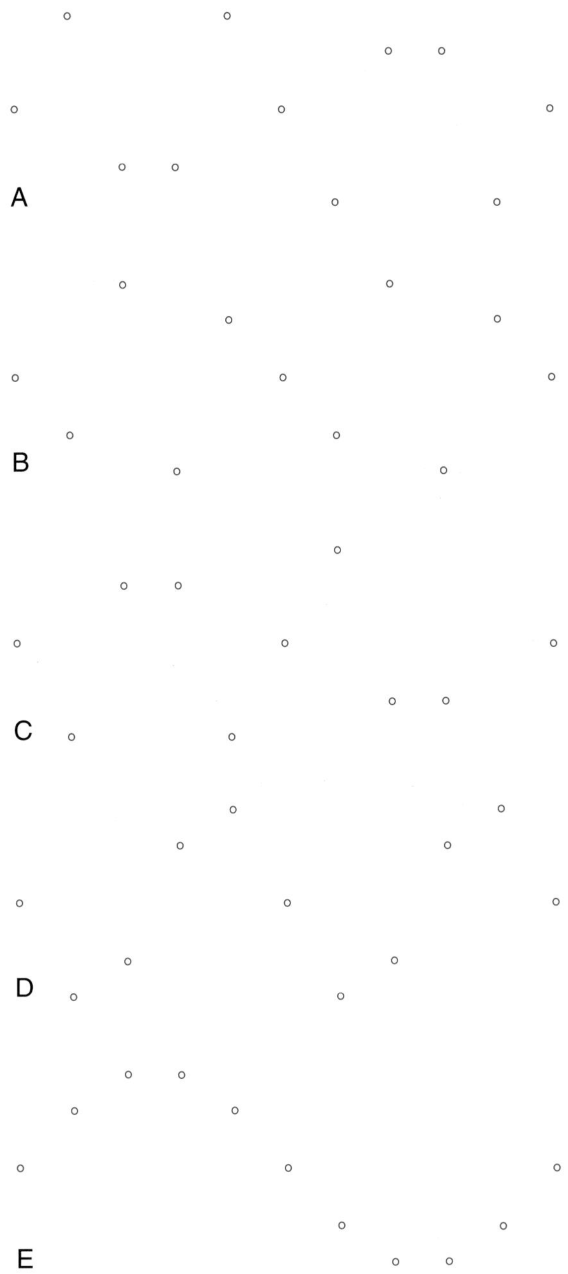

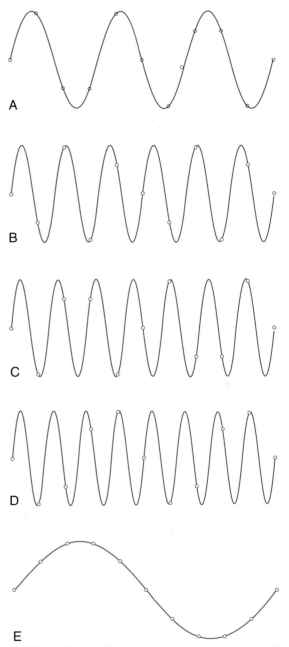

A

B

C

D

E

FIGURE 6-42 **A–E,** Illustrations to accompany Exercise 42.

A

B

C

D

E

FIGURE 6-43 **A–E,** Illustrations to accompany Exercise 43.

34. Range ambiguity produces which error in spectral Doppler studies?
a. Incorrect spectral peaks
b. Incorrect gate location
c. Intensity too high
d. Intensity too low
e. All of the above

35. Range ambiguity produces which error in anatomic imaging?
a. Range too long
b. Range too short
c. Intensity too high
d. Doppler shift too high
e. Doppler shift too low

36. If a pulse is emitted 65 μs after the previous one, echoes returning from beyond _____ cm will produce range ambiguity.
a. 1   d. 4
b. 2   e. 5
c. 3

37. If the maximum imaging depth is 5 cm, the frequency is 2 MHz, and the Doppler angle is zero, what is the maximum flow speed that will avoid aliasing and range ambiguity?
a. 100 cm/s
b. 200 cm/s
c. 300 cm/s
d. 400 cm/s
e. 500 cm/s

38. Does solving aliasing by decreasing operating frequency increase the possibility of range-ambiguity artifact?

39. If operating frequency is increased to decrease the possibility of range ambiguity (by increasing attenuation), does the possibility of aliasing increase?

40. If a pulsed wave Doppler sample volume is located at a depth of 8 cm, the sampled echoes arrive at what time following the emission of the pulse?
   a. 25 µs   d. 104 µs
   b. 50 µs   e. 117 µs
   c. 75 µs

41. In Exercise 40, if the pulse repetition frequency is set at 11 kHz, a second gate would be located at what depth?
   a. 1 cm   d. 4 cm
   b. 2 cm   e. 5 cm
   c. 3 cm

42. Connect the dots (samples) in Figure 6-42 to determine the Doppler shift frequency. How many cycles are in each example?
   a. _____
   b. _____   d. _____
   c. _____   e. _____

43. The frequencies that were sampled in Exercise 42 are shown in Figure 6-43. In which example(s) has aliasing occurred?

44. Which of the following instruments can produce aliasing?
   a. Continuous wave Doppler
   b. Pulsed wave Doppler
   c. Duplex
   d. Color flow
   e. More than one of the above

45. In Figure 6-44 the solid line shows the Doppler shift and the dots are the samples. The dashed line shows the _____ result. To avoid aliasing in this signal, at least _____ samples would be required.

46. In Figure 6-45 (R, red; B, blue), assume the color bar shown in G and give the direction of blood flow (R for from right to the left; L for from left to the right) in each case.

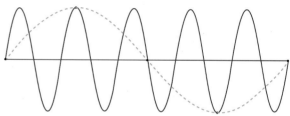

FIGURE 6-44 Illustration to accompany Exercise 45.

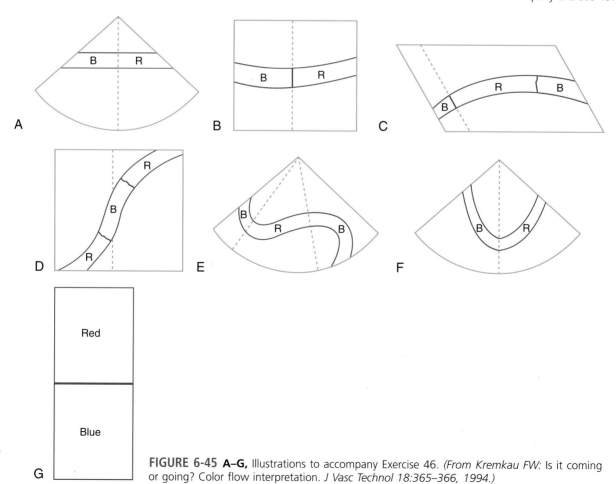

FIGURE 6-45 A–G, Illustrations to accompany Exercise 46. *(From Kremkau FW: Is it coming or going? Color flow interpretation. J Vasc Technol 18:365–366, 1994.)*

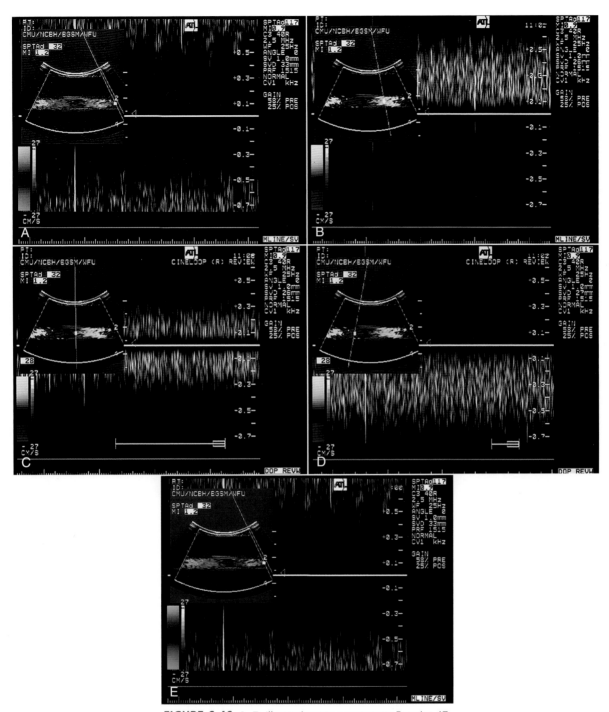

FIGURE 6-46 A–E, Illustrations to accompany Exercise 47.

47. Figure 6-46 shows five regions of different colors in the flow. Match each of the following with the proper region.

a. _____   1. 90-degree Doppler angle
b. _____   2. Unaliased flow toward
c. _____   3. Unaliased flow away
d. _____   4. Aliased flow toward
e. _____   5. Aliased flow away

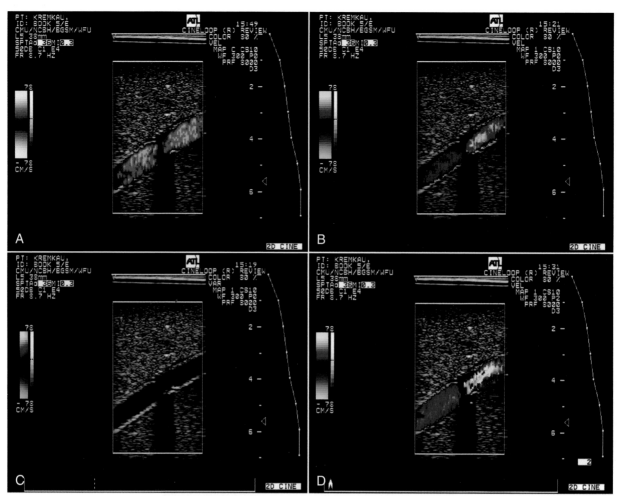

FIGURE 6-47 **A–D,** Illustrations to accompany Exercises 48 to 50.

48. Which part of Figure 6-47 shows a Doppler-power display?

49. Referring to Figure 6-47, B, C, and D, what is the order of figure parts when they are arranged according to increasing flow speed?

50. What artifact appears in all parts of Figure 6-47? What is the additional artifact that appears in Figure 6-47, D?

Performance and Safety

Several devices (Figure 7-1) are available for determining whether sonographic and Doppler ultrasound instruments are operating correctly and consistently. These devices can be divided into two groups:

1. *Those that measure the acoustic output of the instrument:* This group considers only the beam former and the transducer acting together as a source of ultrasound.
2. *Those that test the operation of the instrument (anatomic imaging and flow evaluation performance):* This group takes into account the operation of the entire instrument. Imaging and Doppler performance are important for evaluating the instrument as a diagnostic tool. The acoustic output of an instrument is important when considering bioeffects and safety.

Bioeffects are useful in the therapeutic applications of ultrasound, a subject not considered in this book.[6] Of interest here is what the known bioeffects of ultrasound indicate about the safety or risk of diagnostic ultrasound. We desire knowledge about the probability of damage or injury and under what conditions this probability is maximized (to avoid those conditions) or minimized (to seek those conditions while obtaining useful diagnostic information).

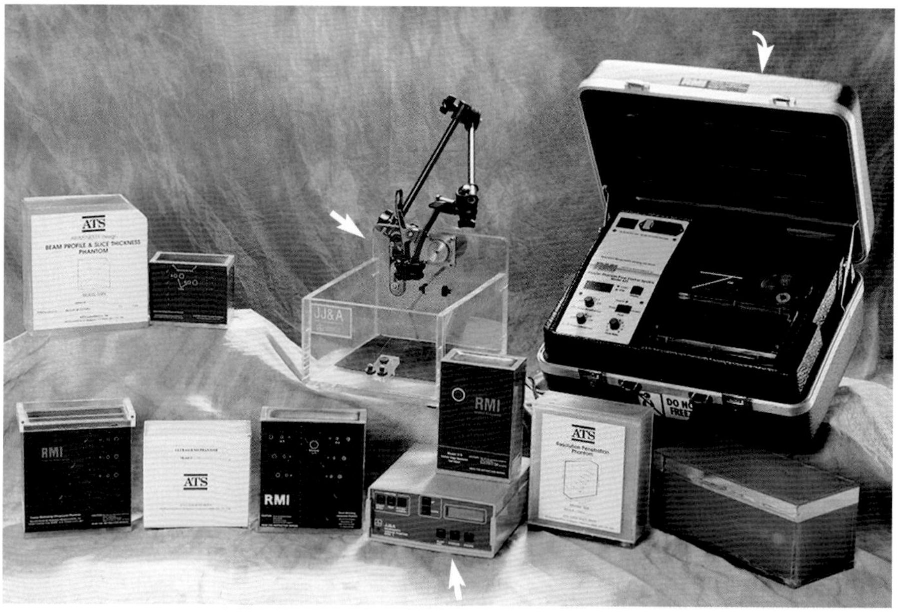

FIGURE 7-1 Several test objects and phantoms. Those intended for Doppler applications are indicated by arrows. The other devices are used to evaluate sonographic instruments.

PERFORMANCE MEASUREMENTS

Imaging performance is determined by measuring primarily the following parameters:

- Detail resolution
- Contrast resolution
- Penetration and dynamic range
- Time gain compensation operation
- Accuracy of depth and distance measurement

Several devices are commercially available for testing imaging performance. These devices fall into two categories: (1) tissue-equivalent **phantoms** and (2) **test objects**. Tissue-equivalent phantoms have some characteristics representative of tissues (such as scattering and attenuation properties); test objects do not. Some devices are combinations of the two (e.g., tissue-equivalent phantoms containing resolution targets). Phantoms and test objects can be used not only by service personnel but also by instrument operators. The American College of Radiology Ultrasound Accreditation Program requires that routine quality control testing occur regularly; the minimum requirement is semiannual testing. The American Institute of Ultrasound in Medicine (AIUM; www.aium.org) Practice Accreditation program requires that equipment maintenance and calibration be regularly performed on all ultrasound equipment.

Gray-Scale Test Objects and Tissue-Equivalent Phantoms

Tissue-equivalent phantoms are made of graphite-filled aqueous gels or urethane rubber materials. Graphite particles act as ultrasound scatterers (echo producers) in materials. Graphite is the soft carbon that is used in pencils and as a lubricant. Attenuation in these materials

is similar to that for soft tissue, and propagation speed is 1.54 mm/μs in gels and 1.45 mm/μs in rubber. Compensation for the latter speed error is accomplished by positioning targets in the rubber material to closer locations. However, errors can still occur because of speed error. Tissue-equivalent phantoms typically contain echo-free (cystic) regions of various diameters and thin nylon lines (about 0.2 mm in diameter) for measuring detail resolution and distance accuracy. Some phantoms contain cones or cylinders containing material of various scattering strengths (various graphite concentrations) that are hyperechoic or hypoechoic compared with the surrounding material. Figures 7-2 to 7-8 give examples of several phantoms.

 Tissue-equivalent phantoms simulate tissue properties, allowing assessment of detail and contrast resolutions, penetration, dynamic range, and time gain compensation operation.

Test objects do not simulate tissue characteristics but do provide some specific measure of instrument performance. The beam-profile slice-thickness test object (Figure 7-9) contains a thin, scattering layer in an echo-free material. The object can be used to show beam width in the scan plane or perpendicular to it (section thickness).

Test objects contain nylon lines and scattering layers to allow evaluation of detail resolution and beam profiles.

Text continued on p. 218

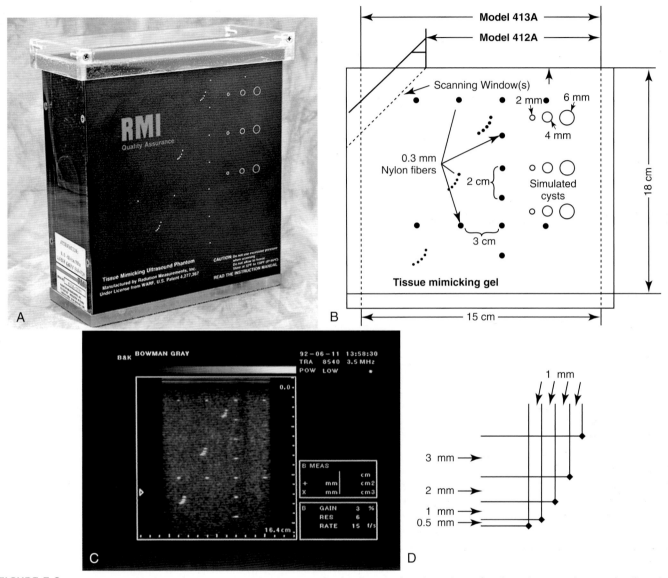

FIGURE 7-2 A, A tissue-equivalent phantom containing groups of nylon lines and cystic regions of various sizes. **B,** Diagram detailing the construction of such a phantom. **C,** Scan of a phantom. **D,** Arrangement of the axial resolution line set in this phantom and in that pictured in Figure 7-3. This set was used in Figure 3-29, *D–F,* to illustrate axial resolution at three frequencies.

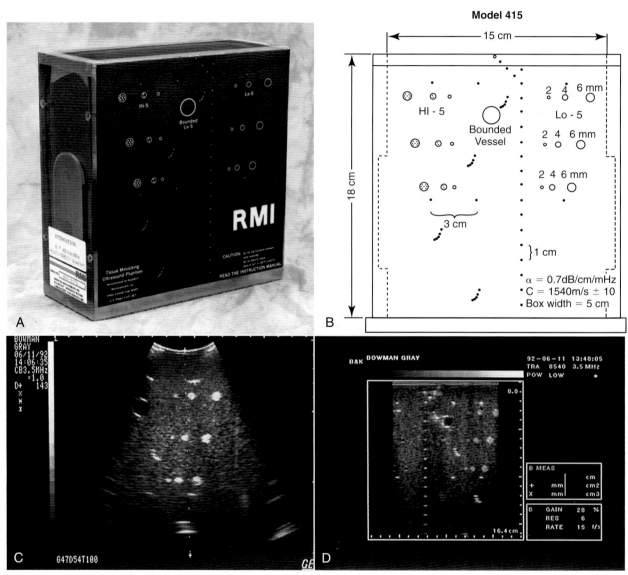

FIGURE 7-3 A, A tissue-equivalent phantom containing nylon lines, simulated cysts, a cystic region with an echogenic rim (simulated bounded vessel), and hyperechoic simulated lesions of various sizes. **B,** Diagram detailing the construction of such a phantom. **C–D,** Scans of phantom.

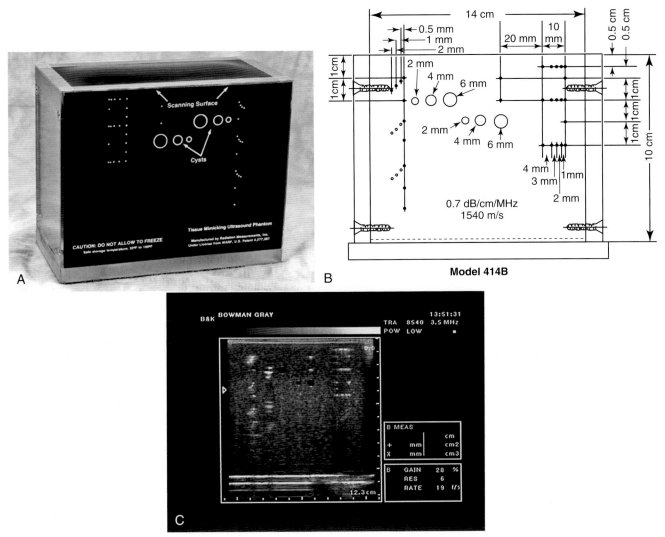

FIGURE 7-4 A, A smaller phantom designed for higher-frequency "small parts" applications. **B,** Diagram detailing the construction of such a phantom. **C,** Scan of phantom.

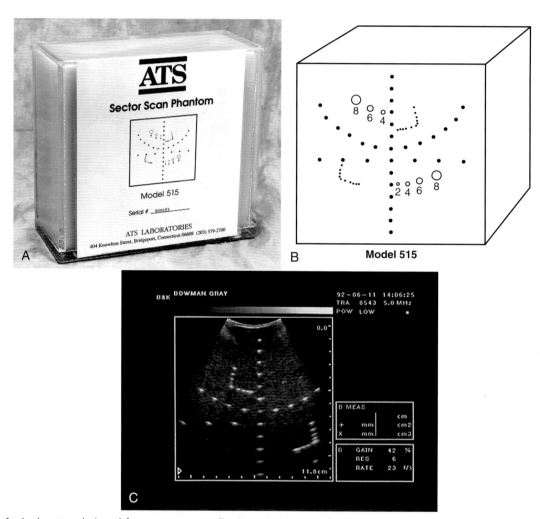

FIGURE 7-5 A, A phantom designed for sector scan applications. **B,** Diagram detailing the construction of such a phantom. **C,** Scan of phantom.

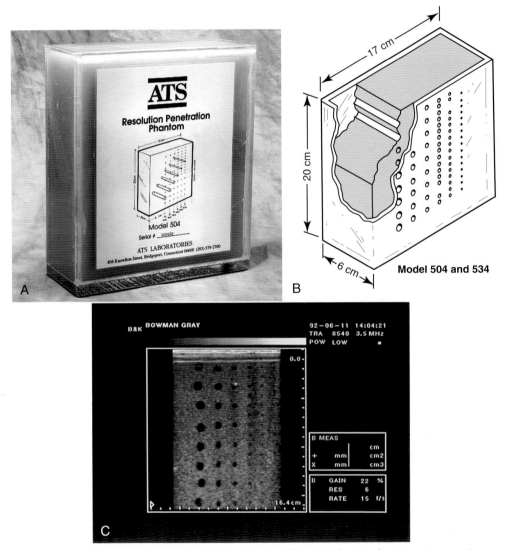

FIGURE 7-6 A, A resolution penetration phantom that contains columns of simulated cysts of various sizes. **B,** Diagram detailing the construction of such a phantom. **C,** Scan of phantom. This phantom was used to illustrate resolution and penetration at two frequencies in Figure 3-34.

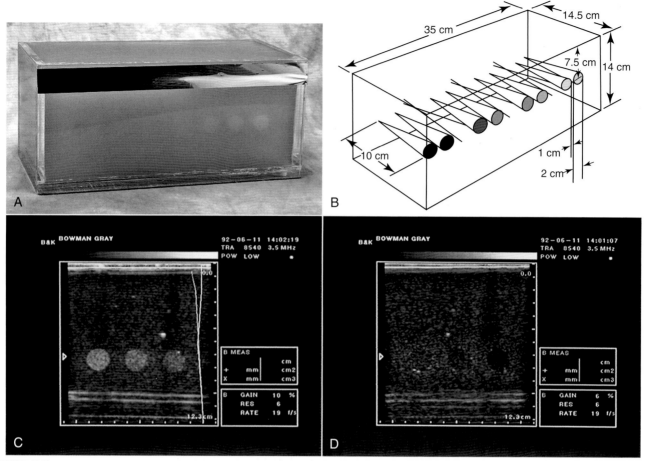

FIGURE 7-7 A, A contrast-detail phantom containing cones of material of various echogenicities. **B,** Diagram detailing the construction of such a phantom. **C,** Scan of hyperechoic sections of phantom. **D,** Scan of hypoechoic sections of phantom.

Doppler Test Objects and Tissue-Equivalent Phantoms

Test objects and tissue- and blood-mimicking phantoms are commercially available for the evaluation of Doppler instruments (Figures 7-10 and 7-11). These objects are useful for testing the effective penetration of the Doppler beam, the ability to discriminate between different flow directions, the accuracy of sample volume location, and the accuracy of the measured flow speed. Doppler flow phantoms use a flowing blood-mimicking liquid. Doppler test objects use a moving solid object (usually a string) for scattering the ultrasound. They can be calibrated and can produce pulsatile and reverse motions.

Doppler phantoms have some disadvantages, such as the presence of bubbles and nonuniform flow, but can simulate clinical conditions, such as tissue attenuation (see Figure 7-11). These phantoms are calibrated with an electromagnetic flow meter or by fluid volume collection over time. Refer back to Figure 5-40, *B–C*, which illustrates the use of a string test object in the evaluation of Doppler angle correction; Figure 6-30, *A–B*, which shows the use of a string test object in evaluating spectral mirror image; Figure 5-43, which illustrates the use of a flow phantom in determining the accuracy of the gate

location indicator on the anatomic display; and Figure 5-29, which shows the use of a flow phantom to illustrate the effect of Doppler angle on Doppler shift.

 Doppler test objects and flow phantoms enable evaluation of spectral calibration and gate location and penetration of spectral and color Doppler instruments.

OUTPUT MEASUREMENTS

Several devices can measure the acoustic output of ultrasound instruments.[7] These devices are normally used by engineers and physicists rather than by instrument operators. Only the **hydrophone** is discussed here. The hydrophone sometimes is called a *microprobe*. It is used in two forms (Figures 7-12 and 7-13):

1. A small transducer element (with a diameter of 1 mm or less) mounted on the end of a hollow needle
2. A large piezoelectric membrane with small metallic electrodes centered on both sides

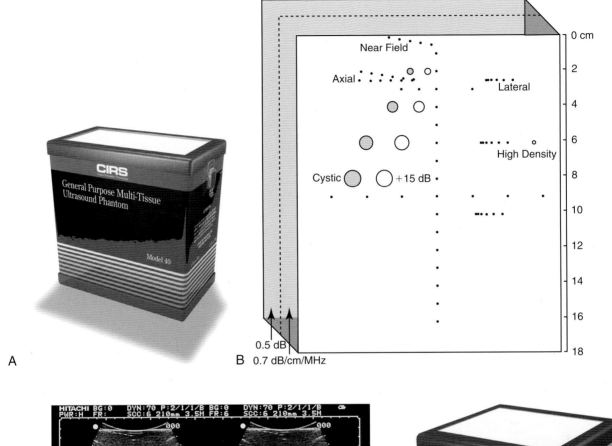

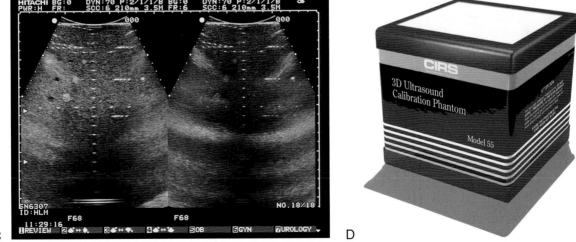

FIGURE 7-8 A, General purpose phantom with two background tissue materials (0.5 and 0.7 dB/cm-MHz). **B,** Construction diagram for the phantom in **A. C,** Image scanned with phantom in **A. D,** Three-dimensional calibration phantom for the assessment of volumetric measurement accuracy.   *Continued*

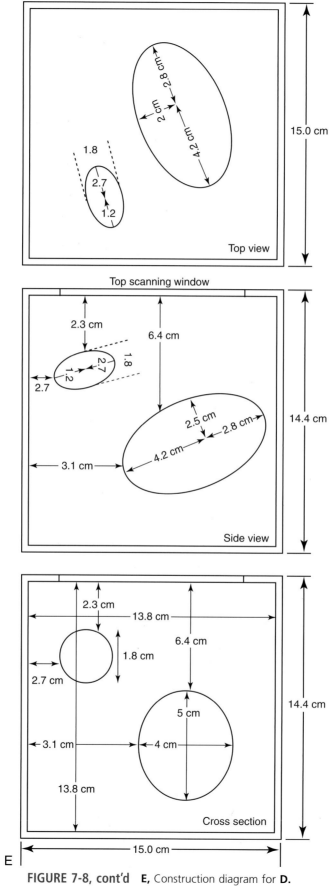

FIGURE 7-8, cont'd   E, Construction diagram for **D.**

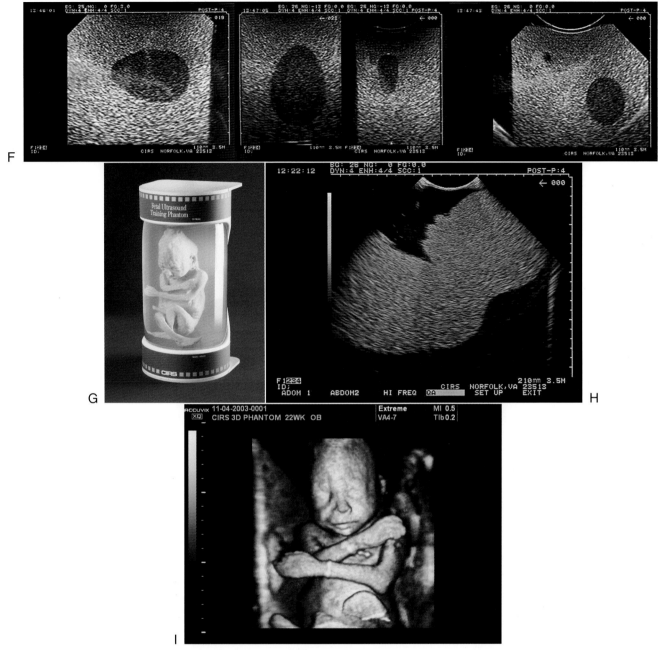

FIGURE 7-8, cont'd **F,** Images obtained by scanning **D. G,** Fetal-training phantom. **H,** Two-dimensional image from **G. I,** Three-dimensional image from **G.**

The membrane is made of **polyvinylidene fluoride** (PVDF). PVDF is used in both types of hydrophones because of its wide bandwidth. Various construction approaches are used for hydrophones, but these are not considered here. Hydrophones receive sound reasonably well from all directions without altering the sound by their presence. In response to the varying pressure of the sound, they produce a varying voltage that can be displayed on an oscilloscope. This produces a picture, from which period, pulse repetition period, and pulse duration can be determined. From these quantities, frequency, pulse repetition frequency, and duty factor can be cal-

culated. Using the hydrophone calibration (relationship between voltage and acoustic pressure), pressure amplitude may also be determined. In addition, wavelength, spatial pulse length, and intensities can be calculated as well.

Using hydrophones, acoustic pressure output levels have been measured, and intensities and output indexes have been calculated for various diagnostic ultrasound instruments and transducers. Generally, sonographic outputs are the lowest and pulsed spectral Doppler outputs are the highest, with M mode and color Doppler imaging outputs falling between the two.

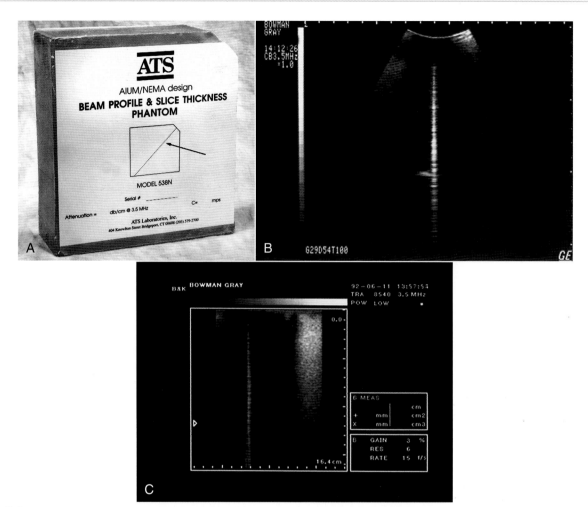

FIGURE 7-9 A, A beam profile and section thickness test object. It contains a thin, scattering layer *(arrow)* in an anechoic material. **B–C,** Scans of beam profiles. Shown in Figure 3-22, *D–F* are beam profiles obtained using this test object.

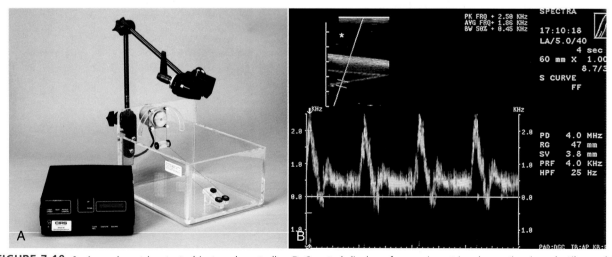

FIGURE 7-10 A, A moving-string test object and controller. **B,** Spectral display of a moving string (operating in pulsatile mode).

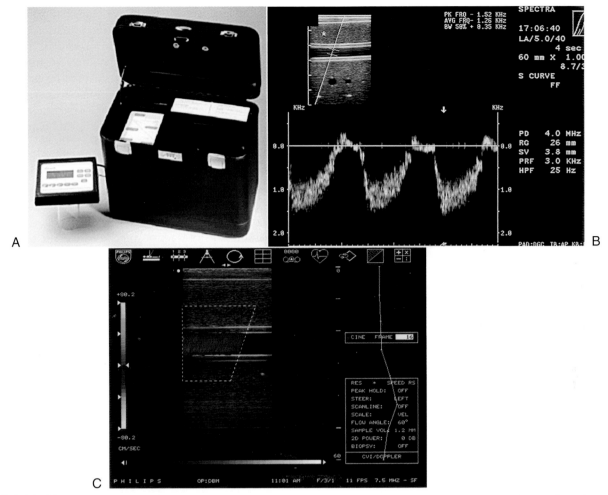

FIGURE 7-11 **A,** Doppler flow phantom. **B,** Spectral display from a flow phantom. **C,** Color Doppler image from a flow phantom.

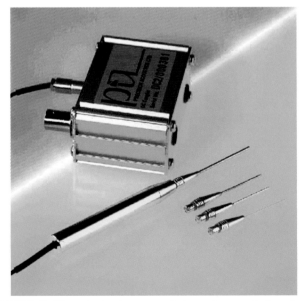

FIGURE 7-12 A hydrophone consisting of a small transducer element mounted on the end of a needle.

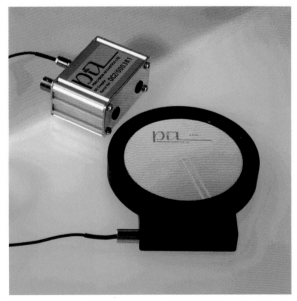

FIGURE 7-13 A hydrophone consisting of a thin membrane with metal electrodes.

Needle and membrane hydrophones are used to measure pressure amplitude and period, from which several other acoustic pulse parameters can be calculated.

BIOEFFECTS

The biological effects and safety of diagnostic ultrasound have received considerable attention. Several review articles, textbooks, and institutional documents have been published. Comprehensive, authoritative publications have been produced by the Bioeffects Committee of the American Institute of Ultrasound in Medicine (AIUM).[8,9]

In the remainder of this chapter, we review knowledge regarding bioeffects in cells, plants, and experimental animals, mechanisms of interaction between ultrasound and biological cells and tissues, regulatory activities, epidemiology, risk and safety considerations, and elements of prudent practice.

As with any diagnostic test, there may be some risk, that is, some probability of damage or injury, with the use of diagnostic ultrasound. This risk, if known, must be weighed against the benefit to determine the appropriateness of the diagnostic procedure. Knowledge of ways to minimize the risk, even if the risk is unidentified, is useful to everyone involved in diagnostic ultrasound. Sources of information used in developing policy regarding the use of diagnostic ultrasound are diagrammed in Figure 7-14, *A*. These sources include (1) bioeffects data from experimental systems, (2) output data from diagnostic instruments, and (3) knowledge and experience with regard to how the diagnostic information obtained is of benefit in patient management. Comparison of the first two components allows an assessment of risk, whereas the combination of the latter two components yields an awareness of the benefit. It seems reasonable to assume that there is some risk (however small) in the use of diagnostic ultrasound because ultrasound is a form of energy and has at least the potential to produce a biological effect that could constitute risk. Even if this risk is so minimal that it is difficult to identify, prudent practice dictates that routine measures be implemented to minimize the risk while obtaining the necessary information to achieve the diagnostic benefit. This is the **ALARA** (*as low as reasonably achievable*) principle of prudent scanning.

Our knowledge of bioeffects resulting from ultrasound exposure comes from several sources (see Figure 7-14, *B*). These sources include experimental observations in cell suspensions and cultures, plants, and experimental animals; epidemiologic studies in human beings; and studies of interaction mechanisms, such as heating and **cavitation**.

 Knowledge of bioeffects is important for the safe and prudent use of sonography.

Cells

Because cells in suspension or in culture are so different from those in the intact patient in a clinical environment, one must exercise restraint in extrapolating in vitro results to clinical significance. Cellular studies are useful in determining mechanisms of interaction and guiding the design of experimental animal studies and epidemiologic studies. The AIUM (http://www.aium.org/publications/statements.aspx) issued the following statement on *in vitro* biological effects in 1997:

It is often difficult to evaluate reports of ultrasonically induced in vitro biological effects with respect to their clinical significance. The predominant physical and biological interactions and mechanisms involved in an in vitro effect may not pertain

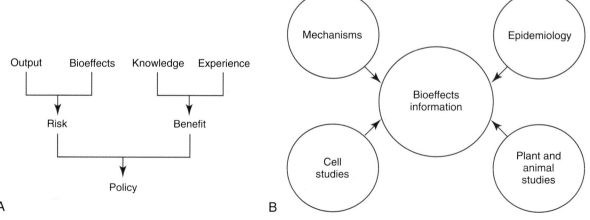

FIGURE 7-14 A, Ultrasound risk and benefit information. Risk information comes from experimental bioeffects (including epidemiology) and instrument output data. Benefit information is derived from knowledge and experience in diagnostic ultrasound use and efficacy. Together, they lead to a policy on the prudent use of ultrasound imaging in medicine. **B,** Bioeffects information sources.

to the in vivo situation. Nevertheless, an in vitro effect must be regarded as a real biological effect.

Results from in vitro experiments suggest new endpoints and serve as a basis for design of in vivo experiments. In vitro studies provide the capability to control experimental variables that may not be controllable in vivo and thus offer a means to explore and evaluate specific mechanisms and test hypotheses. Although they may have limited applicability to in vivo biological effects, such studies can disclose fundamental intercellular or intracellular effects of ultrasound.

While it is valid for authors to place their results in context and to suggest further relevant investigations, reports which do more than that should be viewed with caution.

Studies of the effects of ultrasound on cells in culture or suspension are useful for identifying cellular effects and mechanisms of action. They should not be used directly for risk assessment in clinical scanning.

Plants

The primary components of plant tissues—stems, leaves, and roots—contain gas-filled channels between the cell walls. Thus plants have served as useful biological models for studying the effects of cavitation.

Through this mechanism, normal cellular organization and function can be disturbed. Irreversible effects appear to be limited to cell death. Reversible effects include chromosomal abnormalities, mitotic index reductions, and growth rate reduction. Membrane damage induced by microstreaming shear stress appears to be the cause of cell death in leaves. Intensity thresholds for lysis of leaf cells are much higher with pulsed ultrasound than with continuous wave ultrasound. Apparently, the response of the bubbles within tissues to continuous and pulsed fields is different.

 Plant studies are useful primarily for understanding cavitational effects in living tissue.

Animals

With experimental animals, reported in vivo effects include fetal weight reduction, postpartum mortality, fetal abnormalities, tissue lesions, hind limb paralysis, blood flow stasis, wound repair enhancement, and tumor regression. Many studies on fetal weight reduction in mice and rats have been performed. All rat studies and several mouse studies yielded negative results. Focal lesion production is a well-documented bioeffect that has been observed over a wide range of intensity and exposure duration conditions (Figure 7-15).

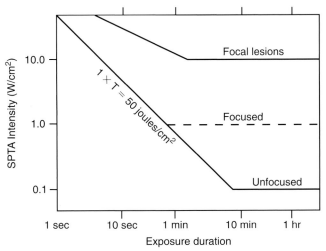

FIGURE 7-15 Comparison of the minimum spatial peak–temporal average (SPTA) intensities required for ultrasonic bioeffects specified in the AIUM Statement on Mammalian Bioeffects. The minimum levels required for focal lesions also are shown in the figure for comparison. Note that logarithmic scaling has been used for the axes of this figure, so the horizontal lines are separated by factors of 10 in intensity. *(From the American Institute of Ultrasound in Medicine:* Bioeffects and safety of diagnostic ultrasound, *Laurel, MD, 1993, The Institute.)*

In 2008, the AIUM (http://www.aium.org/publications/statements.aspx) issued the following statement on mammalian in vivo biological effects:

Information from experiments using laboratory mammals has contributed significantly to our understanding of ultrasonically induced biological effects and the mechanisms that are most likely responsible. The following statement summarizes observations relative to specific diagnostic ultrasound parameters and indices.

In the low-megahertz frequency range there have been no independently confirmed adverse biological effects in mammalian tissues exposed in vivo under experimental ultrasound conditions, as follows:

1. *Thermal Mechanisms: No effects have been observed for an unfocused beam having free-field spatial-peak temporal-average (SPTA) intensities* below 100 mW/cm², or a focused† beam having intensities below 1 W/cm², or thermal index values of less than 2.*

For fetal exposures, no effects have been reported for a temperature increase above the normal physiologic temperature, ΔT, when ΔT < 4.5 − (log₁₀t/0.6), where t is exposure time ranging from 1 to 250 minutes, including off time for pulsed exposure (Miller et al, 2002).

For postnatal exposures producing temperature increases of 6° C or less, no effects have been

---

*Free-field SPTA intensity for continuous wave and pulsed exposures.
†Quarter-power (−6 dB) beam width smaller than 4 wavelengths or 4 mm, whichever is less at the exposure frequency.

reported when $\Delta T < 6 - (\log_{10}t/0.6)$, including off time for pulsed exposure. For example, for temperature increases of 6.0° C and 2.0° C, the corresponding limits for the exposure durations t are 1 and 250 minutes (O'Brien et al, 2008).

For postnatal exposures producing temperature increases of 6° C or more, no effects have been reported when $\Delta T < 6 - (\log_{10}t/0.3)$, including off time for pulsed exposure. For example, for a temperature increase of 9.6° C, the corresponding limit for the exposure duration is 5 seconds (= 0.083 minutes) (O'Brien et al, 2008).

2. Nonthermal Mechanisms: *In tissues that contain well-defined gas bodies, for example, lung, no effects have been observed for in situ peak rarefactional pressures below approximately 0.4 MPa or mechanical index values less than approximately 0.4.*

   In tissues that do not contain well-defined gas bodies, no effects have been reported for peak rarefactional pressures below approximately 4.0 MPa or mechanical index values less than approximately 4.0 (Church et al, 2008).

 Studies of bioeffects in experimental animals have allowed determination of conditions under which thermal and nonthermal bioeffects occur.

Mechanisms

Mechanisms of action by which ultrasound could produce biological effects can be divided into two groups: (1) heating and (2) mechanical. Mechanical is also called *nonthermal*.

Heat. Recall that attenuation in tissue is primarily due to absorption, that is, conversion of ultrasound to heat. Thus ultrasound produces a temperature rise as it propagates through tissues. The extent of the temperature rise produced depends on the applied intensity and frequency (because the absorption coefficient is approximately proportional to frequency) of sound and on beam focusing and tissue perfusion. Heating increases as intensity or frequency is increased. For a given transducer output intensity, with increasing tissue depths, heating is decreased at higher frequencies because of the increased attenuation that reduces the intensity arriving at depth. Temperature rises are considered significant if they exceed 2° C. Intensities greater than a few hundred milliwatts per square centimeter (mW/cm²) can produce such temperature rises. Absorption coefficients are higher in bone than they are in soft tissues. Therefore bone heating, particularly in the fetus, receives special consideration.

Heating has been shown to be an important consideration in some reports on bioeffects. Mathematical models have been developed for calculating temperature rises in tissues. These models have been used to calculate estimated intensities required for a given temperature rise. In 2009, the AIUM (http://www.aium.org/publications/statements.aspx) issued the following conclusions regarding heat:

1. *Excessive temperature increase can result in toxic effects in mammalian systems. The biological effects observed depend on many factors, such as the exposure duration, the type of tissue exposed, its cellular proliferation rate, and its potential for regeneration. Age and stage of development are important factors when considering fetal and neonatal safety. Temperature increases of several degrees Celsius above the normal core range can occur naturally. The probability of an adverse biological effect increases with the duration of the temperature rise.*

2. *In general, adult tissues are more tolerant of temperature increases than fetal and neonatal tissues. Therefore, higher temperatures and/or longer exposure durations would be required for thermal damage. The considerable data available on the thermal sensitivity of adult tissues support the following inferences:*
   For exposure durations up to 50 hours, there have been no significant, adverse biological effects observed due to temperature increases less than or equal to 2° C above normal.

   For temperature increases between 2° C and 6° C above normal, there have been no significant, adverse biological effects observed due to temperature increases less than or equal to $6 - \log_{10}(t/60)/0.6$, where t is the exposure duration in seconds. For example, for temperature increases of 4° C and 6° C, the corresponding limits for the exposure durations t are 16 min and 1 min, respectively.

   For temperature increases greater than 6° C above normal, there have been no significant, adverse biological effects observed due to temperature increases less than or equal to $6 - \log_{10}(t/60)/0.3$, where t is the exposure duration in seconds. For example, for temperature increases of 9.6° C and 6.0° C, the corresponding limits for the exposure durations t are 5 and 60 seconds, respectively.

   For exposure durations less than 5 seconds, there have been no significant, adverse biological effects observed due to temperature increases less than or equal to $9 - \log_{10}(t/60)/0.3$, where t is the exposure duration in seconds. For example, for temperature increases of 18.3° C,

14.9° C, and 12.6° C, the corresponding limits for the exposure durations t are 0.1, 1 and 5 seconds, respectively.

3. *Acoustic output from diagnostic ultrasound devices is sufficient to cause temperature elevations in fetal tissue. Although fewer data are available for fetal tissues, the following conclusions are justified:*

In general, temperature elevations become progressively greater from B-mode to color Doppler to spectral Doppler applications.

For identical exposure conditions, the potential for thermal bioeffects increases with the dwell time during examination.

For identical exposure conditions, the temperature rise near bone is significantly greater than in soft tissues, and it increases with ossification development throughout gestation. For this reason, conditions where an acoustic beam impinges on ossifying fetal bone deserve special attention due to its close proximity to other developing tissues.

The current FDA regulatory limit for $I_{SPTA.3}$ is 720 mW/cm². For this, and lesser intensities, the theoretical estimate of the maximum temperature increase in the conceptus can exceed 2°C.

Although, in general, an adverse fetal outcome is possible at any time during gestation, most severe and detectable effects of thermal exposure in animals have been observed during the period of organogenesis. For this reason, exposures during the first trimester should be restricted to the lowest outputs consistent with obtaining the necessary diagnostic information.

Ultrasound exposures that elevate fetal temperature by 4° C above normal for 5 minutes or more have the potential to induce severe developmental defects. Thermally induced congenital anomalies have been observed in a large variety of animal species. In current clinical practice, using commercially available equipment, it is unlikely that such thermal exposure would occur at a specific fetal anatomic site.

Transducer self-heating is a significant component of the temperature rise of tissues close to the transducer. This may be of significance in transvaginal scanning, but no data for the fetal temperature rise are available.

4. *The temperature increase during exposure of tissues to diagnostic ultrasound fields is dependent upon (a) output characteristics of the acoustic source such as frequency, source dimensions, scan rate, power, pulse repetition frequency, pulse duration, transducer self-heating, exposure time and wave shape and (b)*

tissue properties such as attenuation, absorption, speed of sound, acoustic impedance, perfusion, thermal conductivity, thermal diffusivity, anatomic structure and nonlinearity parameter.

5. *Calculations of the maximum temperature increase resulting from ultrasound exposure in vivo are not exact because of the uncertainties and approximations associated with the thermal, acoustic, and structural characteristics of the tissues involved. However, experimental evidence shows that calculations are generally capable of predicting measured values within a factor of 2. Thus, such calculations are used to obtain safety guidelines for clinical exposures where direct temperature measurements are not feasible. These guidelines, called Thermal Indices,* provide a real-time display of the relative probability that a diagnostic system could induce thermal injury in the exposed subject. Under most clinically relevant conditions, the soft-tissue thermal index, TIS, and the bone thermal index, TIB, either overestimate or closely approximate the best available estimate of the maximum temperature increase (ΔT_{max}). For example, if TIS = 2, then $\Delta T_{max} \leq 2°C$.*

Experimental measurements have shown reasonable confirmation of the mathematical calculations. The biological consequences of hyperthermia include fetal absorption or abortion, growth restriction, microphthalmia, cataract formation, abdominal wall defects, renal agenesis, palatal defects, reduction in brain waves, microencephaly, anencephaly, spinal cord defects, amyoplasia, forefoot hypoplasia, tibial and fibular deformations, and abnormal tooth genesis. About 80 known biological effects are due to hyperthermia. None has occurred at temperatures of less than 39° C. Above that, the occurrence of a biological effect depends on temperature and exposure time, as shown in Figure 7-16.

 Ultrasound is absorbed by tissue, producing a temperature rise. If critical time–temperature values are exceeded, tissue damage occurs.

Mechanical. Nonthermal or mechanical mechanisms of interaction include **radiation force**, streaming, and cavitation. **Radiation force** is the force exerted by a sound beam on an absorber or a reflector. This force can deform

---

*Thermal indices are nondimensional ratios of estimated temperature increases to 1° C for specific tissue models (see the Standard for Real-Time Display of Thermal and Mechanical Acoustic Output Indices on Diagnostic Ultrasound Equipment, Revision 1, AIUM/NEMA, 2001).

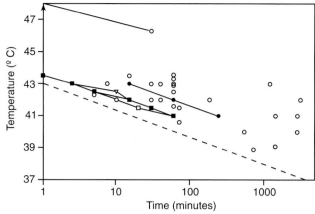

FIGURE 7-16 Thermal bioeffects. A plot of thermally produced biological effects that have been reported in the literature, in which the temperature elevation and exposure durations are provided. Each data point represents the lowest temperature reported for any duration or the shortest duration for any temperature reported for a given effect. Solid lines represent multiple data points relating to a single effect. The dashed line represents a lower boundary ($t_{43} = 1$) for observed, thermally induced biological effects. *(From Miller MV, Ziskin MC: Biological consequences of hyperthermia, Ultrasound Med Biol 15:707–722, 1989. Copyright 1989 by World Federation of Ultrasound in Medicine and Biology.)*

or disrupt structures. Radiation force also can cause flow in an absorbing fluid. This flow can cause shear stresses that can deform or disrupt structure. Some bioeffects observed in experimental studies have been attributed to these nonthermal, noncavitational mechanisms of interaction.

Cavitation is the production and behavior of bubbles in a liquid medium. A propagating sound wave is one means by which cavitation can occur. Two types of cavitation are recognized to occur. *Stable cavitation* is the term used to describe bubbles that oscillate in diameter with the passing pressure variations of the sound wave. Streaming of surrounding liquid can occur in this situation, resulting in shear stresses on suspended cells or intracellular organelles. Detection of cavitation in tissues under continuous wave, high-intensity conditions has been reported. *Transient (collapse) cavitation* occurs when bubble oscillations are so large that the bubble collapses, producing pressure discontinuities (shock waves), localized extremely high temperatures, and light emission in clear liquids. Transient cavitation has the potential for significant destructive effects. Transient cavitation is the means by which laboratory cell disruptors operate. One theory predicts that ultrasound could produce transient cavitation under diagnostically relevant conditions in water. Another theory incorporates a range of bubble sizes that yields a predictable dependence of the cavitation threshold on pressure and frequency. Experimental verification of this dependence has been carried out using stabilized microbubbles in water. Thresholds for cavitation in soft tissue and body liquids have been determined recently.

The AIUM (http://www.aium.org/publications/statements.aspx) has summarized information on the cavitation mechanism in its conclusions regarding gas bodies, which were approved in 2008:

Biologically significant, adverse, nonthermal effects have only been identified with certainty for diagnostically relevant exposures in tissues that have well-defined populations of stabilized gas bodies. Such gas bodies either may occur naturally or may be injected from an exogenous source such as an ultrasound contrast agent. This statement concerns the former, while a separate statement deals with contrast agents.

1. *The outputs of some currently available diagnostic ultrasound devices can generate levels that produce hemorrhage in the lungs and intestines of laboratory animals.*
2. *A mechanical index (MI)* has been formulated to assist users in evaluating the likelihood of cavitation-related adverse biological effects for diagnostically relevant exposures. The MI is a better indicator than single-parameter measures of exposure, for example, derated spatial-peak pulse-average intensity ($I_{SPPA.3}$) or derated peak rarefactional pressure ($p_{r.3}$), for known adverse nonthermal biological effects of ultrasound.*
3. *The threshold value of the current MI for lung hemorrhage in the mouse is approximately 0.4. The corresponding threshold for the intestine is MI = 1.4. The implications of these observations for human exposure are yet to be determined.*
4. *Thresholds for adverse nonthermal effects depend upon tissue characteristics, exposure duration (ED), and ultrasound parameters such as frequency (f_c), pulse duration (PD), and pulse repetition frequency (PRF). For lung hemorrhage in postnatal laboratory animals, an empirical relation for the threshold value of in situ acoustic pressure is*

$$P^r = (2.4\, f_c^{0.28}\, PRF^{0.04})/(PD^{0.27}\, ED^{0.23})\, MPa,$$

where the ranges and units of the variables investigated are (f_c) = 1 to 5.6 MHz, PRF = 0.017 to 1.0 kHz, PD = 1.0 to 11.7 μs, and ED = 2.4 to 180 s. The above relationship differs significantly from the corresponding form used for the MI, and a lung-specific MI is in development.

---

*The MI is equal to the derated peak rarefactional pressure (in MPa) at the point of the maximum derated pulse intensity integral divided by the square root of the ultrasonic center frequency (in MHz) (see Standard for Real-Time Display of Thermal and Mechanical Acoustic Output Indices on Diagnostic Ultrasound Equipment, Revision 2, AIUM/NEMA, 2004).

5. *The worst-case theoretical threshold for bubble nucleation and subsequent inertial cavitation in soft tissue is MI = 3.9 at 1 MHz. The threshold decreases to MI approximately 1.9 at 5 MHz and above, a level equal to the maximum output permitted by the U.S. Food and Drug Administration for diagnostic ultrasound devices. Experimental values for the cavitation threshold correspond to MI >4 for extravasation of blood cells in mouse kidneys, and MI >5.1 for hind limb paralysis in the mouse neonate.*

6. *For diagnostically relevant exposures (MI ≤1.9), no independently confirmed, biologically significant adverse nonthermal effects have been reported in mammalian tissues that do not contain well-defined gas bodies.*

Peak rarefactional pressure is illustrated in Figure 7-17. Experimental measurements have been performed that have shown reasonable confirmation of theoretical calculations (Figure 7-18). The only well-documented mammalian biological consequence of gas bodies in an ultrasound beam is blood cell extravasation in inflated lung. It has not occurred at acoustic pressure amplitudes of less than 0.3 MPa. Above that, its occurrence depends on frequency, exposure time, and pulsing conditions.

 Cavitation can occur in tissues containing gas bubbles with sufficient pressure amplitude and frequency conditions. Damage can result from cavitational activity in tissue.

The development of contrast agents in diagnostic ultrasound introduces a new consideration regarding cavitation effects; that is, these agents introduce bubbles (that normally would not be there) into circulation and into tissues. This decreases the acoustic pressure threshold for, and increases the severity of, cavitation bioeffects. The AIUM (http://www.aium.org/publications/

statements.aspx) issued the following statement on contrast agents in 2008:

Presently available ultrasound contrast agents consist of suspensions of gas bodies (stabilized gaseous microbubbles). The gas bodies have the correct size for strong echogenicity with diagnostic ultrasound and also for passage through the microcirculation. Commercial agents undergo rigorous clinical testing for safety and efficacy before Food and Drug Administration approval is granted, and they have been in clinical use in the United States since 1994. Detailed information on the composition and use of these agents is included in the package inserts. To date, diagnostic benefit has been proven in patients with suboptimal echocardiograms to opacify the left ventricular chamber and to improve the delineation of the left ventricular endocardial border. Many other diagnostic applications are under development or clinical testing.

Contrast agents carry some potential for nonthermal bioeffects when ultrasound interacts with the gas bodies. The mechanism for such effects is related to the physical phenomenon of acoustic cavitation. Several published reports describe adverse bioeffects in mammalian tissue in vivo resulting from exposure to diagnostic ultrasound

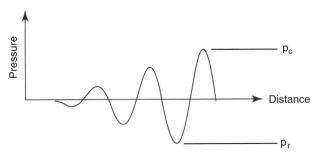

FIGURE 7-17 Pressure versus distance for a three-cycle pulse of ultrasound. *p_c*, Peak compressional pressure; *Pr*, peak rarefactional pressure.

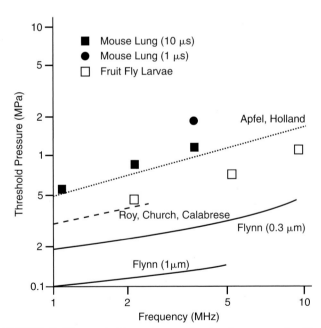

FIGURE 7-18 Threshold (in situ) rarefactional pressures for biological effects In vivo of low-temporal-average-intensity, pulsed ultrasound. Pulse durations are shown in parentheses in the legend. In all cases, the tissues contain identifiable, small, stabilized gas bodies. As in diagnostic ultrasound, all exposures consist of repetitive pulses (at 10 μs). Total exposure times were less than 5 minutes. (*Adapted from the American Institute of Ultrasound in Medicine: Bioeffects and safety of diagnostic ultrasound, Laurel, MD, 1993, The Institute.*)

with gas body contrast agents in the circulation. Induction of premature ventricular contractions by triggered contrast echocardiography in humans has been reported for a noncommercial agent and in laboratory animals for commercial agents. Micro-vascular leakage, killing of cardiomyocytes, and glomerular capillary hemorrhage, among other bioeffects, have been reported in animal studies. Two medical ultrasound societies have examined this potential risk of bioeffects in diagnostic ultra-sound with contrast agents and provide extensive reviews of the topic: the World Federation for Ultrasound in Medicine and Biology (WFUMB) Contrast Agent Safety Symposium (WFUMB, 2007) and the American Institute of Ultrasound in Medicine 2005 Bioeffects Consensus Conference (Miller et al, 2008). Based on review of these reports and of recent literature, the Bioeffects Committee issues the following statement:

> **Statement on Bioeffects of Diagnostic Ultra-sound with Gas Body Contrast Agents**
>
> *Induction of premature ventricular contrac-tions, microvascular leakage with petechiae, glomerular capillary hemorrhage, and local cell killing in mammalian tissue in vivo have been reported and independently confirmed for diag-nostic ultrasound exposure with a mechanical index (MI) above about 0.4 and a gas body contrast agent present in the circulation.*
>
> *Although the medical significance of such microscale bioeffects is uncertain, minimizing the potential for such effects represents prudent use of diagnostic ultrasound. In general, for imaging with contrast agents at an MI above 0.4, practitioners should use the minimal agent dose, MI, and examination time consistent with efficacious acquisition of diagnostic informa-tion. In addition, the echocardiogram should be monitored during high-MI contrast cardiac-gated perfusion echocardiography, particularly in patients with a history of myocardial infarc-tion or unstable cardiovascular disease. Further-more, physicians and sonographers should follow all guidance provided in the package inserts of these drugs, including precautions, warnings and contraindications.*

SAFETY

Information derived from in vitro and in vivo experimen-tal studies has not included any known risks in the use of diagnostic ultrasound. Thermal and mechanical mechanisms have been considered but do not appear to be operating significantly at diagnostic intensities. Cur-rently, there is no known risk associated with the use of diagnostic ultrasound. Experimental animal data have

helped define the intensity-exposure time region in which bioeffects can occur. However, physical and biological differences between the two situations make it difficult to apply the results from one to the risk assessment in the other. In the absence of any known risk—but recog-nizing the possibility that subtle, low-incidence, or delayed bioeffects could be occurring—a conservative approach to the medical use of ultrasound is recom-mended. This approach is described in more detail later in this section.

Instrument Outputs

Several reports and compilations of output data have been published. Instrument output may be expressed in many ways. Intensity has been the most popular quan-tity presented to describe instrument output. Several intensities may be used. Spatial peak–temporal average (SPTA) intensity is used in the AIUM statement on mam-malian bioeffects, and it relates reasonably well to a thermal mechanism of interaction. The SPTA is the output intensity most commonly presented. Imaging instruments dominate the lower portion of the range, whereas spectral Doppler instruments dominate the higher portion. In general, spectral Doppler outputs are the highest, gray-scale imaging outputs are the lowest, and outputs of M mode and color Doppler fall between the two.

These output intensity measurements usually are made with **hydrophones** located in the beam in a water bath. Attenuation in water is low compared with that in tissues, so an intensity at a comparable location within tissues would be considerably less than that in water. Models have been applied to account for the tissue atten-uation. The AIUM (http://www.aium.org/publications/ statements.aspx) issued the following statement on these models in 2007:

1. *Tissue models are necessary to estimate attenu-ation and acoustic exposure levels in situ from measurements of acoustic output made in water. Presently available models are limited in their ability to represent clinical conditions because of varying tissue paths during diagnostic ultra-sound exposures and uncertainties in acoustical properties of soft tissues. No single tissue model is adequate for predicting in vivo exposures in all situations from measurements made in water, and continued improvement and verification of these models is necessary for making exposure assessments for specific applications.*

2. *A homogeneous tissue model with an attenua-tion coefficient of 0.3 dB/cm-MHz throughout the beam path is commonly used when estimat-ing exposure levels. The model is conservative in that it overestimates the in-situ acoustic expo-sure when the path between the transducer and the site of interest is composed entirely of soft*

tissue. When the path contains significant amounts of fluid, as in many first- and second-trimester pregnancies scanned transabdominally, this model may underestimate the in-situ acoustical exposure. The amount of underestimation depends on each specific situation.

3. *"Fixed-path" tissue models, in which soft tissue thickness is held constant, sometimes are used to estimate in situ acoustical exposures when the beam path is greater than 3 cm and consists largely of fluid. When this model is used to estimate maximum exposure to the fetus during transabdominal scans, a value of 1 dB/MHz may be used as a conservative estimate during all trimesters.*

4. *Existing tissue models that are based on linear propagation are not valid when nonlinear acoustic distortion is present.*

 Instrument output data are available that allow comparison with conditions necessary for bioeffects to occur.

U.S. Food and Drug Administration

Manufacturers are required to submit premarket notifications to the U.S. Food and Drug Administration (FDA) before marketing a device for a specific application in the United States. The FDA then reviews this notification to determine whether the device is substantially equivalent, with regard to safety and effectiveness, to instruments on the market before the enactment of the relevant act (1976). If the device is determined to be substantially equivalent, the manufacturer then may market it for that application. Part of the FDA evaluation involves output data for the instrument, which then are compared with maximum values determined for pre-1976 devices. These values are given in the FDA *510(k) Guide for Measuring and Reporting Acoustic Output of Diagnostic Ultrasound Medical Devices* and are presented in Table 7-1. Some of the values have been updated since the 1985 publication of this guide. The current values are shown

TABLE 7-1	510(k) Guide Spatial Peak: Temporal Average In Situ Intensity Upper Limits
Diagnostic Application	**ISPTA (mW/cm²)**
Cardiac	430
Peripheral vessel	20
Ophthalmic	17
Fetal imaging and other*	94

*Abdominal, intraoperative, pediatric, small organ (breast, thyroid, testes), neonatal cephalic, adult cephalic.

in the table. To facilitate another path to device approval, a voluntary output display standard was developed by a joint committee involving the AIUM, the FDA, the National Electrical Manufacturers Association, and several other ultrasound-related professional societies. The goal of this activity was to develop a voluntary standard that would provide a parallel pathway to the current regulatory 510(k) process. The process would allow exemption from the upper limits given in the 510(k) guide (except that an overall upper limit of 720 mW/cm² SPTA still would apply) in exchange for presenting output information on the display. The standard includes two indices that would be displayed: thermal and mechanical. The thermal index (TI) is defined as the transducer acoustic output power divided by the estimated power required to raise tissue temperature by 1° C. The estimated power calculation for the TI involves frequency, aperture, and intensity. Three variations exist on the TI. The TIS (thermal index for soft tissues) applies when the beam travels through soft tissue and does not encounter bone. The TIB (thermal index for bone) applies for bone at or near the beam focus after passing through soft tissue. The TIC (thermal index for cranial tissues) applies when the transducer is close to bone. The mechanical index (MI) is equal to the peak rarefactional pressure (see Figure 7-17) divided by the square root of the center frequency of the pulse bandwidth,

$$MI = \frac{p_r \, (MPa)}{\left[(f)^{1/2} (MHz)^{1/2} \right]}$$

where p_r is pressure amplitude and f is frequency.

Display of any of these indexes would not be required if the instrument were incapable of exceeding index values of 1. Modern instruments incorporate this output display standard (Figure 7-19).

 The Food and Drug Administration regulates ultrasound instruments according to application and output intensities and thermal and mechanical indices.

Epidemiology

A dozen or so epidemiologic studies have been conducted and their results published, but these and other surveys in widespread clinical usage over many years have yielded no evidence of any adverse effect from diagnostic ultrasound. One study included 806 children, approximately half of whom had been exposed to diagnostic ultrasound in utero. The study measured Apgar scores, gestational age, head circumference, birth weight and length, congenital abnormalities, neonatal infection, and congenital infection at birth; it also included conductive and

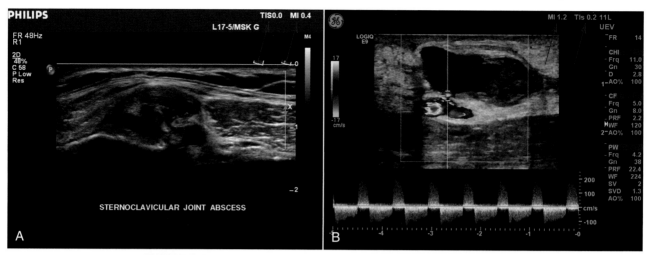

FIGURE 7-19 Displays showing thermal and mechanical indices *(arrows)*.

nerve measurements of hearing, visual acuity, and color vision; cognitive function and behavioral assessments; and complete and detailed neurologic examinations from age 7 to 12 years. No biologically significant differences between exposed and unexposed children were found. Another study measured the head circumference, height, and weight of 149 sibling pairs of the same sex, one of whom had been exposed to diagnostic ultrasound in utero. No statistically significant differences of head circumference at birth or of height and weight between birth and 6 years of age were found between ultrasound-exposed and unexposed siblings.

Although these studies have some limitations and flaws, they have not revealed any risk associated with the clinical use of diagnostic ultrasound. The AIUM http://www.aium.org/publications/statements.aspx) developed and approved in 2005 the following statement regarding epidemiology:

> *Based on the epidemiologic data available and on current knowledge of interactive mechanisms, there is insufficient justification to warrant conclusion of a causal relationship between diagnostic ultrasound and recognized adverse effects in humans. Some studies have reported effects of exposure to diagnostic ultrasound during pregnancy, such as low birth weight, delayed speech, dyslexia and non–right-handedness. Other studies have not demonstrated such effects. The epidemiologic evidence is based on exposure conditions prior to 1992, the year in which acoustic limits of ultrasound machines were substantially increased for fetal/obstetric applications.*

 Epidemiologic studies have revealed no known risk to the use of diagnostic ultrasound.

Prudent Use

As discussed above, epidemiologic studies have revealed no known risk associated with the use of diagnostic ultrasound. Experimental animal studies have shown bioeffects to occur only at intensities higher than those expected at relevant tissue locations during ultrasound imaging and flow measurements with most equipment. Thus a comparison of instrument output data, adjusted for tissue attenuation, with experimental bioeffects data does not indicate any risk. We must be open, however, to the possibility that unrecognized risk may exist. Such risk, if it does exist, may have eluded detection up to this point because it is subtle or delayed, or has incidence rates close to normal values. As more sensitive endpoints are studied over longer periods or with larger populations, such risk may be identified. However, future studies might not reveal any positive effects either, which strengthens the possibility that medical ultrasound imaging has no detectable risk.

In the meantime, with no known risk and with known benefit to the procedure, a conservative approach to imaging should be used; that is, ultrasound imaging should be used when medically indicated, with minimum exposure of the patient and fetus (Figure 7-20). Exposure is limited by minimizing instrument output and exposure time during a study. Instrument outputs for spectral Doppler studies can be significantly higher than those for other applications. It thus seems most likely that the greatest potential for risk in ultrasound diagnosis (although no specific risk has been identified even in this case), is with fetal spectral Doppler studies. These studies involve potentially high-output intensities with stationary beams and a presumably more sensitive fetus.

The AIUM (http://www.aium.org/publications/statements.aspx) first issued its statement on clinical safety in 1982. The statement was last updated in 2007 to the following:

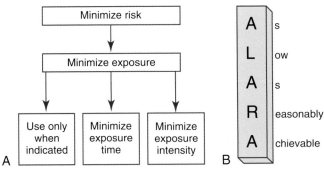

FIGURE 7-20 Minimizing risk by minimizing exposure **(A)** is the cornerstone of the ALARA principle **(B)**.

Diagnostic ultrasound has been in use since the late 1950s. Given its known benefits and recognized efficacy for medical diagnosis, including use during human pregnancy, the American Institute of Ultrasound in Medicine herein addresses the clinical safety of such use:

No independently confirmed adverse effects caused by exposure from present diagnostic ultrasound instruments have been reported in human patients in the absence of contrast agents. Biological effects (such as localized pulmonary bleeding) have been reported in mammalian systems at diagnostically relevant exposures but the clinical significance of such effects is not yet known. Ultrasound should be used by qualified health professionals to provide medical benefit to the patient.

In 2007 the AIUM issued another statement on prudent use:

The AIUM advocates the responsible use of diagnostic ultrasound and strongly discourages the nonmedical use of ultrasound for entertainment purposes. The use of ultrasound without a medical indication to view the fetus, obtain a picture of the fetus, or determine the fetal gender is inappropriate and contrary to responsible medical practice. Ultrasound should be used by qualified health professionals to provide medical benefit to the patient.

 Prudent practice of sonography involves application of the ALARA principle. By requiring medical indication and by using minimum output and exposure time in diagnostic examinations, exposure and risk are minimized.

In conclusion, extensive mechanistic, in vitro, in vivo, and epidemiologic studies have revealed no known risk devolving with the current ultrasound instrumentation

used in medical diagnosis. However, a prudent and conservative approach to ultrasound safety is to assume that there may be unidentified risk, which should be minimized in medically indicated ultrasound studies by minimizing exposure time and output. This is known as the ALARA principle (see Figure 7-20). The AIUM http://www.aium.org/publications/statements.aspx) issued a statement on this principle in 2008:

The potential benefits and risks of each examination should be considered. The ALARA (As Low As Reasonably Achievable) principle should be observed when adjusting controls that affect the acoustical output and by considering transducer dwell times. Further details on ALARA may be found in the AIUM publication Medical Ultrasound Safety.[9]

It is difficult to make a firm statement about the clinical safety of diagnostic ultrasound. The experimental and epidemiologic bases for risk assessment are incomplete. However, much work has been done, and no evidence of clinical harm has been revealed. Patients should be informed that there currently is no basis for concluding that diagnostic ultrasound produces any harmful effects in patients. However, unobserved effects could be occurring. Thus ultrasound should not be used indiscriminately. The AIUM Clinical Safety Statement forms an excellent basis for formulating a response to patient questions and concerns. Prudence in practice is exercised by minimizing exposure time and output. Display of instrument outputs in the forms of thermal and mechanical indices facilitates such prudent use.

In more than five decades of use, there has been no report of injury to patients or to operators from medical ultrasound equipment. Those working in the ultrasound community want to maintain that level of safety. In the past, application-specific output limits and the user's knowledge of equipment controls and patient body characteristics were the means to minimize exposure. Now, more information is available. The mechanical and thermal indices provide users with information that can be applied specifically to the ALARA principle. Values of mechanical and thermal indices eliminate some of the guesswork and provide an indication of what actually may be happening within the patient and what occurs when control settings are changed. These values make it possible for the user to obtain the best image possible while following the ALARA principle and thus maximizing the benefit-risk ratio.

REVIEW

- Phantoms and test objects provide means for measuring the detail resolution, distance accuracy, compensation, sensitivity, and dynamic range of diagnostic instruments.

- Hydrophones are used to measure the acoustic output of diagnostic instruments.
- The AIUM has stated that there have been no independently confirmed, significant bioeffects reported to occur in mammalian tissues exposed to focused SPTA intensities of less than 1 W/cm. Furthermore, no risk has been identified with the use of diagnostic ultrasound in human beings.
- Because there is limited specific knowledge, a conservative approach is justified. Such an approach calls for diagnostic ultrasound to be used, with minimum exposure, when medical benefit is expected to be derived from the procedure.

EXERCISES

1. A tissue-equivalent _____ has an attenuation of about 0.5 dB/cm-MHz and a propagation speed of 1.54 mm/μs. A _____ does not mimic tissue but provides a means for measuring some aspect of instrument performance.
2. Match the parameters measured with the items used (answers may be used more than once):
   1. Nylon fibers
   2. Attenuating scattering material
   3. Simulated cysts
   4. Hyperechoic and hypoechoic simulated lesions
   5. Thin scattering layer
   a. Axial resolution:
   b. Lateral resolution:
   c. Range accuracy:
   d. Caliper accuracy:
   e. Contrast resolution:
   f. Compensation:
   g. Sensitivity:
   h. Dynamic range:
   i. Beam profile:
   j. Section thickness:
3. Match the parameters measured with the correlating types of observation modes (answers may be used more than once):
   1. Gain settings
   2. Deepest scattering material imaged
   3. Fiber distances from the transducer or from each other on the display
   4. Minimum spacing of separately displayed fibers
   5. Lateral smearing of fibers
   a. Axial resolution:
   b. Lateral resolution:
   c. Range accuracy:
   d. Caliper accuracy:
   e. Compensation:
   f. Sensitivity:
   g. Dynamic range:

4. Test objects and phantoms are available commercially. True or false?
5. Test objects and phantoms can be used by the instrument operator. True or false?
6. A moving _____ test object is useful in checking the accuracy of Doppler spectral displays.
7. A _____ phantom is useful in simulating physiologic _____ conditions for a Doppler instrument.
8. Which of the following is used for Doppler sensitivity measurements?
   a. Cyst phantom
   b. Profile test object
   c. String test object
   d. Contrast phantom
   e. None of the above
9. Tissue-equivalent phantoms attempt to represent some acoustic property of _____.
10. The string test object measures volumetric flow rate. True or false?
11. Using a hydrophone, which of the following can be measured or calculated? (more than one correct answer)
    a. Impedance
    b. Amplitude
    c. Period
    d. Pulse duration
    e. Pulse repetition period
12. All hydrophones consist of a small element mounted on the end of a needle. True or false?
13. A needle hydrophone contains a small _____ element.
14. Because of its small size, a hydrophone can measure spatial details of a sound beam. True or false?
15. A hydrophone _____.
    a. interacts with light
    b. produces a voltage
    c. measures intensity directly
    d. measures total energy
    e. none of the above

16. Match the items in column **A** with those in **B** and **C** (answers may be used more than once). (Note: Items in **A** can be calculated from **B** if **C** is known.)

A
a. Frequency: _____, _____
b. Pulse repetition frequency: _____,

_____
c. Duty factor: _____, _____
d. Wavelength: _____, _____
e. Spatial pulse length: _____, _____
f. Energy: _____, _____
g. Intensity: _____, _____

B
1. Wavelength
2. Period
3. Pulse repetition period
4. Frequency
5. Energy
6. Power

C
7. Number of cycles in the pulse
8. Pulse duration
9. Propagation speed
10. Exposure time
11. Beam area
12. Nothing else

17. The piezoelectric material commonly used in hydrophones is
    a. Quartz
    b. PZT
    c. PVDF
    d. PDQ
    e. PVC

18. The important characteristic of the material used in hydrophones (*see Exercise 17*) is _____.
    a. impedance
    b. propagation speed
    c. efficiency
    d. density
    e. bandwidth

19. Heating depends most directly on _____.
    a. SATA intensity
    b. SATP intensity
    c. SPTP intensity
    d. pressure

20. Conditions under which cavitation may occur are best described by _____.
    a. SATA intensity
    b. SATP intensity
    c. SPTP intensity
    d. peak rarefactional pressure

21. Bioeffects have been observed in experimental animals with intensities greater than _____.
    a. 100 mW/cm^2 SPTA
    b. 1 W/cm^2 SPTA
    c. 10 W/cm^2 SPTA
    d. 1 mW/cm^2 SPTP
    e. 10 mW/cm^2 SPTP

22. Bioeffects have been observed in experimental animals with focused intensities greater than _____.
    a. 100 mW/cm SPTA
    b. 1 W/cm SPTA
    c. 10 W/cm SPTA
    d. 1 mW/cm SPTP
    e. 10 mW/cm SPTP

23. Focal lesions have been observed in experimental animals with intensities greater than _____.
    a. 100 mW/cm SPTA
    b. 1 W/cm SPTA
    c. 10 W/cm SPTA
    d. 1 mW/cm SPTP
    e. 10 mW/cm SPTP

24. The available epidemiologic data are sufficient to make a final judgment on the safety of diagnostic ultrasound. True or false?

25. Exposure is minimized by using diagnostic ultrasound _____.
    a. only when indicated
    b. with minimum intensity
    c. with minimum time
    d. all of the above
    e. none of the above

26. Which of the following is (are) used currently to indicate output on the display?
    a. Percent
    b. Decibel
    c. SPTA intensity
    d. Mechanical index
    e. All of the above

27. Which of the following affect(s) exposure of a fetus?
    a. Intensity at the transducer
    b. Distance to the fetus
    c. Frequency
    d. Gain
    e. More than one of the above
    f. All of the above

28. There is no possible hazard involved in the use of diagnostic ultrasound. True or false?

29. Ultrasound should not be used as a diagnostic tool because of the bioeffects it can produce. True or false?

30. No independently confirmed, significant bioeffects in mammalian tissues have been reported at intensities below _____.
    a. 10 W/cm^2 SPTP
    b. 100 mW/cm^2 SPTA
    c. 10 mW/cm^2 SPTA
    d. 10 mW/cm^2 SATA
    e. 1 mW/cm^2 SATP
31. Is there any known risk with the current use of diagnostic ultrasound?
32. Are there any bioeffects that ultrasound produces in small animals under experimental conditions?
33. Which of the following are mechanisms by which ultrasound can produce bioeffects? (more than one correct answer)
    a. Direction ionization
    b. Absorption
    c. Photoelectric effect
    d. Cavitation
    e. Compton effect
34. Which of the following relates to heating?
    a. Impedance
    b. Sound speed
    c. Absorption
    d. Refraction
    e. Diffraction
35. Which of the following endpoints is documented well enough in the scientific literature to allow a risk assessment for diagnostic ultrasound to be based on it?
    a. Fetal weight
    b. Sister-chromatid exchange
    c. Fetal abnormalities
    d. Carcinogenesis
    e. None
36. On which of the following endpoints has more than one epidemiologic study shown a statistically significant effect of ultrasound exposure?
    a. Fetal activity
    b. Birth weight
    c. Fetal abnormalities
    d. Dyslexia
    e. None
37. Which of the following acoustic parameters has (have) been documented in ultrasound epidemiologic studies published thus far?
    a. Frequency
    b. Exposure time
    c. Intensity and pulsing conditions
    d. Scanning patterns
    e. None

38. A device commonly used to measure the output of diagnostic ultrasound instruments is a(n) _____.
    a. hydrophone
    b. optical interferometer
    c. Geiger counter
    d. photoelectric cell
    e. absorption radiometer
39. A typical output intensity (SPTA) for an ultrasound imaging instrument is _____.
    a. 1540 W
    b. 13 kW/mm^2
    c. 3.5 MHz
    d. 1 mW/cm^2
    e. 2 dB/cm
40. Which of the following typically has the highest output intensity?
    a. Fetal monitor Doppler
    b. Duplex pulsed Doppler
    c. Color Doppler shift
    d. Color power Doppler
    e. Phase array, gray scale
41. As far as we know now, which of the following is the most correct and informative response to a patient's question, "Will this hurt me or my baby?"
    a. No.
    b. Yes.
    c. We don't know.
    d. The risks are well understood, but the benefits always outweigh them.
    e. There is no known risk with ultrasound imaging as it is applied currently.
42. To minimize whatever risk there may be with ultrasound imaging, which of the following should be done? (more than one correct answer)
    a. Scan to produce pictures for the family album
    b. Scan to determine fetal sex
    c. Minimize exposure time
    d. Scan for medical indication(s) only
    e. Minimize exposure intensity
43. Which of the following controls affect instrument output intensity?
    a. Dynamic range, compression
    b. Transmit, output
    c. Near gain, far gain
    d. Overall gain
    e. Slope, time gain compensation

44. Which of the following are correct for a duplex, pulsed wave Doppler instrument? (more than one correct answer)
    a. Tissue anywhere in the Doppler beam is exposed to ultrasound.
    b. Tissue anywhere in the imaging plane is exposed to ultrasound.
    c. Imaging intensities are higher than for conventional gray-scale instruments.
    d. Doppler intensities are higher than for continuous-wave fetal monitoring.

45. The tissue of greatest concern regarding bioeffects in an abdominal scan is the _____.
    a. spleen
    b. pancreas
    c. liver
    d. kidney
    e. fetus

46. Would it be wise to substitute a duplex, pulsed-wave Doppler device for an inoperative fetal monitor for long-term (e.g., 24-hour) monitoring in labor?
    a. Yes
    b. No
    c. Depends on frame rate of image
    d. Depends on frequency of Doppler beam
    e. Depends on gate location

47. Which of the following is (are) likely to be exposed to ultrasound during a diagnostic study?
    a. Patient
    b. Sonographer
    c. Sonologist
    d. Observers in the room
    e. More than one of the above

48. No bioeffects have been observed in nonhuman mammalian tissues at thermal index values of less than _____.
    a. 5
    b. 4
    c. 3
    d. 2
    e. 1

49. No bioeffects have been observed in nonhuman mammalian tissues at mechanical index values of less than _____.
    a. 0.5
    b. 0.4
    c. 0.3
    d. 0.2
    e. 0.1

50. No bioeffects have been observed in nonhuman mammalian tissues at peak rarefactional pressure values (megapascals) of less than _____.
    a. 0.5
    b. 0.4
    c. 0.3
    d. 0.2
    e. 0.1

Review

OUTLINE

ARDMS SPI Examination Content Outline
Comprehensive Examination

Diagnostic sonography is medical cross-sectional and three-dimensional anatomic and flow imaging that uses pulse-echo ultrasound. Pulses of ultrasound are generated by a transducer and are sent into the patient, where they produce echoes at organ boundaries and within tissues. These echoes return to the transducer, where they are detected and then presented on the display of a sonographic instrument. Each pulse produces a series of echoes that is displayed as a scan line. An anatomic image is composed of many scan lines. If flowing blood or moving tissues produce echoes, a frequency change, called *Doppler shift*, occurs. Doppler shifts provide motion information that can be presented audibly or as a spectral or two- or three-dimensional color Doppler display.

Ultrasound is sound (a wave of traveling acoustic variables, including pressure, density, and particle motion) having a frequency greater than 20 kHz. Ultrasound is described by frequency, period, wavelength, propagation speed, amplitude, intensity, and attenuation. Pulsed ultrasound is described by additional terms: *pulse repetition frequency* (PRF), *pulse repetition period*, *pulse duration*, *duty factor*, and *spatial pulse length*. Propagation speed and impedance are characteristics of the medium that are determined by density and stiffness. Attenuation increases with frequency and path length. Imaging depth decreases with increasing frequency. The soft tissue propagation speed is 1.54 mm/μs, and the attenuation coefficient is 0.5 dB/cm for each megahertz of frequency. When sound encounters boundaries between media with different impedances, part of the sound is reflected (echo) and part is transmitted. With perpendicular incidence, if the two media have the same impedance, there is no reflection. With oblique incidence, the sound is refracted at a boundary between the media where propagation speeds are different. Incidence and reflection angles are always equal. Scattering occurs at

rough media boundaries and within heterogeneous media. The range equation is used to determine distance to reflectors. Pulse-echo round-trip travel time is 13 μs/cm. Using harmonic echoes improves image quality. Contrast media enhance echo generation and detection.

Ultrasound transducers convert electric energy to ultrasound energy, and vice versa. They operate on the piezoelectric principle. The preferred operating frequency depends on element thickness. Axial resolution is equal to one half the spatial pulse length. Pulsed transducers have damping material to shorten the spatial pulse length for acceptable resolution. Transducers produce sound in the form of beams with near and far zones. Lateral resolution is equal to beam width. Beam width is reduced by focusing to improve resolution. *Linear* and *convex* are types of array construction. *Sequenced*, *phased*, and *vector* are types of array scanning operation. Phasing also enables electronic control of focus.

Diagnostic ultrasound imaging (sonographic) systems are of the pulse-echo type. They use the strength, direction, and arrival time of received echoes to generate A-, B-, and M-mode displays. Imaging systems consist of the transducer, beam former, signal processor, image processor, and display. Beam formers direct the transmitted beam through the imaged tissue cross-section, direct and focus the reception beam, amplify the received echo voltages, compensate for attenuation, and digitize the echo voltages. Signal processors filter, detect, and compress echo signals. Image processors convert scan line signals to image formats, store images in digital form, and perform preprocessing and postprocessing on images. Preprocessing includes persistence, panoramic imaging, spatial compounding, and three-dimensional acquisition. A mode shows echo amplitudes. B and M modes use a brightness display. M mode shows reflector motion in time. B scans show anatomic cross-sections in gray scale through the scanning plane. Image memories store echo amplitude information as numbers in the memory elements. Contrast resolution improves with increasing bits per pixel (layers of memory). Real-time imaging is the rapid sequential display of ultrasound images resulting in a moving presentation. Such imaging requires automatic, rapid, repeatable, sequential scanning of the sound beam through the tissue. This scanning is accomplished by electronic transducer arrays. Rectangular or sector display formats result from such scanning techniques. Displays are flat panel liquid-crystal displays (LCDs). Instruments often are connected to peripheral recording devices and to picture archiving and communications systems (PACS).

Fluids (gases and liquids) are substances that flow. Blood is a liquid that flows through the vascular system under the influence of pulsatile pressure provided by the beating heart. Volume flow rate is proportional to pressure difference at the ends of a tube and inversely proportional to flow resistance. Flow resistance increases with viscosity and tube length and decreases (strongly) with increasing tube diameter. Seven (two temporal and five spatial) flow classifications include *steady*, *pulsatile*, *plug*, *laminar*, *parabolic*, *disturbed*, and *turbulent*. In a stenosis, flow speeds up, pressure drops (Bernoulli effect), and flow is disturbed. If flow speed exceeds a critical value, turbulence occurs. Pulsatile flow is common in arterial circulation. Diastolic flow, flow reversal, or both may occur in some locations within the arterial system. Fluid inertia and vessel compliance are characteristics that are important in determining flow with pulsatile driving pressure.

The Doppler effect is a change in frequency resulting from motion. In most medical ultrasound applications, the motion is that of blood flow in circulation. The change in frequency of the returning echoes with respect to the emitted frequency is called the *Doppler shift*. For flow toward the transducer, Doppler shift is positive; for flow away, it is negative. The Doppler shift depends on the speed of the scatterers of sound, the angle between their direction and that of the sound propagation, and the operating frequency of the Doppler system. A moving scatterer of sound produces a double Doppler shift. Greater flow speeds and smaller Doppler angles produce larger Doppler shifts but not stronger echoes. Higher operating frequencies produce larger Doppler shifts. Typical ranges of flow speeds (10 to 100 cm/s), Doppler angles (30 to 60 degrees), and operating frequencies (2 to 10 MHz) yield Doppler shifts in the range of 100 Hz to 11 kHz for vascular studies. In Doppler echocardiography, where zero angle and speeds of a few meters per second can be encountered, Doppler shifts can be as high as 30 kHz.

Doppler instruments make use of the Doppler shift to yield information regarding motion and flow. Color Doppler imaging acquires Doppler-shifted echoes from a cross-section of tissue scanned by an ultrasound beam.

These echoes then are presented in color and are superimposed on the gray-scale anatomic image of nonshifted echoes that were received during the scan. The flow echoes are assigned colors according to the selected color map. Red, orange, yellow, blue, cyan, and white indicate positive or negative Doppler shifts (i.e., approaching or receding flow). Yellow, cyan, or green is used to indicate variance (disturbed or turbulent flow). Several pulses (the number is called *ensemble length*) are needed to generate a color scan line. Color controls include gain, color map selection, variance on/off, persistence, ensemble length, color/gray priority, scale (PRF), baseline shift, wall filter, and color window angle, location, and size. Color Doppler instruments are pulsed-wave Doppler instruments and are subject to the same limitations—Doppler angle dependence and aliasing—as are other Doppler instruments. Doppler-power displays color encode the strength of the Doppler shifts into a sensitive angle-independent and aliasing-independent presentation of flow information.

Continuous-wave systems provide motion and flow information without depth selection capability. Pulsed-wave Doppler systems have the capability of selecting a depth from which Doppler information is received. Spectral analysis provides quantitative information on the distribution of received Doppler-shift frequencies resulting from the distribution of scatterer velocities (speeds and directions) encountered. In addition to audible output, visual presentation of flow spectra is possible in Doppler systems. Combined (duplex) systems using real-time sonography and continuous-wave and pulsed-wave Doppler are available commercially. The Doppler spectrum is generated by the range of scatterer velocities encountered by the ultrasound beam. The Doppler spectrum is derived electronically using the fast Fourier transform (FFT) and is presented on the display as Doppler shift versus time, with brightness indicating power. Flow conditions at the site of measurement are indicated by the width of the spectrum; spectral broadening indicates disturbed and turbulent flow. Flow conditions downstream, particularly distal flow resistance, are indicated by the relationship between peak systolic and end diastolic flow speeds. Various indexes for quantitatively presenting this information have been developed.

Axial resolution is determined by spatial pulse length, whereas lateral resolution is determined by beam width. The beam width perpendicular to the scan plane causes section thickness artifacts. Apparent resolution close to the transducer is not related directly to tissue texture but is a result of interference effects from a distribution of scatterers in the tissue (speckle). Reverberation produces a set of equally spaced artifactual echoes distal to the real reflector. Refraction displaces echoes laterally. In the mirror-image artifact, objects that are present on one side of a strong reflector are displayed on the other side as well. Shadowing is caused by high-attenuation objects in the sound path. Enhancement results from low-attenuation objects in the sound path. Propagation speed error and refraction can cause objects to be displayed in improper locations or incorrect sizes or both. Refraction also can cause edge shadowing. Artifacts that can occur with Doppler ultrasound include aliasing, range ambiguity, color Doppler image and Doppler signal mirroring, and spectral trace mirroring. Aliasing is the most common artifact. Aliasing occurs when the Doppler-shift frequency exceeds one half the PRF (the Nyquist limit). Aliasing can be reduced or eliminated by increasing the PRF or Doppler angle, shifting the baseline, reducing operating frequency, or switching to continuous-wave operation.

Phantoms and test objects provide means for measuring the detail and contrast resolutions, distance accuracy, compensation, penetration, and dynamic range of diagnostic instruments. Hydrophones are used to measure the acoustic output of diagnostic instruments.

The American Institute of Ultrasound in Medicine (AIUM) has stated that no independently confirmed, significant bioeffects have been reported to occur in mammalian tissues exposed to focused spatial peak–temporal average intensities of less than 1 W/cm^2. Furthermore, no risk has been identified with the use of diagnostic ultrasound in human beings. Because there is limited specific knowledge, a conservative approach is justified; that is, diagnostic ultrasound should be used, with minimum exposure, when medical benefit is expected to be derived from the procedure (ALARA principle).

ARDMS SPI EXAMINATION CONTENT OUTLINE

This American Registry of Diagnostic Medical Sonographers (ARDMS) *Sonography Principles and Instrumentation* (SPI) Examination Content Outline is available at http://www.ardms.org/. It is reproduced here (by permission), indicating chapters in this textbook that cover each topic.

I. Patient care, safety and communication [5%]
   A. Patient identification/documentation
   B. Patient interaction
   C. Verification of requested examination
   D. Emergency situations
   E. Universal precautions
   F. Bioeffects and ALARA [Chapter 7]

II. Physics principles [20%] [Chapter 2]
   A. Properties of ultrasound waves
   B. Interactions of sound with tissue
   C. Power, intensity, and amplitude
   D. Units of measurement

III. Ultrasound transducers [20%] [Chapter 3]
   A. Transducer construction and characteristics
   B. Transducer types (sector, linear, phased arrays, etc.)
   C. Spatial resolution
   D. Transducer selection

IV. Pulse-echo instrumentation [30%] [Chapter 4]
   A. Display modes and their formation (A mode, B mode, M mode, 3-D, etc.)
   B. Transmission of ultrasound
   C. Reception of ultrasound (preprocessing)
   D. Beam former
   E. Postprocessing of ultrasound signals
   F. Pulse-echo imaging artifacts [Chapter 6]
   G. Tissue harmonic imaging
   H. Realtime ultrasound instrumentation
   I. Recording and storage devices

V. Doppler instrumentation and hemodynamics [20%] [Chapter 5]
   A. Ability to acquire color flow image
   B. Ability to acquire a Doppler spectral image
   C. Ability to take measurements from the spectral waveform
   D. Hemodynamics

VI. Quality assurance/quality control of equipment [5%]
   A. Preventive maintenance
   B. Malfunctions
   C. Performance testing with phantoms [Chapter 7]

COMPREHENSIVE EXAMINATION

1. Which of the following frequencies is in the ultrasound range?
   a. 15 Hz
   b. 15 kHz
   c. 15 MHz
   d. 17,000 Hz
   e. 17 km

2. The average propagation speed in soft tissues is _____.
   a. 1.54 mm/μs
   b. 0.501 m/s
   c. 1540 dB/cm
   d. 37.0 km/min
   e. 1 to 10 km/min

3. The propagation speed is greatest in _____.
   a. lung
   b. liver
   c. bone
   d. fat
   e. blood

4. Which of the following has a significant dependence on frequency in soft tissues?
   a. Propagation speed
   b. Density
   c. Stiffness
   d. Attenuation
   e. Impedance

5. The frequencies used in diagnostic ultrasound imaging _____.
   a. are much lower than those used in Doppler measurements
   b. determine imaging depth in tissue
   c. determine detail resolution
   d. all of the above
   e. b and c

6. An echo from a 5-cm deep reflector arrives at the transducer _____ μs after pulse emission.
   a. 13
   b. 154
   c. 65
   d. 5
   e. 77

7. A small (relative to the wavelength) reflector is said to _____ an incident sound beam.
   a. focus
   b. speculate
   c. scatter
   d. shatter
   e. amplify

8. Which of the following determines the operating frequency of an ultrasound transducer?
   a. Element diameter
   b. Element thickness
   c. Speed of sound in tissue
   d. Element impedance
   e. All of the above

9. The fundamental operating principle of medical ultrasound transducers is _____.
   a. Snell's law
   b. Doppler law
   c. magnetostrictive effect
   d. piezoelectric effect
   e. impedance effect

10. The axial resolution of a transducer is primarily determined by _____.
    a. spatial pulse length
    b. the near-field limit
    c. the transducer diameter
    d. the acoustic impedance of tissue
    e. density

11. The lateral resolution of a transducer is primarily determined by _____.
    a. spatial pulse length
    b. the near-field limit
    c. the aperture
    d. the acoustic impedance of tissue
    e. applied voltage

12. Increasing frequency _____.
    a. improves resolution
    b. increases penetration
    c. increases refraction
    d. a and b
    e. a and c

13. Ultrasound bioeffects _____.
    a. do not occur
    b. do not occur with diagnostic instruments
    c. are not confirmed below a spatial peak–temporal average intensity of 100 mW/cm^2
    d. b and c
    e. none of the above

14. Diagnostic ultrasound frequency range is _____.
    a. 2 to 10 mHz
    b. 2 to 10 kHz
    c. 2 to 15 MHz
    d. 5 to 15 kHz
    e. none of the above

15. What determines the lower and upper limits of frequency range useful in diagnostic ultrasound?
    a. Resolution and penetration
    b. Intensity and resolution
    c. Intensity and propagation speed
    d. Scattering and impedance
    e. Impedance and wavelength

16. Reverberation causes us to think there are reflectors that are too great in _____.
    a. impedance
    b. attenuation
    c. range
    d. size
    e. number

17. A flat panel display is composed of a back-lighted rectangular matrix of thousands of _____ display elements.
    a. plasma
    b. television
    c. fluorescent
    d. liquid-crystal
    e. piezo-crystal

18. In an ultrasound imaging instrument, a flat panel display may be used as a _____.
    a. pulser
    b. digitizer
    c. memory
    d. display
    e. scan converter

19. The compensation (time gain compensation) control _____.
    a. compensates for machine instability in the warm-up time
    b. compensates for attenuation
    c. compensates for transducer aging and the ambient light in the examining area
    d. decreases patient examination time
    e. none of the above

20. A scan converter changes signals from _____ to _____ format.
    a. gray-scale, color
    b. radio frequency, amplitude
    c. B mode, M mode
    d. scan line, image
    e. none of the above

21. Enhancement is caused by a _____.
    a. strongly reflecting structure
    b. weakly attenuating structure
    c. strongly attenuating structure
    d. frequency error
    e. propagation speed error

22. Echo intensity is represented in image memory by _____.
    a. positive charge distribution
    b. a number
    c. electron density of the scan converter writing beam
    d. a and c
    e. all of the above

23. Which of the following is (are) performed in a signal processor?
    a. Filtering
    b. Detection
    c. Compression
    d. All of the above
    e. None of the above

24. Increasing the pulse repetition frequency _____.
    a. improves detail resolution
    b. increases maximum unambiguous depth
    c. decreases maximum unambiguous depth
    d. both a and b
    e. both a and c

25. Attenuation is corrected by _____.
    a. demodulation
    b. desegregation
    c. decompression
    d. compensation
    e. remuneration

26. What must be known to calculate distance to a reflector?
    a. Attenuation, speed, density
    b. Attenuation, impedance
    c. Attenuation, absorption
    d. Travel time, speed
    e. Density, speed

27. Which of the following improve(s) sound transmission from the transducer element into the tissue?
    a. Matching layer
    b. Doppler effect
    c. Damping material
    d. Coupling medium
    e. a and d

28. Lateral resolution is improved by _____.
    a. damping
    b. pulsing
    c. focusing
    d. reflecting
    e. absorbing

29. Axial resolution is improved by _____.
    a. damping
    b. pulsing
    c. focusing
    d. reflecting
    e. absorbing

30. An image memory divides the cross-sectional image into _____.
    a. frequencies
    b. bits
    c. pixels
    d. binaries
    e. wavelengths

31. In general, as a reflector approaches a transducer at constant speed, the positive Doppler-shift frequency _____.
    a. increases
    b. decreases
    c. remains constant
    d. b or c
    e. none of the above
32. A reduction in vessel diameter produces a(n) _____.
    a. increase in flow resistance
    b. decrease in area
    c. increase in flow speed
    d. decrease in flow speed
    e. all of the above
33. Which of the following increases vascular flow resistance?
    a. Decreasing vessel length
    b. Decreasing viscosity
    c. Decreasing vessel diameter
    d. Decreasing pressure
    e. Decreasing flow speed
34. The Doppler effect occurs as _____.
    a. leukocytes move through plasma
    b. erythrocytes move through plasma
    c. erythrocytes move through serum
    d. blood moves relative to the vessel wall
    e. all of the above
35. When a reflector is moving toward the transducer, _____.
    a. propagation speed increases
    b. propagation speed decreases
    c. the Doppler shift is positive (higher frequency)
    d. the Doppler shift is negative (lower frequency)
    e. none of the above
36. Doppler sample volume is determined by _____.
    a. beam width
    b. pulse length
    c. frequency
    d. amplifier gate length
    e. all of the above
37. Doppler shift frequencies _____.
    a. are generally in the audible range
    b. are usually above 1 MHz
    c. can be applied to a loudspeaker
    d. a and b
    e. a and c
38. The quantitative presentation of frequencies contained in echoes is called _____.
    a. preamplification
    b. digitizing
    c. optical encoding
    d. spectral analysis
    e. all of the above
39. The Doppler frequency shift is caused by _____.
    a. relative motion between the transducer and the reflector
    b. the patient shivering in a cool room
    c. a high transducer frequency and real-time scanner
    d. small reflectors in the transducer beam
    e. changing transducer thickness
40. The Doppler effect is a change in _____.
    a. intensity
    b. wavelength
    c. frequency
    d. all of the above
    e. b and c
41. The Doppler shift is zero when the angle between the sound direction and the movement (flow) direction is _____ degrees.
    a. 30
    b. 60
    c. 90
    d. 45
    e. none of the above
42. The duplex Doppler presents _____.
    a. anatomic (structural) data
    b. physiologic (flow) data
    c. impedance data
    d. more than one of the above
    e. all of the above
43. The Doppler shift frequencies are usually in a relatively narrow range above 20 kHz. True or false?
44. Continuous wave sound is used in _____.
    a. all ultrasound imaging instruments
    b. only bistable instruments
    c. all Doppler instruments
    d. some Doppler instruments
    e. some M mode instruments
45. An advantage of continuous wave Doppler over pulsed Doppler is _____.
    a. depth information
    b. bidirectionality
    c. no aliasing
    d. b and c
    e. all of the above
46. In color Doppler instruments, hue can represent _____.
    a. sign (+ or −) of Doppler shift
    b. flow direction
    c. magnitude of the Doppler shift
    d. amplitude of the Doppler shift
    e. all of the above

47. The Doppler effect for a scatterer moving toward the sound source causes the scattered sound (compared with incident sound) received by the transducer to have _____.
    a. increased intensity
    b. decreased intensity
    c. increased impedance
    d. increased frequency
    e. decreased impedance

48. Duplex Doppler instruments include _____.
    a. pulsed-wave Doppler
    b. continuous-wave Doppler
    c. B-scan imaging
    d. dynamic imaging
    e. more than one of the above

49. If the Doppler shifts from normal and stenotic arteries are 4 kHz and 10 kHz, respectively, for which will there be aliasing with a pulse repetition frequency of 7 kHz?
    a. Normal artery
    b. Stenotic artery
    c. Both
    d. Neither

50. The signal processor in a Doppler system compares the _____ of the output with the returning echo voltage from the transducer.
    a. wavelength
    b. intensity
    c. impedance
    d. frequency
    e. all of the above

51. In the Doppler equation that follows, which can normally be ignored?

$$f_D = \frac{2fv}{(c-v)}$$

    a. v in the denominator
    b. v in the numerator
    c. f
    d. fD
    e. b and c

52. For which of the following is the reflected frequency less than the incident frequency?
    a. Advancing flow
    b. Receding flow
    c. Perpendicular flow
    d. Laminar flow
    e. All of the above

53. Doppler ultrasound can measure flow speed in the _____.
    a. heart
    b. veins
    c. arterioles
    d. capillaries
    e. a and b

54. Which of the following are fluids?
    a. Gas
    b. Liquid
    c. Solid
    d. a and b
    e. All of the above

55. The mass per unit volume of a fluid is called its _____.
    a. resistance
    b. viscosity
    c. kinematic viscosity
    d. impedance
    e. density

56. The resistance to flow offered by a fluid is called_____.
    a. resistance
    b. viscosity
    c. kinematic viscosity
    d. impedance
    e. density

57. Viscosity divided by density is called _____.
    a. resistance
    b. viscosity
    c. kinematic viscosity
    d. impedance
    e. density

58. If the following is increased, flow increases.
    a. Pressure difference
    b. Pressure gradient
    c. Resistance
    d. a and b
    e. All of the above

59. Flow resistance depends most strongly on_____.
    a. vessel length
    b. vessel radius
    c. blood viscosity
    d. all of the above
    e. none of the above

60. Proximal to, at, and distal to a stenosis, _____ must be constant.
    a. laminar flow
    b. disturbed flow
    c. turbulent flow
    d. volume flow rate
    e. none of the above

61. Added forward flow and flow reversal in diastole are results of _____ flow.
    a. volume
    b. turbulent
    c. laminar
    d. disturbed
    e. pulsatile

62. A broad spectrum indicates _____ flow.
a. pulsatile
b. laminar
c. constant
d. turbulent
e. a and b

63. As diameter at a stenosis decreases, the following pass(es) through a maximum.
a. Flow speed at the stenosis
b. Flow speed proximal to the stenosis
c. Volume flow rate
d. Doppler shift at the stenosis
e. a and d

64. The Doppler shift (kilohertz) for 4 MHz, 50 cm/s, and 60 degrees is _____.
a. 0.5
b. 1.0
c. 1.3
d. 2.6
e. 5.0

65. Physiologic flow speeds can be as much as _____% of the propagation speed in soft tissues.
a. 0.01
b. 0.3
c. 5
d. 10
e. 50

66. Which Doppler angle yields the greatest Doppler shift?
a. −90
b. −45
c. 0
d. 45
e. 90

67. Doppler shift frequency does not depend on _____.
a. amplitude
b. flow speed
c. operating frequency
d. Doppler angle
e. propagation speed

68. The Fourier transform technique is not used in color Doppler operation because it is not _____ enough.
a. slow
b. fast
c. bright
d. cheap
e. none of the above

69. Which of the following on a color Doppler display is (are) presented in real time?
a. Gray-scale anatomy
b. Flow direction
c. Doppler spectrum
d. a and b
e. All of the above

70. For a 5-MHz instrument and a 60-degree Doppler angle, a 100-Hz filter eliminates flow speeds below _____.
a. 1 cm/s
b. 2 cm/s
c. 3 cm/s
d. 4 cm/s
e. 5 cm/s

71. For a 7.5-MHz instrument and a 0-degree Doppler angle, a 100-Hz filter eliminates flow speeds below _____.
a. 1 cm/s
b. 2 cm/s
c. 3 cm/s
d. 4 cm/s
e. 5 cm/s

72. The functions of a Doppler detector include _____.
a. amplification
b. phase quadrature detection
c. demodulation
d. all of the above
e. none of the above

73. A later amplifier gate time means a(n) _____ sample volume depth.
a. earlier
b. shallower
c. deeper
d. stronger
e. none of the above

74. The Doppler shift is typically _____ the source frequency.
a. one thousandth
b. one hundredth
c. one tenth
d. 10 times
e. 100 times

75. Approximately _____ pulses are required to obtain one line of color Doppler information.
a. 1
b. 10
c. 100
d. 1000
e. 1,000,000

76. There are approximately _____ samples per line on a color Doppler display.
a. 2
b. 20
c. 200
d. 2000
e. 2,000,000

77. Which of the following Doppler instruments can produce aliasing?
a. Continuous wave
b. Pulsed
c. Duplex
d. Color
e. More than one of the above

78. For normal flow in a large vessel, a _____ range of Doppler shift frequencies is received.
a. narrow
b. broad
c. steady
d. disturbed
e. all of the above

79. Doppler signal power is proportional to _____.
a. the volume flow rate
b. flow speed
c. the Doppler angle
d. cell density
e. more than one of the above

80. Stenosis affects _____.
a. peak systolic flow speed
b. end diastolic flow speed
c. spectral broadening
d. window
e. all of the above

81. Spectral broadening is a _____ of the spectral trace.
a. vertical thickening
b. horizontal thickening
c. brightening
d. darkening
e. horizontal shift

82. As stenosis is increased, _____ increase(s).
a. vessel diameter
b. systolic Doppler shift
c. diastolic Doppler shift
d. spectral broadening
e. more than one of the above

83. Flow reversal in diastole (normal flow) indicates _____.
a. stenosis
b. aneurysm
c. high distal flow resistance
d. low distal flow resistance
e. more than one of the above

84. About _____ fast Fourier transforms are performed per second on a spectral display.
a. 3
b. 10
c. 100 to 1000
d. 700 to 7000
e. 17,000

85. Each fast Fourier transform appears on a spectral display as a _____.
a. dot
b. circle
c. horizontal line
d. vertical line
e. none of the above

86. Hue is _____.
a. color seen
b. light frequency
c. brightness
d. mix with white
e. more than one of the above

87. A component not included in a continuous-wave Doppler instrument is a(n) _____.
a. loudspeaker
b. wall filter
c. oscillator
d. demodulator
e. gate

88. On a spectral display, amplitude is indicated by _____.
a. brightness
b. horizontal position
c. vertical position
d. b and c
e. none of the above

89. Doppler shift can change because of changes in _____.
a. velocity
b. speed
c. direction
d. frequency
e. all of the above

90. A gate-open time of 10 μs corresponds to a sample volume length (millimeters) of _____.
a. 10.0
b. 7.7
c. 3.8
d. 3.3
e. 2.0

91. Sample volume width is determined by _____.
a. gate-open time
b. pulse duration
c. pulse repetition frequency
d. pulse repetition period
e. beam width

92. What problem(s) is (are) encountered if pulse repetition frequency is 10 kHz, sample volume is located at 10-cm depth, and the Doppler shift is 4 kHz?
    a. Aliasing
    b. Mirror image
    c. Refraction
    d. Range ambiguity
    e. More than one of the above

93. What problem(s) is (are) encountered if pulse repetition frequency is 10 kHz, sample volume is located at a 5-cm depth, and the Doppler shift is 6 kHz?
    a. Aliasing
    b. Mirror image
    c. Refraction
    d. Range ambiguity
    e. More than one of the above

94. What problem(s) is (are) encountered if pulse repetition frequency is 10 kHz, sample volume is located at a 10-cm depth, and the Doppler shift is 6 kHz?
    a. Aliasing
    b. Mirror image
    c. Refraction
    d. Range ambiguity
    e. More than one of the above

95. The functions of a color Doppler signal processor include _____.
    a. amplification
    b. phase quadrature detection
    c. demodulation
    d. autocorrelation
    e. all of the above

96. If all cells in a vessel were moving at the same constant speed, the spectral trace would be a _____ line.
    a. thin horizontal
    b. thick horizontal
    c. thin vertical
    d. thick vertical
    e. none of the above

97. Doppler power displays _____.
    a. are independent of Doppler angle
    b. are more sensitive than Doppler-shift displays
    c. are independent of aliasing
    d. show uniform flow presentations
    e. all of the above.

98. For a physiologic flow speed, a 5-MHz beam could produce a Doppler shift of about _____.
    a. 5 kHz
    b. 5 MHz
    c. 5 Hz
    d. depends on the mode (continuous-wave or pulsed-wave)
    e. none of the above

99. Spectral analysis is performed in a Doppler instrument _____.
    a. electronically
    b. mathematically
    c. acoustically
    d. mechanically
    e. more than one of the above

100. The Doppler shift is proportional to _____.
    a. the volume flow rate
    b. flow speed
    c. the Doppler angle
    d. cell density
    e. more than one of the above

101. Which of the following can be used to evaluate the performance of a Doppler instrument?
    a. Contrast detail phantom
    b. String test object
    c. Flow phantom
    d. b and c
    e. All of the above

102. Place the following instruments in general order of increasing acoustic output: (1) spectral Doppler, (2) sonographic, (3) color Doppler.
    a. 1, 2, 3
    b. 2, 3, 1
    c. 3, 1, 2
    d. 3, 2, 1
    e. 2, 1, 3

103. If operating frequency is 5 MHz, Doppler angle is 60 degrees, pulse repetition frequency is 9 kHz, and the Doppler shift is 2 kHz, what problem is encountered if the angle is changed to zero?
    a. Aliasing
    b. Range ambiguity
    c. Mirror image
    d. Refraction
    e. None

104. When angle correction is applied on a color Doppler display, the Nyquist limits (in centimeters per second) on the color map _____.
    a. increase
    b. decrease
    c. do not change
    d. are irrelevant
    e. are ambiguous

105. When angle correction is applied on a color Doppler display, the Nyquist limits (in kilohertz) on the color map _____.
    a. increase
    b. decrease
    c. do not change
    d. are irrelevant
    e. are ambiguous

106. Flow is _____ if it appears red on a color Doppler display.
    a. approaching
    b. receding
    c. turbulent
    d. disturbed
    e. undetermined (depends on color map)
107. Two different colors in the same vessel indicate _____.
    a. flow reversal
    b. sector scan
    c. vessel curvature
    d. aliasing
    e. any of the above
108. The following increase(s) the amount of color appearing in a vessel.
    a. Increased color gain
    b. Increased wall filter
    c. Increased priority
    d. Increased pulse repetition frequency
    e. More than one of the above
109. The following decrease(s) the amount of color appearing in a vessel.
    a. Increased wall filter
    b. Increased pulse repetition frequency
    c. Increased ensemble length
    d. Baseline shift
    e. More than one of the above
110. Which of the following on a color Doppler display is (are) presented as a two-dimensional, cross-sectional display?
    a. Gray-scale anatomy
    b. Flow direction
    c. Doppler spectrum
    d. a and b
    e. All of the above
111. Comparing gray with white is an example of _____.
    a. hue
    b. luminance
    c. saturation
    d. b and c
    e. all of the above
112. Comparing red with green is an example of _____.
    a. hue
    b. luminance
    c. saturation
    d. b and c
    e. all of the above
113. There are about _____ frames per second produced by a color Doppler instrument.
    a. 10
    b. 20
    c. 40
    d. 80
    e. more than one of the above

114. The autocorrelation technique yields _____.
    a. the mean Doppler shift
    b. a sign of the Doppler shift
    c. a spread around the mean (variance)
    d. all of the above
    e. none of the above
115. Increasing ensemble length _____ color sensitivity and accuracy and _____ frame rate.
    a. improves, increases
    b. degrades, increases
    c. degrades, decreases
    d. improves, decreases
    e. none of the above
116. Which control can be used to help with clutter?
    a. Wall filter
    b. Gain
    c. Baseline shift
    d. Pulse repetition frequency
    e. Smoothing
117. Doubling the width of a color window produces a(n) _____ frame rate.
    a. doubled
    b. quadrupled
    c. unchanged
    d. halved
    e. quartered
118. Steering the color window to the right or left changes the _____.
    a. frame rate
    b. pulse repetition frequency
    c. the Doppler angle
    d. the Doppler shift
    e. more than one of the above
119. Lack of color in a vessel may be due to_____.
    a. low color gain
    b. low wall filter setting
    c. small Doppler angle
    d. low baseline shift
    e. more than one of the above
120. Which control(s) can help with aliasing?
    a. Wall filter
    b. Gain
    c. Smoothing
    d. Pulse repetition frequency
    e. More than one of the above
121. Pulse duration is the _____ for a pulse to occur.
    a. space
    b. time
    c. delay
    d. pressure
    e. reciprocal

122. Spatial pulse length equals the number of cycles in the pulse multiplied by _____.
    a. period
    b. impedance
    c. beam width
    d. resolution
    e. wavelength

123. If pulse duration is 1 μs and the pulse repetition period is 100 μs, duty factor is _____.
    a. 1%
    b. 10%
    c. 50%
    d. 90%
    e. 100%

124. The attenuation of 5-MHz ultrasound in 4 cm of soft tissue is _____.
    a. 5 dB/cm
    b. 10 dB
    c. 2.5 MHz/cm
    d. 2 cm
    e. 5 dB/MHz

125. If the maximum value of an acoustic variable in a sound wave is 10 units and the normal (no sound) value is 7 units, the amplitude is _____ units.
    a. 1
    b. 3
    c. 7
    d. 10
    e. 17

126. Impedance equals propagation speed multiplied by _____.
    a. density
    b. stiffness
    c. frequency
    d. attenuation
    e. path length

127. Which of the following cannot be determined from the others?
    a. Frequency
    b. Amplitude
    c. Intensity
    d. Power
    e. Beam area

128. For perpendicular incidence, in medium 1, density equals 1 and propagation speed equals 3; in medium 2, density equals 1.5 and propagation speed equals 2. What is the intensity reflection coefficient?
    a. 0
    b. 1
    c. 2
    d. 3
    e. 4

129. For perpendicular incidence, if the intensity transmission coefficient is 96%, what is the intensity reflection coefficient?
    a. 2%
    b. 4%
    c. 6%
    d. 8%
    e. 10%

130. The colors presented on a Doppler-power display represent the _____ of the spectrum.
    a. mean Doppler shift
    b. variance
    c. area
    d. angle
    e. all of the above

131. For oblique incidence and a medium 2 speed that is equal to twice the speed of medium 1, the transmission angle will be about _____ times the incidence angle.
    a. 0.5
    b. 17
    c. 2
    d. 4
    e. 5

132. The range equation describes the relationship of _____.
    a. reflector distance, propagation time, and sound speed
    b. distance, propagation time, and reflection coefficient
    c. number of cows and sheep on a ranch
    d. propagation time, sound speed, and transducer frequency
    e. dynamic range and system sensitivity

133. Axial resolution in a system equals _____.
    a. four times the spatial pulse length
    b. the ratio of reflector size to transducer frequency
    c. the maximum reflector separation expected to be displayed
    d. the minimum reflector separation expected to be displayed
    e. spatial pulse length

134. In soft tissue, two boundaries that generate reflections are separated in axial distance (depth) by 1 mm. With a two-cycle pulse of ultrasound, the minimum frequency that will axially resolve these boundaries is _____.
    a. 1.0 MHz
    b. 2.0 MHz
    c. 3.0 MHz
    d. 4.0 MHz
    e. 5.0 MHz

135. Transducers operating properly in pulse-echo imaging systems have a quality factor of approximately _____.
    a. 1 to 3
    b. 7 to 10
    c. 25 to 50
    d. 100
    e. 500

136. Which of the following quantities varies most with distance from the transducer face?
    a. Axial resolution
    b. Lateral resolution
    c. Frequency
    d. Wavelength
    e. Period

137. The near-zone length for an unfocused, 5-MHz, circular transducer with a 13-mm diameter is greater than that for a 5-MHz transducer with a diameter of _____.
    a. 19 mm
    b. 15 mm
    c. 9 mm
    d. depends on impedance
    e. none of the above

138. If the near-zone length of an unfocused transducer that is 13 mm in diameter extends (in soft tissue) 6 cm from the transducer face, at which of the following distances from the face can the lateral resolution be improved by focusing the sound from this transducer?
    a. 13 cm
    b. 8 cm
    c. 3 cm
    d. 9 cm
    e. None of the above

139. The lateral resolution of an ultrasound system depends on _____.
    a. the aperature
    b. the transducer frequency
    c. the speed of sound in soft tissue
    d. the memory and the display
    e. all of the above

140. Which of the following is a characteristic of a medium through which sound is propagating?
    a. Impedance
    b. Intensity
    c. Amplitude
    d. Frequency
    e. Period

141. Which of the following cannot be determined from the others?
    a. Frequency
    b. Period
    c. Amplitude
    d. Wavelength
    e. Propagation speed

142. For perpendicular incidence, if the impedances of two media are the same, there will be no _____.
    a. inflation
    b. reflection
    c. refraction
    d. calibration
    e. b and c

143. What is the transmitted intensity if the incident intensity is 1 and the impedances are 1.00 and 2.64?
    a. 0.2
    b. 0.4
    c. 0.6
    d. 0.8
    e. 1.0

144. Increasing the intensity produced by the transducer _____.
    a. is accomplished by increasing pulser voltage
    b. increases the sensitivity of the system
    c. increases the possibility of biological effects
    d. all of the above
    e. none of the above

145. If the propagation speeds of two media are equal, incidence angle equals _____.
    a. the reflection angle
    b. the transmission angle
    c. the Doppler angle
    d. a and b
    e. b and c

146. If no reflection occurs at a boundary, it always means that media impedances are equal in the case of _____.
    a. perpendicular incidence
    b. oblique incidence
    c. refraction
    d. a and b
    e. b and c

147. Increasing spatial pulse length _____.
    a. accompanies increased transducer damping
    b. is accompanied by decreased pulse duration
    c. improves axial resolution
    d. all of the above
    e. none of the above

148. Place the following media in order of increasing sound propagation speed.
    a. Gas, solid, liquid
    b. Solid, liquid, gas
    c. Gas, liquid, solid
    d. Liquid, solid, gas
    e. Solid, gas, liquid

149. What is the wavelength of 1-MHz ultrasound in tissue with a propagation speed of 1540 m/s?
    a. 1×10^6 m
    b. 1.54 mm
    c. 1540 m
    d. 1.54 cm
    e. 0.77 cm

150. What is the spatial pulse length for two cycles of ultrasound having a wavelength of 2 mm?
    a. 4 cm
    b. 4 mm
    c. 7 mm
    d. 1.5 mm
    e. 3 mm
151. Increased damping produces _____.
    a. increased bandwidth
    b. shorter pulses
    c. decreased efficiency
    d. all of the above
    e. none of the above
152. If no refraction occurs as an oblique sound beam passes through the boundary between two materials, what is unchanged as the boundary is crossed?
    a. Impedance
    b. Propagation speed
    c. Intensity
    d. Sound direction
    e. b and d
153. If the spatial average intensity in a beam is 1 W/cm^2 and the transducer is 5 cm^2 in area, what is the total acoustic power?
    a. 1 W
    b. 2 W
    c. 3 W
    d. 4 W
    e. 5 W
154. How does the propagation speed in bone compare with that in soft tissue?
    a. Lower
    b. The same
    c. Higher
    d. Cannot say unless soft tissue is specified
    e. b and c
155. Attenuation along a sound path is a decrease in_____.
    a. frequency
    b. amplitude
    c. intensity
    d. b and c
    e. impedance
156. A focused transducer that is 13 mm in diameter has a lateral resolution at the focus of better than (i.e., smaller than) _____.
    a. 26 mm
    b. 13 mm
    c. 6.5 mm
    d. depends on frequency
    e. none of the above

157. An important factor in the selection of a transducer for a specific application is the ultrasonic attenuation of tissue. Because of this attenuation, a 7.5-MHz transducer generally should be used for _____.
    a. imaging deep structures
    b. imaging superficial structures
    c. imaging deep and shallow structures
    d. imaging adult intracranial structures
    e. all of the above
158. A real-time scan _____.
    a. consists of many frames produced per second
    b. depends on how short a time the sonographer takes to make a scan
    c. is made only between 8 AM and 5 PM
    d. yields a gray-scale image, whereas other scans yield only an M-mode display
    e. none of the above
159. Which of the following is determined by the pulser in an instrument?
    a. Amplitude
    b. Pulse repetition frequency
    c. Length of time required for a pulse to reach a specific reflector and return to the instrument
    d. More than one of the above
    e. None of the above
160. If the power at the output of an amplifier is 1000 times the power at the input, the gain is _____.
    a. 60 dB
    b. 30 dB
    c. 1000 dB
    d. 1000 volts
    e. none of the above
161. The dynamic range of an ultrasound system is defined as _____.
    a. the speed with which ultrasound examination can be performed
    b. the range over which the transducer can be manipulated
    c. the ratio of the maximum to the minimum intensity that can be displayed
    d. the range of pulser voltages applied to the transducer
    e. none of the above
162. The display generally will have a dynamic range _____ than other portions of the ultrasound instrument.
    a. larger
    b. smaller
163. The number 30 in the binary system is _____.
    a. 0110
    b. 1110
    c. 1001
    d. 1111
    e. none of the above

164. An ultrasound instrument that could represent 64 shades of gray would require an 8-bit memory. True or false?

165. Imaging systems consist of a beam former, display, and _____ and _____ processors.
a. beam
b. image
c. signal
d. a and b
e. b and c

166. Phased array systems involve the sequential switching of a small group of elements along the array. True or false?

167. For a two-cycle pulse of 5 MHz in soft tissue, the axial resolution is _____.
a. 0.1 mm
b. 0.3 mm
c. 0.5 mm
d. 0.7 mm
e. 0.9 mm

168. Postprocessing is the process of assigning numbers to be placed in the memory. True or false?

169. The minimum displayed axial dimension of a reflector is approximately equal to _____.
a. the beam diameter
b. half the beam diameter
c. twice the beam diameter
d. the spatial pulse length
e. half the spatial pulse length
f. twice the spatial pulse length

170. The minimum displayed lateral dimension of a reflector is approximately equal to _____.
a. the beam diameter
b. half the beam diameter
c. twice the beam diameter
d. the spatial pulse length
e. half the spatial pulse length
f. twice the spatial pulse length

171. M-mode recordings have _____ dimension(s).
a. two spatial
b. one spatial and one temporal
c. one Doppler and one temporal
d. one Doppler and one spatial
e. b and c

172. Nonlinear propagation of ultrasound in tissue generates _____.
a. speckle
b. attenuation
c. harmonics
d. refraction
e. reverberations

173. The operation in the signal processor that reduces noise is _____.
a. filtering
b. time gain compensation
c. scan conversion
d. compression
e. detection

174. The binary number 01001 is _____ in the decimal system.
a. 1
b. 3
c. 5
d. 7
e. 9

175. Reflectors may be added to the display because of _____.
a. reverberation
b. propagation speed error
c. enhancement
d. oblique reflection
e. the Doppler shift

176. If the propagation speed in a soft tissue path is 1.60 mm/μs, a diagnostic instrument assumes a propagation speed too _____ and will show reflectors too _____ the transducer.
a. high, close to
b. high, far from
c. low, close to
d. low, far from
e. none of the above

177. The reflector information that can be obtained from an M-mode display includes _____.
a. distance and motion pattern
b. transducer frequency, reflection coefficient, and distance
c. acoustic impedance, attenuation, and motion pattern
d. all of the above
e. none of the above

178. Increasing gain generally produces the same effect as _____.
a. decreasing attenuation
b. increasing compression
c. increasing rectification
d. both b and c
e. all of the above

179. A gray-scale display shows _____.
a. gray color on a white background
b. reflections with one brightness level
c. a white color on a gray background
d. a range of reflection amplitudes or intensities
e. none of the above

180. Electric pulses from the pulser are applied through the delays and transmit/receive switch to the _____.
    a. pulser
    b. transducer
    c. demodulator
    d. display
    e. memory
181. Peak detection is part of _____.
    a. amplipression
    b. rejection
    c. a and b
    d. compression
    e. amplitude demodulation
182. Multiple focus is not used with color Doppler instruments because of _____.
    a. ensemble length
    b. wall filter
    c. priority
    d. low frame rate
    e. a and d
183. If the gain of an amplifier is reduced by 3 dB and input power is unchanged, the output power of the amplifier is _____ what it was before.
    a. equal to
    b. twice
    c. one half
    d. greater than
    e. none of the above
184. If gain was 30 dB and output power is reduced by one half, the new gain is _____ dB.
    a. 15
    b. 60
    c. 33
    d. 27
    e. none of the above
185. If four shades of gray are shown on a display, each twice the brightness of the preceding one, the brightest shade is _____ times the brightness of the dimmest shade.
    a. 2
    b. 4
    c. 8
    d. 16
    e. 32
186. The dynamic range displayed in Exercise 185 is _____ dB.
    a. 100
    b. 9
    c. 5
    d. 2
    e. 0

187. Phantoms with nylon lines measure _____.
    a. resolution
    b. pulse duration
    c. spatial average–temporal average intensity
    d. wavelength
    e. all of the above
188. The following may be used to measure acoustic output.
    a. Hydrophone
    b. Optical encoder
    c. 100-mm test object
    d. All of the above
    e. None of the above
189. Real-time imaging is made possible by _____.
    a. scan converters
    b. single-element transducers
    c. gray-scale display
    d. transmit/receive switches
    e. arrays
190. Gain and attenuation are usually expressed in _____.
    a. decibels
    b. decibels per centimeter
    c. centimeters
    d. centimeters per decibel
    e. none of the above
191. Gray-scale display requires _____.
    a. array transducers
    b. cathode-ray storage tubes
    c. more than one bit per pixel
    d. b and c
    e. all of the above
192. With which of the following is time represented on one axis?
    a. B mode
    b. B scan
    c. M mode
    d. A la mode
    e. None of the above
193. Analog voltages occur at the output of the _____.
    a. beam former
    b. transducer
    c. signal processor
    d. display
    e. a and b
194. Digital signals occur at the output of the _____.
    a. beam former
    b. transducer
    c. signal processor
    d. display
    e. a and c

195. Which of the following produce(s) a rectangular image format?
a. Vector array
b. Convex array
c. Phased array
d. Linear array
e. All of the above

196. The piezoelectric effect describes how _____ is converted into _____ by a _____.
a. electricity, an image, display
b. incident sound, reflected sound, boundary
c. ultrasound, electricity, transducer
d. ultrasound, heat, tissue
e. none of the above

197. Propagation speed in soft tissues _____.
a. is directly proportional to frequency
b. is inversely proportional to frequency
c. is directly proportional to intensity
d. is inversely proportional to intensity
e. none of the above

198. Doppler-power imaging indicates (with color) the _____ of flow.
a. presence
b. direction
c. speed
d. character
e. more than one of the above

199. As frequency is increased, _____.
a. wavelength increases
b. a three-cycle ultrasound pulse decreases in length
c. imaging depth decreases
d. propagation speed decreases
e. b and c

200. Focusing _____.
a. improves lateral resolution
b. improves axial resolution
c. increases beam width in the focal region
d. shortens pulse length
e. increases duty factor

All of the key terms that were listed at the beginning of the individual chapters are compiled and defined here. More detailed and complete compilations of terminology are available.[10]

A mode A display presentation of echo amplitude versus depth (used in ophthalmology).

absorption Conversion of sound to heat.

acoustic Having to do with sound.

acoustic variables Pressure, density, and particle vibration; sound wave quantities that vary in space and time.

ALARA Acronym for "as low as reasonably achievable"; the principle that it is prudent to obtain diagnostic information with the least amount possible of energy exposure to the patient.

aliasing Improper Doppler-shift information from a pulsed-wave Doppler or color Doppler instrument when the true Doppler shift exceeds one half the pulse repetition frequency.

amplification The process by which small voltages are increased to larger ones.

amplifier A device that accomplishes amplification.

amplitude Maximum variation of an acoustic variable or voltage.

analog Related to a procedure or system in which data are represented by proportional, continuously variable, physical quantities (e.g., electric voltage).

analog-to-digital converter A device that converts voltage amplitude to a number. Abbreviated ADC.

anechoic Echo free.

aperture Size of a transducer element (for a single-element transducer) or group of elements (for an array).

apodization Nonuniform (i.e., involving different voltage amplitudes) driving of elements in an array to reduce grating lobes.

array A transducer assembly containing several piezoelectric elements.

attenuation Decrease in amplitude and intensity with distance as a wave travels through a medium.

attenuation coefficient Attenuation per centimeter of wave travel.

autocorrelation A rapid technique, used in most color Doppler instruments, for obtaining mean Doppler-shift frequency.

axial In the direction of the transducer axis (sound travel direction).

axial resolution The minimum reflector separation along the sound path that is required to produce separate echoes (i.e., to distinguish between two reflectors).

B mode Mode of operation in which the display presents a spot of appropriate brightness for each echo received by the transducer.

B scan A B-mode image that represents an anatomic cross-section through the scanning plane.

backscatter Sound scattered back in the direction from which it originally came.

bandwidth Range of frequencies contained in an ultrasound pulse; range of frequencies within which a material, device, or system can operate.

baseline shift Movement of the zero Doppler-shift frequency or zero flow speed line up or down on a spectral display.

beam Region containing continuous wave sound; region through which a sound pulse propagates.

beam former The part of an instrument that accomplishes electronic beam scanning, apodization, steering, focusing, and aperture with arrays.

Bernoulli effect Pressure reduction in a region of high-flow speed.

bidirectional Indicating Doppler instruments capable of distinguishing between positive and negative Doppler shifts (forward and reverse flow).

bistable Having two possible states (e.g., on or off, white or black).

bit Binary digit.

cathode-ray tube A display device that produces an image by scanning an electron beam over a phosphor-coated screen. Abbreviated CRT.

cavitation Production and dynamics of bubbles in sound.

channel A single one- or two-way path for transmitting electric signals, in distinction from other parallel paths; an independent transmission delay line and transducer element path; an independent reception transducer element, amplifier, analog-to-digital converter, and delay line path.

cine loop Sequential display of all the frames stored in memory at a controllable frame rate.

clutter Noise in the Doppler signal that generally is caused by high-amplitude, Doppler-shifted echoes from the heart or vessel walls.

coded excitation A sophisticated form of transmission in which the driving voltage pulses have intrapulse variations in amplitude, frequency, and/or phase.

color-Doppler display The presentation of two-dimensional, real-time Doppler-shift information superimposed on a real-time, gray-scale, anatomical, cross-sectional image. Flow directions toward and away from the transducer (i.e., positive and negative Doppler shifts) are presented as different colors on the display.

comet tail A series of closely spaced reverberation echoes.

compensation Equalization of received echo amplitude differences caused by different attenuations for different reflector depths; also called *depth gain compensation* or *time gain compensation*.

compliance Distensibility; nonrigid stretchability of vessels.

composite Combination of a piezoelectric ceramic and a nonpiezoelectric polymer.

compression Reduction in differences between small and large amplitudes. Region of high density and pressure in a compressional wave.

constructive interference Combination of positive or negative pressures.

continuous wave A wave in which cycles repeat indefinitely; not pulsed. Abbreviated CW.

continuous-wave doppler A Doppler device or procedure that uses continuous-wave ultrasound.

contrast agent A suspension of bubbles or particles introduced into circulation to enhance the contrast between anatomical structures, thereby improving their imaging.

contrast resolution Ability of a gray-scale display to distinguish between echoes of slightly different intensities.

convex array Curved linear array.

cosine The cosine of angle A in Figure 5-20, C, is the length of side b divided by the length of side c. Abbreviated cos.

coupling medium A gel used to provide a good sound path between a transducer and the skin by eliminating the air between the two.

critical Reynolds number The Reynolds number above which turbulence occurs.

cross-talk Leakage of strong signals in one direction channel of a Doppler receiver into the other channel; can produce the Doppler mirror-image artifact.

crystal Element.

Curie point Temperature at which an element material loses its piezoelectric properties.

cycle One complete variation of an acoustic variable.

damping Material attached to the rear face of a transducer element to reduce pulse duration; the process of pulse duration reduction.

decibel Unit of power or intensity ratio; the number of decibels is 10 times the logarithm (to the base 10) of the power or intensity ratio. Abbreviated dB.

demodulation Detection.

density Mass divided by volume.

depth gain compensation See *compensation*. Abbreviated DGC.

destructive interference Combination of positive and negative pressures.

detail resolution The ability to image fine detail and to distinguish closely spaced reflectors. (See *axial resolution* and *lateral resolution*.)

detection Conversion of voltage pulses from radio frequency to video form. Also called *demodulation, amplitude detection*, and *envelope detection*.

digital Related to a procedure or system in which data are represented by numeric digits.

digital-to-analog converter A device that converts a number to a proportional voltage amplitude. Abbreviated DAC.

disk A thin, flat, circular object.

display A device that presents a visual image derived from voltages received from an image processor.

disturbed flow Flow that cannot be described by straight, parallel streamlines.

Doppler angle The angle between the sound beam and the flow direction.

Doppler effect A change in frequency caused by motion of reflectors.

Doppler equation The mathematical description of the relationship between the Doppler shift, frequency, Doppler angle, propagation speed, and reflector speed.

Doppler-power display Color Doppler display in which colors are assigned according to the strength (amplitude, power, intensity, energy) of the Doppler-shifted echoes.

Doppler shift Reflected frequency minus incident frequency; a change in frequency that occurs as a result of motion.

Doppler spectrum The range of frequencies present in Doppler-shifted echoes.

duplex instrument An ultrasound instrument that combines gray-scale sonography with pulsed Doppler and, possibly, continuous-wave Doppler.

duty factor Fraction of time that pulsed ultrasound is on.

dynamic aperture Aperture that increases with increasing focal length (to maintain constant focal width).

dynamic focusing Continuously variable reception focusing that follows the increasing depth of the transmitted pulse as it travels.

dynamic range Ratio (in decibels) of largest to smallest power that a system can handle; ratio of the largest to smallest intensity of echoes encountered.

echo Reflection.

eddies Regions of circular flow patterns present in turbulence.

elastography Imaging tissue stiffness by tracking movement under mechanical stress.

element The piezoelectric component of a transducer assembly.

elevational resolution The detail resolution in the direction perpendicular to the scan plane. It is equal to the section thickness and is the source of section thickness artifact.

energy Capability of doing work.

enhancement Increase in echo amplitude from reflectors that lie behind a weakly attenuating structure.

ensemble length Number of pulses used to generate one color Doppler image scan line.

far zone The region of a sound beam in which the beam diameter increases as the distance from the transducer increases; also called *far field*.

fast Fourier transform Digital computer implementation of the Fourier transform.

filter An electric circuit that passes frequencies within a certain range.

flat-panel display A back-lighted rectangular matrix of thousands of liquid crystal display elements.

flow To move in a stream; volume flow rate.

fluid A material that flows and conforms to the shape of its container; a gas or liquid.

focal length Distance from a focused transducer to the center of a focal region or to the location of the spatial peak intensity.

focal region Region of minimum beam diameter and area.

focal zone Length of the focal region.

focus The concentration of the sound beam into a smaller beam area than would exist otherwise.

Fourier transform A mathematical technique for obtaining a Doppler frequency spectrum.

fractional bandwidth Bandwidth divided by operating frequency.

frame A single image produced by one complete scan of the sound beam.

frame rate   Number of frames of echo information stored each second.

Fraunhofer zone   Far zone.

freeze-frame   Constant display of one of the frames in memory.

frequency   Number of cycles per second.

frequency spectrum   The range of Doppler-shift frequencies present in the returning echoes.

Fresnel zone   Near zone.

fundamental frequency   The primary frequency in a collection of frequencies that can include odd and even harmonics and subharmonics.

gain   Ratio (in decibels) of amplifier output to input electric power.

gate   A device that allows only echoes from a selected depth (arrival time) to pass.

grating lobes   Additional weaker beams of sound traveling out in directions different from the primary beam as a result of the multielement structure of transducer arrays.

gray scale   Range of brightnesses between white and black.

harmonics   Frequencies that are even and odd multiples of another, commonly called *fundamental* or *operating frequency*.

hertz   Unit of frequency, one cycle per second; unit of pulse repetition frequency, one pulse per second. Abbreviated Hz.

hue   The color perceived based on the frequency of light.

hydrophone   A small transducer element mounted on the end of a narrow tube; a piezoelectric membrane with small metallic electrodes.

hypoechoic   Having relatively weak echoes. Opposite of hyperechoic (having relatively strong echoes).

image   A reproduction, representation, or imitation of the physical form of a person or thing.

image memory   The part of the image processor where echo information is stored in image format.

image processor   An electronic device that manipulates and prepares images for visual presentation.

impedance   Density multiplied by the sound propagation speed.

incidence angle   Angle between incident sound direction and a line perpendicular to the boundary of a medium.

inertia   Resistance to acceleration.

instrument   An electronic system that electrically drives a transducer, receives returning echoes, and presents them on a visual display as an anatomical image, Doppler spectrum, or color Doppler presentation.

intensity   Power divided by area.

intensity reflection coefficient   Reflected intensity divided by incident intensity; the fraction of incident intensity reflected.

intensity transmission coefficient   Transmitted intensity divided by incident intensity; the fraction of incident intensity transmitted into the second medium.

interference   Combinations of positive and/or negative pressures.

kilohertz   One thousand hertz. Abbreviated kHz.

laminar flow   Flow in which fluid layers slide over each other in a smooth, orderly manner, with no mixing between layers.

lateral   Perpendicular to the direction of sound travel.

lateral gain control   Gain controls that enable different gain values to be applied laterally across an image to compensate for differing attenuation values in different anatomical regions.

lateral resolution   Minimum reflector separation perpendicular to the sound path that is required to produce separate echoes.

lead zirconate titanate   A ceramic piezoelectric material. Abbreviated PZT.

lens   A curved material that focuses a sound or light beam.

linear   Adjectival form of *line*.

linear array   Array made of rectangular elements arranged in a line.

linear image   An anatomical image presented in a rectangular format.

linear phased array   Linear array operated by applying voltage pulses to all elements, but with small time differences (phasing) to direct ultrasound pulses out in various directions.

linear sequenced array   Linear array operated by applying voltage pulses to groups of elements sequentially.

longitudinal wave   Wave in which the particle motion is parallel to the direction of wave travel (compressional wave).

luminance   Brightness of a presented hue and saturation.

M mode   A B-mode presentation of changing reflector position (motion) versus time (used in echocardiography).

mass   Measure of the resistance of an object to acceleration.

matching layer   Material attached to the front face of a transducer element to reduce the reflections at the transducer surface.

mechanical index   An indicator of nonthermal mechanism activity; equal to the peak rarefactional pressure divided by the square root of the center frequency of the pulse bandwidth.

medium   Material through which a wave travels.

megahertz   One million hertz. Abbreviated MHz.

mirror image   An artifactual gray-scale, color flow, or Doppler signal appearing on the opposite side (from the real structure or flow) of a strong reflector.

multiple reflection   Several reflections produced by a pulse encountering a pair of reflectors; reverberation.

natural focus   The narrowing of a sound beam that occurs with an unfocused flat transducer element.

near zone   The region of a sound beam in which the beam diameter decreases as the distance from the transducer increases; also called *near field*.

nonlinear propagation   Sound propagation in which the propagation speed depends on pressure causing the wave shape to change and harmonics to be generated.

Nyquist limit   The Doppler-shift frequency above which aliasing occurs; one half the pulse repetition frequency.

oblique incidence   Sound direction that is not perpendicular to media boundaries.

operating frequency   Preferred (maximum efficiency) frequency of operation of a transducer.

panoramic imaging   An expansion of the field of view beyond the normal limits of a transducer scan plane.

parabolic flow   Laminar flow with a profile in the shape of a parabola.

penetration   Imaging depth.

period   Time per cycle.

perpendicular   Geometrically related by 90 degrees.

perpendicular incidence   Sound direction that is perpendicular to the boundary between media.

persistence   Averaging sequential frames together.

phantom   Tissue-equivalent device that has characteristics that are representative of tissues (e.g., scattering, propagation speed, and attenuation).

phase   A description of progress through a cycle; one full cycle is divided into 360 degrees of phase.

phase quadrature   Two signals differing by one fourth of a cycle.

phased array   An array that steers and focuses the beam electronically (with short time delays).

phased linear array   Linear sequenced array with phased focusing added; linear sequenced array with phased steering of pulses to produce a parallelogram-shaped display.

picture archiving and communications system   The system provides means for electronically communicating images and associated information to work stations and devices external to the sonographic instrument, the examining room and even the building in which the scanning is done. Abbreviated PACS.

piezoelectricity   Conversion of pressure to electric voltage.

pixel   Picture element; the unit into which imaging information is divided for storage and display in a digital instrument.

plug flow   Flow with all fluid portions traveling with the same flow speed and direction.

poise   Unit of viscosity.

Poiseuille's equation   The mathematical description of the dependence of volume flow rate on pressure, vessel length and radius, and fluid viscosity.

polyvinylidene fluoride   A piezoelectric thin-film material.

postprocessing   Image processing done after storage in the memory.

power   Rate at which work is done; rate at which energy is transferred.

preprocessing   Signal and image processing accomplished before storage in the memory.

pressure   Force divided by the area in a fluid.

priority   The gray-scale echo strength below which color Doppler information is shown preferentially on a display.

probe   Transducer assembly.

propagation   Progression or travel.

propagation speed   Speed at which a wave moves through a medium.

pulsatile flow   Flow that accelerates and decelerates with each cardiac cycle.

pulsatility index   A description of the relationship between peak systolic and end diastolic flow speeds or Doppler shifts.

pulse   A brief excursion of a quantity from its normal value; a few cycles.

pulse duration   Interval of time from beginning to end of a pulse.

pulse repetition frequency   Number of pulses per second; sometimes called *pulse repetition rate*. Abbreviated PRF.

pulse repetition period   Interval of time from the beginning of one pulse to the beginning of the next.

pulsed Doppler   A Doppler device or procedure that uses pulsed-wave ultrasound.

pulsed ultrasound   Ultrasound produced in pulsed form by applying electric pulses or voltages of one or a few cycles to the transducer.

pulse-echo technique   Ultrasound imaging in which pulses are reflected and used to produce a display.

radiation force   The force exerted by a sound beam on an absorber or a reflector.

radio frequency   Voltages representing echoes in cyclic form. Abbreviated RF.

range ambiguity   An artifact produced when echoes are placed too close to the transducer because a second pulse was emitted before they were received.

range equation   Relationship between round-trip pulse travel time, propagation speed, and distance to a reflector.

range gating   Selection of the depth from which echoes are accepted based on echo arrival time.

rarefaction   Region of low density and pressure in a compressional wave.

rayl   Unit of impedance.

real time   Imaging with a rapid frame sequence display.

real-time display   A display that, with a sufficient frame rate, appears to image moving structures or a changing scan plane continuously.

reflection   Portion of sound returned from a media boundary; echo.

reflection angle   Angle between the reflected sound direction and a line perpendicular to the media boundary.

reflector   Media boundary that produces a reflection; reflecting surface.

refraction   Change of sound direction on passing from one medium to another.

refresh rate   The number of times each second that information is sent from the image memory to the display. The number of times per second that a computer monitor redraws the information found in the memory.

resistance (flow)   Pressure difference divided by volume flow rate for steady flow.

resolution   The ability to distinguish echoes in terms of space, time, or strength (called *detail*, *temporal*, and *contrast resolutions*, respectively).

resonance   The condition in which a driven mechanical vibration is of a frequency similar to a natural vibration frequency of the structure.

resonance frequency   Operating frequency.

reverberation   Multiple reflection.

Reynolds number   A number that depends on flow speed and viscosity to predict the onset of turbulence.

sample volume   The anatomical region from which pulsed Doppler echoes are accepted.

saturation   The amount of hue present in a mix with white.

scan converter   An electronic device that reformats echo data into an image form for image processing, storage, and display.

scan line A line produced on a display that represents ultrasonic echoes returning from the body. A sonographic image is composed of many such lines.

scanhead Transducer assembly.

scanning The sweeping of a sound beam through the anatomy to produce an image.

scatterer An object that scatters sound because of its small size or its surface roughness.

scattering Diffusion or redirection of sound in several directions upon encountering a particle suspension or a rough surface.

sector A geometric figure bounded by two radii and the arc of the circle included between them.

sector image An anatomic image presented in a pie slice–shaped format.

sensitivity Ability of an imaging system to detect weak echoes.

shadowing Reduction in echo amplitude from reflectors that lie behind a strongly reflecting or attenuating structure.

side lobes Weaker beams of sound traveling out from a single element in directions different from those of the primary beam.

signal Information-bearing voltages in an electric circuit; an acoustic, visual, electric, or other conveyance of information. The physical representation of a message or information.

signal processor An electronic device that manipulates electric signals in preparation for appropriate presentation of information contained in them.

slice thickness Thickness of the scanned tissue volume perpendicular to the scan plane; also called *section thickness*.

sonography Medical two-dimensional, cross-sectional, and three-dimensional anatomical and flow imaging using ultrasound.

sound Traveling wave of acoustic variables.

sound beam The region of a medium that contains virtually all of the sound produced by a transducer.

source An emitter of ultrasound; transducer.

spatial compounding Averaging of frames that view the anatomy from different angles.

spatial pulse length Length of space over which a pulse occurs.

speckle The granular appearance of images and spectral displays that is caused by the interference of echoes from the distribution of scatterers in tissue.

spectral analysis Separation of frequencies in a Doppler signal for display as a Doppler spectrum; the application of the Fourier transform to determine the frequency components present in a Doppler signal.

spectral broadening The widening of the Doppler-shift spectrum; that is, the increase in the range of Doppler-shift frequencies present that occurs because of a broadened range of flow velocities encountered by the sound beam. This occurs for disturbed and turbulent flow.

spectral-Doppler display The presentation of Doppler information in a quantitative form. Visual display of a Doppler spectrum.

spectrum analyzer A device that derives a frequency spectrum from a complex signal.

specular reflection Reflection from a large (relative to wavelength), flat, smooth boundary.

speed error Propagation speed that is different from the assumed value (1.54 mm/μs).

stenosis Narrowing of a vessel.

stiffness Property of a medium; applied pressure divided by the fractional volume change produced by the pressure.

streamline A line representing the path of motion of a particle of fluid.

strength Nonspecific term referring to amplitude or intensity.

temporal resolution Ability to distinguish closely spaced events in time; improves with increased frame rate.

test object A device without tissue-like properties that is designed to measure some characteristic of an imaging system.

thermal index An indicator of thermal mechanism activity (estimated temperature rise); a value equal to transducer acoustic output power divided by the estimated power required to raise tissue temperature by 1°C.

time gain compensation Equalization of echo amplitude differences caused by different attenuations for different reflector depths; also called *depth gain compensation*. Abbreviated TGC.

transducer A device that converts energy from one form to another.

transducer assembly Transducer element(s) with damping and matching materials assembled in a case.

transmission angle Angle between the transmitted sound direction and a line perpendicular to the media boundary.

turbulence Random, chaotic, multidirectional flow of a fluid with mixing between layers; flow that is not laminar.

ultrasound Sound having a frequency greater than what humans can hear, that is, greater than 20 kHz.

ultrasound transducer A device that converts electric energy to ultrasound energy, and vice versa.

variance Square of standard deviation; one of the outputs of the autocorrelation process; a measure of spectral broadening (i.e., spread around the mean).

vector array Linear sequenced array that emits pulses from different starting points and (by phasing) in different directions.

viscosity Resistance of a fluid to flow.

volume imaging Three-dimensional imaging.

volumetric flow rate Volume of fluid passing a point per unit of time (i.e., per second or minute).

wall filter An electric filter that passes frequencies above a set level and eliminates strong, low-frequency Doppler shifts from pulsating heart or vessel walls.

wave Traveling variation of one or more quantities.

wavelength Length of space over which a cycle occurs.

window An anechoic region appearing beneath echo frequencies presented on a Doppler spectral display.

work Force multiplied by displacement.

zero-crossing detector An analog detector that yields mean Doppler shift as a function of time.

CHAPTER 1

1. d
2. a
3. a
4. c
5. c
6. d
7. a
8. b
9. c
10. a
11. c
12. a
13. b
14. d
15. d
16. b
17. d
18. d
19. a
20. c
21. a
22. d
23. e
24. c
25. b

CHAPTER 2

1. b
2. d
3. c
4. d
5. d
6. b
7. a
8. a
9. c
10. c
11. b
12. a
13. a
14. d
15. d
16. b
17. d
18. c
19. c
20. b
21. a
22. c
23. d (fastest in solids)
24. b
25. a

26. Mechanical, longitudinal or compressional
27. Doubled
28. Unchanged (determined by the medium)
29. 1
30. Information or energy
31. c
32. True
33. 6
34. d
35. c
36. e (c and d)
37. Frequencies, even, odd, fundamental, harmonics
38. 1,540,000
39. True
40. True
41. Density, propagation speed
42. Continuous wave
43. Pulses
44. Period
45. Decreases
46. Time
47. Length, space
48. Duty factor
49. Period
50. Wavelength
51. 1 (100%)
52. 6
53. 0.6 (Soft tissue propagation speed is 1.54 mm/μs; wavelength is 0.3 mm.)
54. 0.4 (Period is 0.2 μs; soft tissue is irrelevant.)
55. 1 (1000 pulses per second; $\frac{1}{1000}$ second from one pulse to the next)
56. 0.0004 (0.04%)
57. d
58. e (50,000)
59. c
60. Less than
61. a
62. Variation
63. Power, area
64. W/cm^2 or mW/cm^2
65. Amplitude
66. Doubled
67. Halved
68. Unchanged
69. Quadrupled
70. 5
71. Amplitude, intensity
72. Absorption, reflection, scattering
73. Centimeter
74. dB, dB/cm
75. 0.5
76. 1.5 dB/cm
77. Increases
78. Doubled, doubled, quadrupled

79. Unchanged
80. Sound, heat
81. No
82. Higher
83. Decreases
84. 0.32 (Attenuation is 8 dB, and intensity ratio is 0.16.)
85. 0.00000002 (Attenuation is 80 dB, and intensity ratio is 0.00000001.
86. c (0.5×7.5 MHz $\times$ 0.8 cm = 3 dB)
87. Impedances
88. Impedances, intensity
89. Impedances
90. 0.0008, 1.9992
91. True, for perpendicular incidence
92. d (difference in numerator; sum in denominator)
93. Direction, propagation speed
94. Perpendicular incidence, equal media propagation speeds
95. 32
96. Scattering
97. True
98. d
99. Impedances
100. False

CHAPTER 3

1. Energy
2. Electric, ultrasound
3. Piezoelectric
4. Disks
5. Thickness
6. Element, assembly
7. Element, assembly
8. Pulse, frequency
9. Thickness
10. Decreases
11. Cycles, axial resolution, bandwidth
12. Efficiency, sensitivity
13. Two, three
14. 0.2
15. e
16. Reflection
17. Air
18. False
19. False
20. Back
21. Front
22. Intermediate
23. Rectangles
24. f (a, b, c)
25. Resonance frequency
26. Composites
27. Broad bandwidth
28. No (because these frequencies are outside the bandwidth [4.5 to 5.5 MHz])

29. No (because these frequencies are outside the 2.5-MHz bandwidth [3.75 to 6.25 MHz])
30. Near, far
31. Near zone
32. Aperture
33. Aperture, frequency
34. c
35. Longer
36. Shorter
37. False (can focus only in the near zone)
38. c
39. d (all of the above)
40. False (See Figure 3-14.)
41. Focal length
42. Elements
43. Sequencing
44. One (the lateral dimension in the scan plane)
45. Curved, lens
46. Elements
47. a. 1; b. 2; c. 1
48. b
49. c
50. a, e
51. b, c, d
52. c
53. The same, different
54. Different, origin
55. Convex, vector
56. Sound travel or scan lines, echoes
57. Spatial pulse length
58. True
59. 1.5
60. 1
61. Wavelength, 0.3
62. Halved
63. Doubled
64. False
65. False
66. 2
67. 15 (less than 15 MHz in many applications)
68. Wavelength, spatial pulse length
69. Attenuation
70. Separation, echoes
71. Beam width
72. e
73. True
74. True
75. False, in general (only true near the transducer)
76. b, c, e, f
77. a. 4; b. 3; c. 2; d. 1
78. a, d
79. a. 10; b. 0.15; c. 14; d. 6.5; e. 13; f. 14
80. c
81. Half, near-zone
82. Focal
83. 6.5 (frequency not needed)
84. 0.7 (size not needed)

85. True
86. False
87. Focal
88. True
89. False
90. a. 1, 2, 3; b. 2; c. 2; d. 1
91. e
92. a
93. b, c, d
94. True (axial resolution 0.3 mm)
95. Resolution, penetration
96. 2, 15
97. 1, 1.5
98. 3 mm, 2 mm
99. 4 cm
100. a. 1; b. 4; c. 3; d. 5; e. 2

CHAPTER 4

1. Pulse
2. Amplitude, intensity
3. a (A minimum echo reception time of 130 μs is required.)
4. Filtering, detection, compression
5. a. 2; b. 4; c. 5; d. 1; e. 3
6. 10, 100, 20
7. 1
8. 10
9. b
10. Depth
11. Times
12. Dynamic, display, vision
13. 2.0
14. Radio frequency, amplitude
15. False
16. c
17. Zero, maximum, values, higher, weakest, strongest
18. 30
19. 50, 75, 87.5
20. 20
21. 10
22. 40
23. 32
24. 45, 32,000
25. −2, 2, 0.63
26. a. 6; b. 9; c. 10; d. 13; e. 14
27. a (43/32)
28. c (45/64)
29. a. 5; b. 3; c. 2; d. 6; e. 1; f. 4
30. e
31. a. 4; b. 5; c. 6; d. 7; e. 8
32. 50,000
33. c
34. e
35. a
36. Two (0 and 1)
37. Bit

38. Two, on, off
39. a. 3; b. 7; c. 8; d. 5; e. 4; f. 2; g. 1; h. 6
40. 25
41. 1101
42. a. 5; b. 10; c. 3; d. 1; e. 9; f. 2; g. 8; h. 7; i. 4; j. 6
43. a. 1 (0); b. 1 (1); c. 3 (101); d. 4 (1010); e. 5 (11001); f. 5 (11110); g. 6 (111111); h. 7 (1000000); i. 7 (1001011); j. 7 (1100100)
44. a. 3 (111); b. 4 (1111); c. 2 (11); d. 9 (111111111); e. 10 (1111111111); f. 6 (111111); g. 8 (11111111); h. 1 (1); i. 7 (1111111); j. 5 (11111)
45. a. 1 (0, 1); b. 2 (00, 01, 10, 11); c. 3 (000, 001, 010, 011, 100, 101, 110, 111); d. 4; e. 4; f. 5; g. 5; h. 6; i. 7; j. 7
46. B (brightness), M (motion), A (amplitude), all, cardiac, ophthalmic
47. M
48. Scan
49. Gray-scale, B mode
50. Image memory
51. a. 1; b. 2; c. 2; d. 2
52. 40
53. 1200
54. True (10 × 1 × 100 × 30 = 30,000 < 77,000)
55. c
56. Transducer, beam former, signal processor, image processor, display
57. a
58. b
59. d
60. c
61. Scan converter
62. c
63. b
64. d
65. Echoes
66. Pulse-echo
67. Brightness
78. Strength, direction, time
69. b
70. Display, voltages
71. Beam former
72. Beam former
73. Signal processor
74. a
75. a
76. Transducer
77. b
78. c
79. d
80. c
81. b
82. a
83. False
84. A, M
85. B
86. Electronic

87. Frame
88. Pulsed
89. Lines, frame
90. Frame rate
91. Increase
92. Improved, decreases, increased
93. $256 \times 512 = 131,072$; $512 \times 512 = 262,144$
94. b; e (a, c, d)
95. $1000/20 = 50$ lines per frame (one scan line for each pulse)
96. d
97. b
98. e (approaching the focus)
99. d
100. b

CHAPTER 5

1. a, c, d, e, g, h
2. Capillaries
3. a, b, f
4. Stream
5. b
6. Viscosity
7. Force
8. c
9. Difference, gradient
10. a
11. Pressure, resistance
12. d
13. Decreases
14. d
15. c
16. d
17. b
18. b
19. e
20. e
21. e
22. c
23. Disturbed
24. Turbulent
25. Distal
26. Stenosis
27. d
28. a
29. Decrease
30. Increase
31. a
32. e
33. e
34. b
35. d
36. e
37. d
38. Doppler, flow
39. Frequency
40. 0.02, 1.02
41. 0.026
42. −0.026
43. Received, emitted
44. Cosine
45. 0.01, 1.01 (The Doppler shift is cut in half.)
46. 0, 1.00 (no Doppler shift at 90 degrees)
47. 0.26 kHz
48. 1.95 kHz
49. Constant
50. c
51. Doppler angle
52. Doubled
53. Doubled
54. Decreased
55. Flow or motion, anatomy
56. d
57. Autocorrelation
58. Mean, sign, variance, power
59. True (Power displays have no angle dependence.)
60. No
61. False
62. b
63. e (a, b, or c)
64. False
65. False (It also can mean aliasing or changing Doppler angle.)
66. False (Remember the Doppler angle.)
67. Decreases
68. Autocorrelation
69. a and c
70. a, b, c
71. d
72. a
73. b
74. d
75. c
76. b, c
77. e (c and d)
78. b
79. e
80. False
81. e
82. a
83. e (a, b, c, d)
84. e
85. b
86. d
87. False
88. e
89. a
90. a
91. False
92. False
93. e (b, c, d)
94. False (Remember the Doppler angle.)
95. c

96. a
97. b
98. d
99. 50
100. c

CHAPTER 6

1. Range ambiguity
2. 11, 1
3. c (assumes 1.54 mm/μs, lower than the actual speed)
4. False
5. a
6. e (a, b, d)
7. False (This is the display of the interference pattern [speckle] of scattered sound from the distribution of scatterers within the ultrasound pulse in the tissue.)
8. Slice or section thickness
9. c, d, e, f
10. True (edge shadowing)
11. Figure 6-40, A (Figure 6-40, B, shows a comet tail artifact originating as reverberations within a structure.)
12. a. 1; b. 2, 3; c. 3; d. 4, 5; e. 4, 5
13. Separation
14. Weaker
15. b
16. d
17. True
18. b
19. b
20. b
21. c
22. Refraction (double image)
23. e
24. e (c and d)
25. e
26. a
27. True
28. Continuous wave
29. Red, blue, blue, red
30. Range ambiguity
31. d
32. b
33. b
34. b
35. b
36. e
37. c
38. Yes (less attenuation, greater penetration, later echoes)
39. Yes (Doppler shift increases with increasing frequency.)
40. d
41. a
42. a. 3; b. 4; c. 3; d. 2; e. 1
43. b, c, d

44. e (b, c, d)
45. Aliased, 10
46. a. R (Color changes at a 90-degree angle because scan lines go in different directions; they are heading upstream on the right and downstream on the left.); b. L (Vessel curvature causes flow to be away from the transducer on the left and toward the transducer on the right.); c. R (The blue area at right is aliasing.); d. L (The blue in the center is aliasing.); e. L; f. L (The color changes because the vessel is curved; flow is away from the transducer on the left and toward the transducer on the right.)
47. a. 4; b. 2; c. 1; d. 3; e. 5
48. a
49. c, b, d
50. Shadowing, aliasing

CHAPTER 7

1. Phantom, test object
2. a. 1, 3; b. 1, 3; c. 1; d. 1; e. 4; f. 2; g. 2; h. 2; i. 5; j. 5
3. a. 4; b. 5; c. 3; d. 3; e. 1; f. 2; g. 1, 2
4. True
5. True
6. String
7. Flow, flow
8. e
9. Tissues
10. False
11. b, c, d, e
12. False
13. Transducer or piezoelectric
14. True
15. b
16. a. 2, 12; b. 3, 12; c. 3, 8; d. 4 or 2, 9; e. 1, 7; f. 6, 10; g. 6, 11
17. c
18. e
19. a
20. d
21. a
22. b
23. c
24. False
25. d
26. e
27. e (a, b, c)
28. False
29. False
30. b
31. No
32. Yes
33. b and d
34. c
35. e

36. e
37. e
38. a
39. d
40. b
41. e
42. c, d, e
43. b
44. a, b, d
45. e (pregnancy possibility in fertile female)
46. b
47. a
48. d
49. c
50. c

CHAPTER 8

Following each answer is the chapter number in which the subject is discussed. Most answers also have explanatory comments.

1. c. Ultrasound is sound of frequency greater than 20 kHz (0.02 MHz). (Chapter 2)
2. a. Propagation speeds in soft tissues are in the range of about 1.4 to 1.6 mm/μs. Answer c is not in speed units. (Chapter 2)
3. c. Solid; high stiffness. (Chapter 2)
4. d. Propagation speed and impedance increase only slightly with frequency. (Chapter 2)
5. e. (Chapters 2 and 3)
6. c. Round-trip travel time is 13 μs/cm. (Chapter 2)
7. c. Scattering occurs with rough surfaces and with heterogeneous media (made up of small particles relative to the wavelength). Large, flat, smooth surfaces produce specular reflections. (Chapter 2)
8. b. The operating frequency of a transducer is such that its thickness is equal to one half the wavelength in the transducer element material. (Chapter 3)
9. d. Transducer elements expand and contract when a voltage is applied; conversely, when returning echoes apply pressure to the element, a voltage is generated. (Chapter 3)
10. a. Axial resolution is equal to one half the spatial pulse length. (Chapter 3)
11. c. Lateral resolution is equal to beam width. Beam width depends on the aperture (size of the element or group of elements generating the beam). (Chapter 3)
12. a. Penetration decreases with increasing frequency, and frequency has no effect on refraction. (Chapters 2 and 3)
13. c. This is part of the American Institute of Ultrasound in Medicine "Statement on Mammalian In Vivo Ultrasonic Biological Effects." (Chapter 7)

14. c. Frequencies lower than this range do not provide the needed resolution, whereas frequencies higher than this range do not allow for adequate penetration for medical purposes. (Chapters 2 and 3)
15. a. See answer to question 14. (Chapters 2 and 3)
16. e. Reverberation adds additional reflectors on the display that are deeper than the true ones. (Chapter 6)
17. d. (Chapter 4)
18. d. (Chapter 4)
19. b. (Chapter 4)
20. d. (Chapter 4)
21. b. (Chapter 6)
22. b. (Chapter 4)
23. d. (Chapter 4)
24. c. Pulse repetition frequency has no direct effect on detail resolution. (Chapters 4 and 6)
25. d. (Chapter 4)
26. d. Distance equals one half the speed multiplied by the round-trip time. (Chapter 2)
27. e. The matching layer improves sound transmission by reducing the reflection at the transducer–skin boundary. The coupling medium improves it by removing the air layer between the transducer and the skin. (Chapter 3)
28. c. (Chapter 3)
29. a. (Chapter 3)
30. c. (Chapter 4)
31. d. If the transducer is in the path of the reflector, answer c is correct because the Doppler angle is zero. If this is not the case, then b is correct because the Doppler angle will increase (decreasing the Doppler shift) as the reflector approaches. (Chapter 5)
32. e. The diameter referred to can be the entire vessel diameter or the diameter of a small portion of it (stenosis). For the former, d is correct. For the latter, c is correct at the stenosis. In either case, a and b are correct. (Chapter 5)
33. c. Poiseuille's equation shows that resistance increases with increasing vessel length, increasing fluid viscosity, or decreasing vessel diameter. (Chapter 5)
34. d. The blood cells move along with the plasma, not through it. (Chapter 5)
35. c. Propagation speed is determined by the medium, not by motion. (Chapters 2 and 5)
36. e. (Chapter 5)
37. e. (Chapter 5)
38. d. Spectral comes from spectrum, referring to color spectrum. A prism is an optical spectrum analyzer that breaks down white light into its component colors. (Chapter 5)
39. a. (Chapter 5)
40. e. If frequency changes, wavelength changes also. (Chapters 2 and 5)
41. c. (Chapter 5)

42. d. Answers a and b are correct. Anatomical data are provided by the real-time B scan, and physiologic data are provided by the pulsed Doppler portion of the operation. (Chapter 5)
43. False. Physiologic Doppler-shift frequencies are usually in the audible frequency range. (Chapter 5)
44. d. All imaging instruments and some Doppler instruments use pulsed ultrasound. (Chapter 4)
45. c. (Chapter 5)
46. e. (Chapter 5)
47. d. (Chapter 5)
48. e. They include pulsed Doppler (and sometimes continuous-wave Doppler) and dynamic B-scan imaging. (Chapter 5)
49. c. Both Doppler shifts exceed one half the pulse repetition frequency. (Chapter 5)
50. d. (Chapter 5)
51. a. This is because physiologic speeds (v) are small compared with the speed of sound (c) in tissues. (Chapter 5)
52. b. (Chapter 5)
53. e. Arterioles and capillaries are too small. (Chapter 5)
54. d. (Chapter 5)
55. e. (Chapter 5)
56. b. (Chapter 5)
57. c. (Chapter 5)
58. d. This is Poiseuille's law. Increasing resistance decreases flow. (Chapter 5)
59. b. It depends on radius to the fourth power. (Chapter 5)
60. d. This is the continuity rule. (Chapter 5)
61. e. (also results of distensible vessels) (Chapter 5)
62. d. (Chapter 5)
63. e. See Figure 5-9. (Chapter 5)
64. c. (assuming a reflector moving at 50 cm/s) (Table 5-5)
65. b. (that is, about 5 m/s) (Chapter 5)
66. c. (smaller angle, larger cosine, larger shift) (Chapter 5)
67. a. (Chapter 5)
68. e. Spectrum is not needed; it cannot be displayed in a pixel. (Chapter 5)
69. d. The spectrum can be shown in addition to the color Doppler display. (Chapter 5)
70. c. (Chapter 5)

$$v = \frac{77 \times 0.100}{(5 \times 0.5)} = 3.08$$

71. a. (Chapter 5)

$$v = \frac{77 \times 0.100}{7.5} = 1.03$$

72. d. (Chapter 5)
73. c. (13 μs of delay per centimeter of depth) (Chapter 5)

74. a. This is because flow speeds are typically one thousandth the speed of sound in tissues. (Chapter 5)
75. b. The range is about 4 to 32. (Chapter 5)
76. c. The range is about 40 to 400. (Chapter 5)
77. e. Any pulsed instrument (b, c, d) can. (Chapter 5)
78. a. This is called near-plug flow. (Chapter 5)
79. d. (Chapter 5)
80. e. A stenosis generally increases a, b, and c and decreases d. (Chapter 5)
81. a. (that is, a widening of the spectrum) (Chapter 5)
82. e. Items b, c, and d are increased; a is decreased. (Chapter 5)
83. c. The blood flows back out of the high-impedance vascular bed during the low-pressure portion of the cardiac cycle. (Chapter 5)
84. c. (Chapter 5)
85. d. (Chapter 5)
86. e. (a resulting from b) (Chapter 5)
87. e. (Chapter 5)
88. a. (gray level or, sometimes, color) (Chapter 5)
89. e. (a = b + c) (Chapter 5)
90. b. (Chapter 5)
91. e. Items a and b determine sample volume length. (Chapter 5)
92. d. Echoes from the sample volume arrive after another pulse is emitted. (Chapter 5)
93. a. The shift exceeds the Nyquist limit (5 kHz). (Chapter 5)
94. e. (a and d) (Chapter 5)
95. e. (Chapter 5)
96. a. (Chapter 5)
97. e. (Chapter 5)
98. a. Because physiologic flow speeds are about one thousandth the ultrasound propagation speed (1540 m/s), Doppler shifts are about one thousandth the operating frequency. (Chapter 5)
99. e. (a and b) (Chapter 5)
100. b. (also proportional to the cosine of the Doppler angle) (Chapter 5)
101. d. Item a is for gray-scale instruments. (Chapter 5)
102. b. (Chapter 7)
103. e. Shift increases to 4 kHz, which is still less than the Nyquist limit (4.5 kHz). (Chapter 5)
104. a. A nonzero Doppler angle increases calculated equivalent flow speed. (Chapter 5)
105. c. The Nyquist limit is still one half of the pulse repetition frequency. (Chapter 5)
106. e. (Chapter 5)
107. e. (Chapters 5 and 6)
108. e. (a and c) (Chapter 5)
109. e. (a and b; c increases the amount of color) (Chapter 5)
110. d. Item c is not strictly part of the color flow display. Also, it is not a cross-sectional display but rather a frequency-versus-time presentation. (Chapter 5)

111. b. White is brighter than gray. (Chapter 5)
112. a. Red and green are different hues, representing different light wave frequencies. (Chapter 5)
113. e. (a, b, c; about 5 to 50 frames per second are displayed) (Chapter 5)
114. d. (Chapter 5)
115. d. (Chapter 5)
116. a. The wall filter removes the lower-frequency clutter Doppler shifts. (Chapter 5)
117. d. (twice as many scan lines per frame) (Chapter 5)
118. e. Items c and d change because the scan line (pulse path) orientation changes. (Chapter 5)
119. a. Items b and c increase the amount of color. (Chapter 5)
120. d. Increasing pulse repetition frequency increases the Nyquist limit, reducing aliasing. (Chapter 5)
121. b. (Chapter 2)
122. e. The wavelength is the length of each cycle in a pulse. (Chapter 2)
123. a. Duty factor is pulse duration divided by pulse repetition period. (Chapter 2)
124. b. The attenuation coefficient of 5-MHz ultrasound is approximately 2.5 dB/cm. The attenuation coefficient multiplied by the path length yields the attenuation (in decibels). Only answer b is given in attenuation (decibel) units. (Chapter 2)
125. b. Amplitude is the maximum amount that an acoustic variable varies from the normal value (in this case, 10 - 7 units). (Chapter 2)
126. a. (Chapter 2)
127. a. Amplitude, intensity, power, and beam area are related to one another. If two of these are known, the others can be found. Frequency is independent of these. All four of them can be known, and yet frequency remains undetermined. (Chapter 2)
128. a. Impedance 1 equals 3, which equals impedance 2; thus there is no reflection. (Chapter 2)
129. b. If 96% of the intensity is transmitted, 4% is reflected because what is not reflected is transmitted (i.e., the two must add up to 100%). (Chapter 2)
130. c. (Chapter 5)
131. c. If the second speed is twice the first speed, then the transmission angle is approximately twice the incidence angle. (Chapter 2)
132. a. Reflector distance = $\frac{1}{2}$ × speed × time. (Chapter 2)
133. d. If reflectors are separated by less than the axial resolution, they are not separated on the display. (Chapter 3)
134. b. Axial resolution is equal to one half the spatial pulse length. Spatial pulse length is equal to the number of cycles in the pulse multiplied by wavelength. Wavelength is equal to propagation speed divided by frequency. For 1 MHz, wavelength is

1.54 mm, spatial pulse length is 2 × 1.54, and axial resolution is 1.54 mm, so two reflectors separated by 1 mm would not be resolved. For 2 MHz, the resolution is 0.77, and the reflectors would be resolved. (Chapter 3)
135. a. For highly damped transducers the quality factor (Q) is approximately equal to the number of cycles in the pulse. (Chapter 3)
136. b. Beam width changes with distance from transducer and thus so does lateral resolution. (Chapter 3)
137. c. Near-zone length increases with transducer diameter so that the only transducer that would have a shorter near-zone length would be a transducer of smaller diameter. (Chapter 3)
138. c. Focusing can be accomplished only in the near zone of a beam. (Chapter 3)
139. e. Answers a, b, and c affect the beam. Resolution of the system also is affected by the electronics of the instrument. (Chapter 3)
140. a. All the others are characteristics of the sound. (Chapter 2)
141. c. Frequency, period, wavelength, and propagation speed are related to one another. However, all four of these can be known, and yet the amplitude is undetermined. (Chapter 2)
142. e. For perpendicular incidence, there is no refraction. For equal impedances, there is no reflection. (Chapter 2)
143. d. (Chapter 2)

$$\text{IRC} = \left(\frac{2.64 - 1.00}{2.64 + 1.00}\right)^2 = \left(\frac{1.64}{3.64}\right)^2 = (0.45)^2 = 0.2$$

For an intensity reflection coefficient (IRC) of 0.2 and an incident intensity of 1, the reflected intensity is 0.2 and the transmitted intensity is 0.8. (Chapter 2)
144. d. (Chapters 4 and 7)
145. d. Incidence angle always equals reflection angle. For equal propagation speeds, incidence angle equals transmission angle as well. (Chapter 2)
146. a. For oblique incidence, it is possible to have no reflection, even if the media impedances are unequal. (Chapter 2)
147. e. Increased transducer damping decreases the spatial pulse length. Increasing spatial pulse length is accompanied by increased pulse duration and degraded axial resolution. (Chapters 2 and 3)
148. c. (Chapter 2)
149. b. Wavelength is equal to propagation speed divided by frequency. (Chapter 2)
150. b. Spatial pulse length is equal to wavelength multiplied by the number of cycles in the pulse. (Chapter 2)
151. d. (Chapter 3)
152. e. No refraction means that there is no change in sound direction. This is a result of no change in

propagation speed (i.e., equal propagation speeds on both sides of the boundary). (Chapter 2)

153. e. If there is 1 W in each square centimeter of area, then there are 5 W in 5 cm^2 of area. (Chapter 2)

154. c. Speeds in solids are higher than in liquids. Soft tissue behaves acoustically as a liquid (as it is mostly water). (Chapter 2)

155. d. (Chapter 2)

156. c. An unfocused 13-mm transducer has a beam width of 6.5 mm at the near-zone length. Focusing would reduce the lateral resolution below this value (i.e., improve it). (Chapter 3)

157. b. A 7.5-MHz transducer can image to a depth of only a few centimeters in tissue. (Chapter 2)

158. a. The other answers make little sense. (Chapter 4)

159. d. (a and b) (Chapter 4)

160. b. For each 10 dB, there is a factor of 10 increase in power. (Chapter 4)

161. c. (Chapter 4)

162. b. (Chapter 4)

163. e. Decimal numbers greater than 15 require at least five bits in a binary number. The number 30 in binary is 11110. (Chapter 4)

164. False. Sixty-four shades require a 6-bit memory. (Chapter 4)

165. e. (Chapter 4)

166. False. This is a description of a linear sequenced array rather than a phased array. (Chapter 3)

167. b. (Chapter 3)

$$AR = \frac{1}{2} SPL = 0.5 \times n \times c/f = \left(\frac{1}{2}\right)(2)(1.54/5) = 0.3$$

168. False. Postprocessing is the assignment of display brightness to numbers coming out of memory. (Chapter 4)

169. e. (Chapter 3)

170. a. (Chapter 3)

171. b. In M mode, echo depth is displayed as a function of time. (Chapter 4)

172. c. (Chapter 2)

173. a. (Chapter 4)

174. e. (1 + 8 = 9) (Chapter 4)

175. a. (Chapter 6)

176. c. The instrument assumes a speed of 1.54 mm/μs. Echoes will arrive sooner because of their higher propagation speed and will be placed closer to the transducer than they should be. (Chapters 2 and 6)

177. a. (Chapter 4)

178. a. Increasing gain or decreasing attenuation increases echo intensity. (Chapters 2 and 4)

179. d. (Chapter 4)

180. b. (Chapters 3 and 4)

181. e. (Chapter 4)

182. e. Multiple pulses per scan line (ensemble length) are required for color Doppler imaging. More pulses per scan line for multiple foci would make the frame rate unacceptably low. (Chapter 5)

183. c. A reduction of 3 dB is a 50% reduction. (Chapter 4)

184. d. See answer to Exercise 183. (Chapter 4)

185. c. (Chapter 4)

186. b. A factor of 8 is three doublings (i.e., 3 + 3 + 3 dB). (Chapter 4)

187. a. (Chapter 7)

188. a. (Chapter 7)

189. e. (Chapter 3)

190. a. (Chapters 2 and 4)

191. c. (Chapter 4)

192. c. (Chapter 4)

193. e. Transmission output side (to the transducer) of a beam former is analog. (Chapters 3 and 4)

194. e. Reception output side of a beam former (to the signal processor) is digital. (Chapter 4)

195. d. (Chapter 3)

196. c. (Chapter 3)

197. e. Propagation speed is independent of frequency and intensity. (Chapter 2)

198. a. (Chapter 5)

199. e. (Chapter 2)

200. a. (Chapter 3)

APPENDIX A

Lists of Symbols

TABLE A-1 | Listed By Symbol

Symbol	Represents	Symbol	Represents
A	area	LR	lateral resolution
a	attenuation	n	number of cycles per pulse; number of foci; ensemble length
a_c	attenuation coefficient	NL	Nyquist limit
a_p	aperture	P	power
AR	axial resolution	p	pressure amplitude
c	propagation speed	PD	pulse duration
cos	cosine	pen	penetration
c_t	element propagation speed	PRF	pulse repetition frequency
d	diameter; distance to reflector; distance from transducer	PRP	pulse repetition period
DF	duty factor	Q	volumetric flow rate
d_f	focal beam diameter	R	flow resistance
f	frequency	r	radius
f_D	Doppler-shift frequency	SPL	spatial pulse length
fl	focal length	T	period
f_o	operating frequency	th	element thickness
FR	frame rate	v	flow speed, scatterer speed
f_R	received (echo) frequency	v_a	average flow speed
FR_m	maximum frame rate	w_b	beam width
f_T	transmitted (operating) frequency	z	impedance
I	intensity	ΔP	pressure difference; pressure drop
I_i	incident intensity	η	viscosity
I_r	reflected intensity	θ_D	Doppler angle
IRC	intensity reflection coefficient	θ_i	incidence angle
I_t	transmitted intensity	θ_r	reflection angle
ITC	intensity reflection coefficient	θ_t	transmission angle
L	path length; tube length	λ	wavelength
LPF	lines per frame	ρ	density

TABLE A-2 | **Listed By Parameter**

Parameter	Represented by	Parameter	Represented by
aperture	a_p	maximum frame rate	FR_m
area	A	number of cycles per pulse	n
attenuation	a	number of foci	n
attenuation coefficient	a_c	Nyquist limit	NL
average flow speed	v_a	operating frequency	f_o
axial resolution	AR	path length	L
beam width	w_b	penetration	pen
cosine	cos	period	T
density	ρ	power	P
diameter	d	pressure amplitude	p
distance from transducer	d	pressure difference	ΔP
distance to reflector	d	pressure drop	ΔP
Doppler angle	θ_D	propagation speed	c
Doppler-shift frequency	f_D	pulse duration	PD
duty factor	DF	pulse repetition frequency	PRF
element propagation speed	c_t	pulse repetition period	PRP
element thickness	th	radius	r
ensemble length	n	received (echo) frequency	f_R
flow resistance	R	receiver speed	v_r
flow speed	v	reflected intensity	I_r
focal beam diameter	d_f	reflection angle	θ_r
focal length	fl	Reynolds number	R_e
frame rate	FR	scatterer speed	v
frequency	f	source speed	v_s
impedance	z	spatial pulse length	SPL
incidence angle	θ_i	transmission angle	θ_t
incident intensity	I_i	transmitted intensity	I_t
intensity	I	tube length	L
intensity reflection coefficient	IRC	viscosity	η
intensity transmission coefficient	ITC	volumetric flow rate	Q
lateral resolution	LR	wavelength	λ
lines per frame	LPF		

Compilation of Equations

For convenient reference, the equations in this book, excepting those in Advanced Concepts sections on the accompanying Evolve site, are compiled here.

Chapter 2

$$T\,(\mu s) = \frac{1}{f\,(MHz)}$$

$$\lambda\,(mm) = \frac{c\,(mm/\mu s)}{f\,(MHz)}$$

$$PRP\,(ms) = \frac{1}{PRF\,(kHz)}$$

$$PD\,(\mu s) = n \times T\,(\mu s)$$

$$DF = \frac{PD\,(\mu s)}{PRP\,(\mu s)} = \frac{PD\,(\mu s) \times PRF\,(kHz)}{1000}$$

$$SPL\,(mm) = n \times \lambda\,(mm)$$

$$I\,(mW/cm^2) = \frac{P\,(mW)}{A\,(cm^2)}$$

$$a\,(dB) = a_c\,(dB/cm) \times L\,(cm)$$

$$a\,(dB) = \frac{1}{2}\,(dB/cm\text{-}MHz) \times f\,(MHz) \times L\,(cm)$$

$$z\,(rayls) = \rho\,(kg/m^3) \times c\,(m/s)$$

$$IRC = \frac{I_r\,(W/cm^2)}{I_i\,(W/cm^2)} = \left[\frac{(z_2 - z_1)}{(z_2 + z_1)}\right]^2$$

$$ITC = \frac{I_t\,(W/cm^2)}{I_i\,(W/cm^2)} = 1 - IRC$$

$$\theta_i\,(degrees) = \theta_r\,(degrees)$$

$$d\,(mm) = \frac{1}{2}\left[c\,(mm/\mu s) \times t\,(\mu s)\right]$$

Chapter 3

$$f_o\,(MHz) = \frac{c_t\,(mm/\mu s)}{2 \times th\,(mm)}$$

$$AR\,(mm) = \frac{SPL\,(mm)}{2}$$

$$LR\,(mm) = w_b\,(mm)$$

Chapter 4

$$pen\,(cm) \times PRF\,(kHz) \le 77\,(cm/ms)$$

$$PRF\,(Hz) = n \times LPF \times FR\,(Hz)$$

$$pen\,(cm) \times n \times LPF \times FR\,(Hz) \le 77,000\,cm/s$$

Chapter 5

$$Q\,(mL/s) = \frac{\Delta P\,(dyne/cm^2)}{R\,(poise)}$$

$$R\,(g/cm^4\text{-}s) = 8 \times L\,(cm) \times \frac{\eta\,(poise)}{\pi \times [r^4\,(cm^4)]}$$

$$Q\,(mL/s) = \frac{\Delta P\,(dyne/cm^2) \times \pi \times d^4\,(cm^4)}{128 \times L\,(cm) \times \eta\,(poise)}$$

$$\Delta P = 4\,(v_2)^2$$

$$f_D\,(kHz) = f_R\,(kHz) - f_o\,(kHz) = f_o\,(kHz) \times \frac{[2 \times v\,(cm/s)]}{c\,(cm/s)}$$

$$v\,(cm/s) = \frac{77\,(cm/ms) \times f_D\,(kHz)}{f_o\,(MHz)}$$

$$f_D\,(kHz) = \frac{[f_o\,(kHz) \times 2 \times v\,(cm/s) \times (\cos\theta)]}{c\,(cm/s)}$$

$$v\,(cm/s) = \frac{[77\,(cm/ms) \times f_D\,(kHz)]}{[f_o\,(MHz) \times \cos\theta]}$$

$$FR_m\,(Hz) = \frac{77,000\,(cm/s)}{pen\,(cm) \times LPF \times n}$$

Chapter 6

$$NL\,(kHz) = \frac{1}{2} \times PRF\,(kHz)$$

Chapter 7

$$MI = \frac{p_r\,(MPa)}{\left[(f)^{1/2}\,(MHz)^{1/2}\right]}$$

Mathematics Review

Algebra and trigonometry are used in the discussion of ultrasound and Doppler principles. Logarithms are involved in decibels, and binary numbers are involved in digital electronics. Mathematical concepts that are applicable to the material in this book are reviewed in this appendix. Relevant aspects of algebra, trigonometry, logarithms, scientific notation, binary numbers, units, and statistics are covered.

First, we review some mathematical terminology. In algebraic equations such as

$$x + y = z$$

$$x - y = z$$

x and y are called *terms*. Terms are connected with each other by addition or subtraction. With addition, the result is called the *sum*. With subtraction, the result is called the *difference*.

In the equations,

$$x \times y = z$$

$$\frac{x}{y} = z$$

x and y are called *factors*. Factors are connected with each other by multiplication or division. When multiplied, the result is called the *product*. When divided, the result is called the *quotient*.

The inverse or reciprocal of x is 1/x, sometimes described as "one over" x.

Algebra. Transposition of quantities in algebraic equations is accomplished by performing identical mathematical operations on both sides.

Example C-1
For the equation,

$$x + y = z$$

transpose to get x alone (solve for x). To do this, subtract y from both sides:

$$x + y - y = z - y$$

Because $y - y = 0$, the left-hand side of the equation is

$$x + y - y = x + 0 = x$$

so that

$$x = z - y$$

Example C-2
For the equation,

$$x - y = z$$

solve for x. Add y to both sides:

$$x - y + y = z + y$$

$$x + 0 = z + y$$

$$x = z + y$$

Example C-3
For the equation,

$$xy = z$$

solve for x. Divide both sides by y:

$$\frac{xy}{y} = \frac{z}{y}$$

Since y/y = 1

$$\frac{xy}{y} = x(1) = x$$

and

$$x = \frac{z}{y}$$

Example C-4
For the equation,

$$\frac{x}{y} = z$$

solve for x. Multiply both sides by y:

$$\left(\frac{x}{y}\right)y = zy$$

$$x(1) = zy$$

$$x = zy$$

Example C-5
Using some numbers, and combining the previous examples, consider the equation

$$\left(\frac{5x + 3}{2}\right) - 3 = 1$$

and solve for x. First, add 3 to both sides:

$$\left(\frac{5x + 3}{2}\right) - 3 + 3 = 1 + 3$$

$$\frac{5x+3}{2} = 4$$

Multiply by 2:

$$\left(\frac{5x+3}{2}\right) \times 2 = 4 \times 2$$

$$5x + 3 = 8$$

Subtract 3:

$$5x + 3 - 3 = 8 - 3$$

$$5x = 5$$

Divide by 5:

$$x = 1$$

Substitution of the answer into the original equation shows that the equality is satisfied and the answer is correct:

$$\left[\frac{5(1)+3}{2}\right] - 3 = 1$$

$$\left(\frac{8}{2}\right) - 3 = 1$$

$$4 - 3 = 1$$

$$1 = 1$$

Example C-6

For the equation,

$$c = f \times \lambda$$

solve for wavelength. Divide by frequency:

$$\frac{c}{f} = \frac{f \times \lambda}{f}$$

$$\frac{c}{f} = \lambda$$

Example C-7

If the intensity reflection coefficient *(IRC)* is 0.1 and the reflected intensity *(I_r)* is 5 mW/cm^2, find the incident intensity *(I_i)*, given that

$$IRC = \frac{I_r}{I_i}$$

Multiply by incident intensity:

$$IRC \times I_i = \frac{I_r}{I_i} \times I_i$$

Divide by intensity reflection coefficient:

$$\frac{IRC \times I_i}{IRC} = \frac{I_r}{IRC}$$

$$I_i = \frac{I_r}{IRC} = \frac{5\ mW/cm^2}{0.1} = 50\ mW/cm^2$$

Example C-8

If the intensity reflection coefficient *(IRC)* is 0.01 and the impedance for medium 1 *(z_1)* is 4.5, find the medium 2 impedance *(z_2)*, given that

$$IRC = \left(\frac{z_2 - z_1}{z_2 + z_1}\right)^2$$

Take the square root of each side:

$$IRC^{1/2} = \frac{z_2 - z_1}{z_2 + z_1}$$

Multiply by the sum of z_2 and z_1:

$$IRC^{1/2} \times (z_2 + z_1) = (z_2 - z_1)$$

Add z_1:

$$IRC^{1/2} \times (z_2 + z_1) + z_1 = z_2$$

Subtract $IRC^{1/2} \times z_2$:

$$(IRC^{1/2} \times z_1) + z_1 = z_2 - (IRC^{1/2} \times z_2)$$

$$z_1(1 + IRC^{1/2}) = z_2(1 - IRC^{1/2})$$

Divide by (1 − IRC$^{1/2}$) and interchange sides of the equation:

$$z_2 = z_1\left[\frac{(1 + IRC^{1/2})}{(1 - IRC^{1/2})}\right]$$

$$= 4.5\left[\frac{1 + (0.01)^{1/2}}{1 - (0.01)^{1/2}}\right]$$

$$= 4.5\left(\frac{1 + 0.1}{1 - 0.1}\right) = 4.5\left(\frac{1.1}{0.9}\right) = 4.5(1.22) = 5.5$$

Trigonometry. If the sides and angles of a right triangle ("right" means one of the angles equals 90 degrees) are labeled as in Figure C-1, the sine of angle A (sin A), the cosine of angle A (cos A), and the tangent of angle A (tan A) are defined as follows:

$$\sin A = \frac{\text{length of side a}}{\text{length of side c}}$$

$$\cos A = \frac{\text{length of side b}}{\text{length of side c}}$$

$$\tan A = \frac{\text{length of side a}}{\text{length of side b}}$$

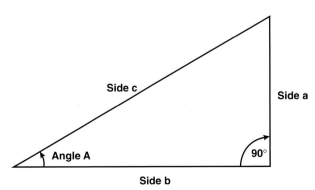

FIGURE C-1 If the sides and angles of a right triangle are labeled as in this figure, the cosine of angle A (cos A) is equal to the length of side b divided by the length of side c. Sine A is equal to the length of side a divided by the length of side c.

Example C-9
If the lengths of the sides a, b, and c are 1, $\sqrt{3}$, and 2, respectively, what are sin A and cos A?

$$\sin A = \frac{1}{2} = 0.5$$

$$\cos A = \frac{\sqrt{3}}{2} = 0.87$$

If the sine or cosine is known, angle A may be found using a calculator or a table such as Table C-1.

Example C-10
If sin A is 0.5, what is A? From Table C-1, A = 30 degrees.

Example C-11
If cos A is 0.87, what is A? From Table C-1, A = 30 degrees.

If angle A is known, sin A or cos A may be found using a calculator or a table such as Table C-1.

Example C-12
If A = 45 degrees, what are the sin A and cos A? From Table C-1, sin A = 0.71 and cos A = 0.71.

Logarithms. The logarithm to the base 10 (log) of a number is equal to the number of tens that must be multiplied together to result in that number. More generally, the logarithm is the power to which 10 must be raised to give a particular number.

Example C-13
What is the logarithm of 1000? To obtain 1000, three tens must be multiplied together:

$$10 \times 10 \times 10 = 1000$$

Three tens then yield the logarithm (log) of 1000.

$$\log 1000 = 3$$

The logarithm of the reciprocal of a number is equal to the negative of the logarithm of the number.

Example C-14
What is the logarithm of 0.01?

$$0.01 = \frac{1}{100}$$

$$\log 100 = 2$$

TABLE C-1			
Angle (°)	**Sine**	**Cosine**	**Tangent**
0	0	1.00	0
30	0.50	0.87	0.58
45	0.71	0.71	1.00
60	0.87	0.50	1.73
90	1.00	0	∞

Note: The symbol ∞ indicates infinity or indeterminate; that is, dividing by zero can be executed an unlimited number of times.

$$\log 0.01 = \log \frac{1}{100} = -2$$

Decibels are quantities that result from taking 10 times the logarithm of the ratio of two powers or intensities.

Example C-15
Compare the following two powers in decibels: power 1 = 1 W; power 2 = 10 W.

$$10 \log \left(\frac{\text{power 1}}{\text{power 2}} \right) = 10 \log \left(\frac{1}{10} \right) = 10 (-\log 10) = 10 (-1) = -10 \text{ dB}$$

Power 1 is 10 dB less than power 2, or power 1 is 10 dB below power 2. Also

$$10 \log \left(\frac{\text{power 2}}{\text{power 1}} \right) = 10 \log \left(\frac{10}{1} \right) = 10 (\log 10) = 10 (1) = 10 \text{ dB}$$

Power 2 is 10 dB more than power 1, or power 2 is 10 dB above power 1.

Example C-16
An amplifier has a power output of 100 mW when the input power is 0.1 mW. What is the amplifier gain in decibels?

$$\text{amplifier gain (dB)} = 10 \log \left(\frac{\text{power out}}{\text{power in}} \right)$$

$$= 10 \log \left(\frac{100}{0.1} \right) = 10 \log 1000 = 10 (3) = 30 \text{ dB}$$

Example C-17
An electric attenuator has a power output of 0.01 mW when the input power is 100 mW. What is the attenuation of the attenuator in decibels?

$$\text{attenuator attenuation (dB)} = -10 \log \left(\frac{\text{power out}}{\text{power in}} \right)$$

$$= -10 \log \left(\frac{0.01}{100} \right) = -10 \log \left(\frac{1}{10,000} \right)$$

$$= -10 (-\log 10,000)$$

$$= -10 (-4) = 40 \text{ dB}$$

The first minus sign is used in the equation to give the attenuation as a positive number. If the minus number had not been used, the "gain" of the attenuator would have been calculated, which would have turned out to be −40 dB. A gain of −40 dB is the same as an attenuation of 40 dB.

Example C-18
Compare intensity 2 with intensity 1; intensity 1 = 10 mW/cm^2; intensity 2 = 0.01 mW/cm^2.

$$10 \log \left(\frac{\text{intensity 2}}{\text{intensity 1}} \right) = 10 \log \left(\frac{0.01}{10} \right)$$

$$= 10 \log \left(\frac{1}{1000} \right) = 10 (-\log 1000)$$

$$= 10 (-3) = -30 \text{ dB}$$

Intensity 2 is 30 dB less than or below intensity 1.

Example C-19

As sound passes through a medium, its intensity at one point is 1 mW/cm^2 and at a point 10 cm farther along is 0.1 mW/cm^2. What are the attenuation and attenuation coefficient? (See Chapter 2.)

$$\text{attenuation (dB)} = -10\log\left(\frac{\text{intensity at second point}}{\text{intensity at first point}}\right)$$
$$= -10\log\left(\frac{0.1}{1}\right) = -10\log\left(\frac{1}{10}\right)$$
$$= -10(-\log 10) = -10(-1) = 10\text{ dB}$$

See Example C-17 for comment on the first minus sign. The attenuation coefficient is the attenuation (dB) divided by the separation between the two points:

$$\text{attenuation coefficient (dB/cm)} = \frac{\text{attenuation (dB)}}{\text{separation (cm)}}$$
$$= \frac{10\text{ dB}}{10\text{ cm}} = 1\text{ dB/cm}$$

Example C-20

Show by example that log x^2 is equal to 2 log x.
Let $x = 5$.
Then log $x = 0.70$ and 2 log $x = 1.40$.
Thus $x = 5^2 = 25$ and log 25 = 1.40.

Example C-21

Power and intensity are proportional to amplitude squared. A power or intensity ratio expressed in decibels is calculated using the definition

$$10\log\left(\frac{\text{power 1}}{\text{power 2}}\right)$$

This is equivalent to

$$20\log\left(\frac{\text{amplitude 1}}{\text{amplitude 2}}\right)$$

as seen with the following values:
Amplitude 1 = 4
Amplitude 2 = 3
Power 1 = 4^2 = 16
Power 2 = 3^2 = 9

$$\text{power ratio (dB)} = 10\log\left(\frac{\text{power 1}}{\text{power 2}}\right)$$
$$= 10\log\left(\frac{16}{9}\right) = 2.5$$

$$\text{amplitude ratio (dB)} = 20\log\left(\frac{\text{amplitude 1}}{\text{amplitude 2}}\right)$$
$$= 20\log\left(\frac{4}{3}\right) = 2.5$$

Table C-2 lists various values of power or intensity ratio with corresponding decibel values of gain or attenuation.

Some authors put output or end-of-path values in the numerator of the equation used for calculating decibels. If the numerator value is less than the denominator value (e.g., attenuation) a negative decibel value is calculated.

TABLE C-2	Decibel Values of Attenuation or Gain for Various Values of Power or Intensity Ratio*	
Decibel Gain or Attenuation	**Attenuation**	**Gain**
1	0.79	1.3
3	0.50	2.0
6	0.25	4.0
10	0.10	10.0
30	0.001	1000
100	0.0000000001	10,000,000,000

*The ratio is output power or intensity divided by input power or intensity.

For example, if the input and output powers for an electrical attenuator were 2 W and 1 W, respectively, −3 dB results; that is, this attenuator has −3 dB of gain. In this book, only positive decibel values are considered with clarification regarding whether attenuation or gain is considered. In this example, the result would be given as 3 dB of attenuation.

Scientific Notation. Scientific notation uses factors of 10, expressed in exponential form, to shorten the expression of very large or very small numbers. For example, 1,540,000 mm/s can be expressed as 1.54×10^6. In the expression x^y, x is called the base and y is called the exponent. When multiplying factors in scientific notation, the exponents are added. When dividing, the exponents are subtracted.

Example C-22

$$\frac{(1.54 \times 10^6 \text{ mm/s}) \times (3.60 \times 10^3 \text{ s/hr})}{(1.61 \times 10^6 \text{ mm/mile})} = 3.44 \times 10^3 \text{ mph}$$

Here, the multiplication result is 5.54×10^9. Then the division by 1.61×10^6 yields 3.44×10^3.

Binary Numbers. The use of digital memories in ultrasound imaging instruments presents a need for understanding the binary numbering system. Digital (computer) memories and data processors use binary numbers in carrying out their functions because they contain electronic components that operate in only two states, off (0) and on (1).

Binary digits (bits) consist of only zeros and ones, represented by the symbols 0 and 1. As in the decimal numbering system, with which we are so familiar, other numbers must be represented by moving these symbols to different positions (columns). In the decimal system, where there are ten symbols (0 through 9), there is no symbol for the number ten (nine is the largest number for which there is a symbol). To represent ten in symbolic form, the symbol for one is used, moving it to the second (from the right) column. A zero is placed in the right column to clarify this so that ten is, symbolically, 10. The symbols for one and zero have been used in such a way that they no longer represent one or zero, but rather ten.

A similar procedure is used in the binary numbering system. The symbol 1 represents the largest number (one) for which there is a symbol in the system. To represent the next number (2), the same thing is done as in the decimal system; that is, the symbol 1 is placed in the next column to represent the number 2. Columns in the two systems represent values as follows:

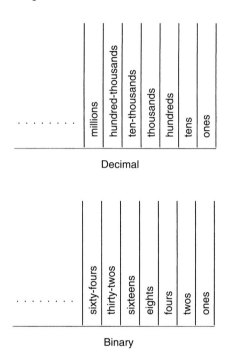

Decimal

Binary

In the decimal system, each column represents 10 times the column to the right. In the binary system each column represents two times the column to the right.

The decimal number 1234 represents (reading from right to left) four ones, three tens, two hundreds, and one thousand; that is, 4 + 30 + 200 + 1000 = 1234. Likewise, the decimal number 10,110 represents zero ones, one ten, one hundred, zero thousands, and one ten thousand. The binary number 10110 represents zero ones, one two, one four, zero eights, and one sixteen, or 0 + 2 + 4 + 0 + 16 = 22 in decimal form. This represents a straightforward way of converting a number from the binary system to the decimal system.

Example C-23
Convert the binary number 101010 to decimal form. This number represents 0 + 2 + 0 + 8 + 0 + 32, or 42 in decimal form.

To convert a number from decimal to binary form, one must successively subtract the largest possible multiples of 2, which are the binary column values, in succession from the decimal number.

Example C-24
Convert the decimal number 60 to binary form:
  a. Can 64 be subtracted from 60? No. (Enter 0 in the 64 column of the binary number.)
  b. Can 32 be subtracted from 60? Yes. (Enter 1 in the 32 column.)
     60 − 32 = 28 (the difference)
  c. Can 16 be subtracted from 28? Yes. (Enter 1 in the 16 column.)
     28 − 16 = 12 (the difference)
  d. Can 8 be subtracted from 12? Yes. (Enter 1 in the 8 column.)
     12 − 8 = 4 (the difference)
  e. Can 4 be subtracted from 4? Yes. (Enter 1 in the 4 column.)
     4 − 4 = 0 (the difference)
  f. Can 2 be subtracted from 0? No. (Enter 0 in the 2 column.)
  g. Can 1 be subtracted from 0? No. (Enter 0 in the 1 column.)

Therefore the decimal 60 equals 0111100 in the binary system. As in the decimal system, we normally drop leading zeroes, that is, those to the left of the first nonzero digit. The result is 111100. To check this answer, convert it back to decimal form. This number, 111100, reading from the right, represents 0 + 0 + 4 + 8 + 16 + 32, or 60 in decimal form.

Table C-3 lists the binary forms of the decimal numbers 0 to 63. Numbers 64 to 127 would have one additional digit, and so forth with higher multiples of 2.

Units. Units for the physics and acoustics quantities discussed in this book are presented in this section. They are drawn primarily from the international system of units (SI).

Table C-4 lists units for the quantities discussed in this book. Table C-5 gives equivalent units. Table C-6 lists prefixes for units, and Table C-7 gives conversion factors between common units.

In algebraic equations involving these units, the units for the quantity solved for are determined by manipulation of the units for the other quantities in the equation.

Example C-25
Determine the unit for frequency in the equation

$$\text{frequency} = \frac{\text{propagation speed (m/s)}}{\text{wavelength (m)}}$$

The units on the right-hand side of the equation are

$$\frac{\text{m/s}}{\text{m}} = \frac{1}{\text{s}}$$

From Table C-5, it can be found that

$$\frac{1}{\text{s}} = \text{Hz}$$

Therefore, the frequency unit is hertz.

TABLE C-3	Binary and Decimal Number Equivalents		
Decimal	**Binary**	**Decimal**	**Binary**
0	000000	32	100000
1	000001	33	100001
2	000010	34	100010
3	000011	35	100011
4	000100	36	100100
5	000101	37	100101
6	000110	38	100110
7	000111	39	100111
8	001000	40	101000
9	001001	41	101001
10	001010	42	101010
11	001011	43	101011
12	001100	44	101100
13	001101	45	101101
14	001110	46	101110
15	001111	47	101111
16	010000	48	110000
17	010001	49	110001
18	010010	50	110010
19	010011	51	110011
20	010100	52	110100
21	010101	53	110101
22	010110	54	110110
23	010111	55	110111
24	011000	56	111000
25	011001	57	111001
26	011010	58	111010
27	011011	59	111011
28	011100	60	111100
29	011101	61	111101
30	011110	62	111110
31	011111	63	111111

Example C-26

Determine the unit for frequency in the equation

$$\text{frequency} = \frac{\text{propagation speed}\,(\text{m/s})}{\text{wavelength}\,(\text{mm})}$$

The units on the right-hand side of the equation are

$$\frac{\text{m/s}}{\text{mm}}$$

From Table C-6, it can be found that 1 mm equals 0.001 m, so that

$$\frac{\text{m/s}}{0.001\,\text{m}} = 1000\,\text{1/s}$$

and from Tables C-5 and C-6,

$$1000\,\text{1/s} = 1000\,\text{Hz} = 1\,\text{kHz}$$

Therefore, the frequency unit is kilohertz. To convert a frequency given in kilohertz to megahertz, multiply by 0.001. To convert a frequency given in kilohertz to hertz, multiply by 1000.

TABLE C-4	Units and Unit Symbols for Physics and Acoustic Quantities	
Quantity	**Unit**	**Unit Symbol or Abbreviation**
Acceleration	meters/second^2	m/s^2
Angle	degrees	°
Area	Meters^2	m^2
Attenuation	decibels	dB
Attenuation coefficient	decibels/meter	dB/m
Beam area	meters^2	m^2
Current	amperes	A
Density	kilograms/meter^3	kg/m^3
Displacement	meters	m
Doppler shift	hertz	Hz
Energy	joules	J
Force	newtons	N
Frequency	hertz	Hz
Gain	decibels	dB
Heat	joules	J
Impedance	rayls	—
Intensity	watts/meter^2	W/m^2
Mass	kilograms	kg
Period	seconds	s
Power	watts	W
Pressure	newtons/meter^2	N/m^2
Propagation speed	meters/second	m/s
Pulse duration	seconds	s
Pulse repetition frequency	hertz	Hz
Pulse repetition period	seconds	s
Resistance	ohms	Ω
Spatial pulse length	meters	m
Speed	metes/second	m/s
Stiffness	newtons/meter^2	N/m^2
Temperature	degrees Kelvin	K
Time	seconds	s
Velocity	meters/second	m/s
Voltage	volts	V
Volume	meters^3	m^3
Wavelength	meters	m
Work	joules	J

TABLE C-5	Equivalent Units for Physics and Acoustics Quantities	
Unit Given in Table C-4	**Equivalent Unit**	**Equivalent Unit Abbreviation**
Hertz	1/second	1/s
Joules	newton-meters	N-m
Joules	watt-seconds	W-s
Rayls	kilograms/meter^2-second	kg/m^2-s
Newtons	kilogram-meters/second^2	kg-m/s^2
Newtons/meter	pascals	Pa
Watts	joules/second	J/s

TABLE C-6	Unit Prefixes	
Prefix	Factor*	Symbol or Abbreviation
mega	1,000,000	M
kilo	1,000	k
centi	0.01	c
milli	0.001	m
micro	0.000001	μ

*Factor is the number of unprefixed units in a unit with the prefix. For example, there are 1000 Hz in 1 kHz, and there is 0.001 m in 1 mm.

TABLE C-7	Conversion Factors Among Common Units		
To Convert	From	To	Multiply by
Area	m^2	cm^2	10,000
	cm^2	m^2	0.0001
Displacement	m	mm	1,000
	m	cm	100
	m	km	0.001
	mm	m	0.001
	mm	km	0.000001
	km	mm	1,000,000
Frequency	Hz	kHz	0.001
	Hz	MHz	0.000001
	kHz	MHz	0.001
	MHz	kHz	1,000
	kHz	Hz	1,000
	MHz	Hz	1,000,000
Intensity	W/cm^2	W/m^2	10,000
	W/cm^2	kW/m^2	10
	W/cm^2	mW/cm^2	1,000
	W/m^2	W/cm^2	0.0001
	W/m^2	mW/cm^2	0.1
	W/m^2	kW/m^2	0.001
Speed	m/s	km/s	0.001
	km/s	m/s	1,000
	km/s	mm/μs	1

Example C-27

Determine the unit for intensity in the equation

$$\text{intensity} = \frac{\text{power (W)}}{\text{area}\,(cm^2)}$$

The units on the right-hand side of the equation are W/cm^2; therefore the intensity unit is watts per centimeter squared.

Example C-28

Determine the unit for impedance in the equation

$$\text{impedance} = \text{density}\,(kg/m^3) \times \text{propagation speed}\,(km/s)$$

The units on the right-hand side of the equation are

$$kg/m^3 \times km/s$$

From Table C-6,

$$kg/m^3 \times km/s = kg/m^3 \times 1000\,m/s = 1000\,kg/m^2{\cdot}s$$

TABLE C-8	Definitions of Numbers in Groups Tested*		
Test Result	Disease	Nondiseased	Total
Positive	TPV	FPV	TP
Negative	FNV	TNV	TN
Total	TD	TND	TOT

*A positive test indicates *disease*. A negative test indicates *disease-free*. FNV (false-negative value), the number of diseased persons testing negative; FPV (false-positive value), the number of nondiseased persons who tested positive; TD, the total number of diseased persons; TN, the total number of persons testing negative; TND, the total number of nondiseased persons; TNV (true-negative value), the number of disease-free persons testing negative; TOT, the total number of persons in the study; TP, the total number of persons testing positive; TPV (true-positive value), the number of diseased persons (in the study) testing positive.

From Table C-5,

$$1000\,kg/m^2{\cdot}s = 1000\,\text{rayls}$$

From Table C-6,

$$1000\,\text{rayls} = 1\,\text{krayl}$$

Therefore, the impedance unit is kilorayl. Because this is uncommon, it would be better to keep the result in rayls.

Statistics. Several concepts are used in evaluating the usefulness of diagnostic tests. These tests can be qualitative, as in the case of interpreting an anatomical image, or they can be quantitative, as with Doppler flow values. Diagnoses are positive and negative; that is, the test indicates the presence or absence of disease. Table C-8 defines the various groups involved in testing for disease.

The sensitivity (SENS) of a test is the proportion of those having the disease (TD) who test positive (TPV):

$$\text{SENS} = \frac{\text{TPV}}{\text{TD}}$$

The specificity (SPEC) of a test is the proportion of those who are disease-free (TND) who test negative (TNV):

$$\text{SPEC} = \frac{\text{TNV}}{\text{TND}}$$

The positive predictive value (PPV) of a test is the proportion of all positive (TP) test results that are correct, that is, the number of true positive results (TPV):

$$\text{PPV} = \frac{\text{TPV}}{\text{TP}}$$

The positive predictive value is the probability that a person who tests positive actually has the disease.

The negative predictive value (NPV) of a test is the proportion of all negative (TN) test results that are correct, that is, the number of true negative results (TNV):

$$\text{NPV} = \frac{\text{TNV}}{\text{TN}}$$

The negative predictive value is the probability that a person who tests negative is actually disease-free.

The accuracy (ACC) of a test is the proportion of all tests in the study (TOT) that have the correct result

$$ACC = \frac{(TPV + TNV)}{TOT}$$

Example C-29

Given the following table, calculate TD, TND, TP, TN, TOT, SENS, SPEC, PPV, NPV, and ACC.

Test Result	Disease	Nondiseased	Total
Positive	8	2	TP
Negative	5	85	TN
Total	TD	TND	TOT

Test Result	Disease	Nondiseased	Total
Positive	8	2	10
Negative	5	85	90
Total	13	87	100

$$SENS = \frac{8}{13} = 0.62$$

$$SPEC = \frac{85}{87} = 0.98$$

$$PPV = \frac{8}{10} = 0.80$$

$$NPV = \frac{85}{90} = 0.94$$

$$ACC = \frac{(8 + 85)}{100} = 0.93$$

EXERCISES

1. Solve each of the following for x:
   a. $x + y + 2 = z$
   b. $x - y = z - 1$
   c. $2xy = z$
   d. $\frac{x}{y} = 3z$
   e. $\frac{(x + 5)}{4} - 2 = 4$
   f. $\frac{(3x + 3)}{2} - 2 = 4$

2. Solve each of the following for the quantity with the asterisk:
   a. propagation speed = frequency* × wavelength
   b. intensity = $\frac{power}{beam\ area*}$
   c. period = $\frac{1}{frequency*}$

3. The age of an ultrasound instrument is equal to 3 times its age 3 years from now minus 3 times its age 3 years ago. What is its present age?

4. Let
$$y + x = \frac{1}{2}(7y - 3x)$$
   a. Subtract 2x from both sides so that
   $$y - x = \frac{1}{2}(7y - 3x) - 2x$$
   b. Divide both sides by (y − x):
   $$\frac{(y - x)}{(y - x)} = \frac{(7y - 3x)}{2(y - x)} - \frac{2x}{(y - x)}$$
   c. Combine right side into single fraction:
   $$\frac{(y - x)}{(y - x)} = \frac{(7y - 3x - 4x)}{2(y - x)} = \frac{7(y - x)}{2(y - x)}$$
   d. Multiply both sides by 2:
   $$2\left[\frac{(y - x)}{(y - x)}\right] = 7\left[\frac{(y - x)}{(y - x)}\right]$$
   Therefore 2 = 7. What went wrong?

5. If side a, b, and c in Figure C-1 have lengths of 3, 4, and 5, respectively, then sin A is _____ and cos A is _____.

6. If angle A is 90 degrees, sin A is _____ and cos A is _____.

7. If sin A is 0.17, angle A is _____ degrees.

8. If cos A is 0.94, angle A is _____ degrees.

9. Give the logarithms of the following numbers:
   a. 10 _____
   b. 0.1 _____
   c. 100 _____
   d. 0.001 _____

10. One watt is _____ dB below 100 W.

11. One watt is _____ dB above 100 mW.

12. If the input power is 1 mW and the output is 10,000 mW, the gain is _____ dB.

13. If the input power is 1 W and the output is 100 mW, the gain is _____ dB. The attenuation is _____ dB.

14. If the intensities of traveling sound are 10 mW/cm² and 0.1 mW/cm² at two points 5 cm apart, the attenuation between the two points is _____ dB. The attenuation coefficient is _____ dB/cm.

15. If an amplifier has a gain of 33 dB, the ratio of output power to input power is _____. (Use Table C-2.)

16. If an attenuator has an attenuation of 26 dB, the ratio of output power to input power is _____. (Use Table C-2.)

17. If the intensity at the start of a path is 3 mW/cm² and the attenuation over the path is 13 dB, the intensity at the end of the path is _____ mW/cm². (Use Table C-2.)

18. If the output of a 22-dB gain amplifier is connected to the input of a 24-dB gain amplifier, the total gain is _____ dB. The overall power ratio is _____. (Use Table C-2.)

19. If a 17-dB attenuator is connected to a 14-dB amplifier, the net gain is _____ dB. The net attenuation is _____ dB. For a 1-W input, the output is _____ W. (Use Table C-2.)

20. In binary numbers, how many symbols are used? _____

21. The term binary digit commonly is shortened into the single word _____.

22. Each binary digit in a binary number is represented in memory by a memory element, which at any time is in one of _____ states.

23. Match the following:
Column in a binary number hgfedcba:
a. _____
b. _____
c. _____
d. _____
e. _____
f. _____
g. _____
h. _____
Decimal number represented by a 1 in the column:
1. 64
2. 32
3. 1
4. 16
5. 8
6. 128
7. 2
8. 4

24. The binary number 10110 represents zero ones, one two, one four, zero eights, and one sixteen, that is, $0 + 2 + 4 + 0 + 16 = 22$. What decimal number is represented by the binary number 11001? _____

25. The decimal number 13 is made up of one one, zero twos, one four, and one eight ($8 + 4 + 0 + 1 = 13$). The decimal number therefore is represented by the binary number _____.

26. Match the following:
a. 1 _____   1. 0001111
b. 5 _____   2. 0011001
c. 10 _____   3. 0001010
d. 15 _____   4. 0110010
e. 20 _____   5. 0000001
f. 25 _____   6. 1100100
g. 30 _____   7. 0101000
h. 40 _____   8. 0011110
i. 50 _____   9. 0010100
j. 100 _____   10. 0000101

27. How many binary digits are required in the binary numbers representing the following numbers?
a. 0 _____
b. 1 _____
c. 5 _____
d. 10 _____
e. 25 _____
f. 30 _____
g. 63 _____
h. 64 _____
i. 75 _____
j. 100 _____

28. Match the following:
Largest decimal number that can be represented by a binary number with this many bits:
a. 7 _____   1. 1
b. 15 _____   2. 2
c. 3 _____   3. 3
d. 511 _____   4. 4
e. 1023 _____   5. 5
f. 63 _____   6. 6
g. 255 _____   7. 7
h. 1 _____   8. 8
i. 127 _____   9. 9
j. 31 _____   10. 10

29. How many bits are required to store numbers representing each number of different gray shades?
a. 2 _____
b. 4 _____
c. 8 _____
d. 15 _____
e. 16 _____
f. 25 _____
g. 32 _____
h. 64 _____
i. 65 _____
j. 128 _____

30. The unit of frequency in the equation

$$\text{frequency} = \frac{\text{propagation speed (km/s)}}{\text{wavelength (mm)}}$$

is _____. To convert frequency in this unit to frequency in kilohertz, multiply by _____.

31. A frequency of 50 kHz is equal to _____ MHz and _____ Hz.

32. A speed of 1.5 mm/μs is equal to _____ km/s, _____ m/s, _____ cm/s, and _____ mm/s.

33. If the frequency is 2 MHz and

$$\text{period} = \frac{1}{\text{frequency}}$$

the period is _____ μs, _____ ms, or _____ s.

34. Mass is given in units of _____.
 a. megahertz
 b. kilogram
 c. degrees Kelvin
 d. watt
 e. none of the above

35. Displacement is given in _____.
 a. megahertz
 b. decibel
 c. ohm
 d. meter
 e. all of the above

36. Attenuation is given in _____.
 a. decirayl
 b. deciwatt
 c. decibel
 d. decimeter
 e. decihertz

37. Given the following table, calculate TD, TND, TP, TN, TOT, SENS, SPEC, PPV, NPV, and ACC.

Test Result	Disease	Nondiseased	Total
Positive	80	20	TP
Negative	50	850	TN
Total	TD	TND	TOT

38. Solve the following for x and y:

$$x + y = 1 \quad x - y = 2$$

ANSWERS

1. a. $z - y - 2$; b. $y + z - 1$; c. $z/2y$; d. $3yz$; e. 19; f. 3

2.
 a. $\dfrac{\text{propagation speed}}{\text{wavelength}}$

 b. $\dfrac{\text{power}}{\text{intensity}}$

 c. $\dfrac{1}{\text{period}}$

3. 18

4. Division by zero is what went wrong. Note that

$$y + x = \frac{1}{2}(7y - 3x)$$

yields

$$2(y + x) = 7y - 3x$$

$$2y + 2x = 7y - 3x$$

$$5x = 5y$$

$$x = y$$

so that dividing by $(y - x)$ is dividing by zero (not allowed in algebra).

5. 0.6, 0.8

6. 1, 0

7. 10
8. 20
9. a. 1; b. –1; c. 2; d. –3
10. 20
11. 10
12. 40
13. –10, 10
14. 20, 4
15. 2000
16. 0.0025
17. 0.15
18. 46, 40,000
19. –3, 3, 0.50
20. Two (0, 1)
21. Bit
22. Two (off, on)
23. a. 3; b. 7; c. 8; d. 5; e. 4; f. 2; g. 1; h. 6
24. 25
25. 1101
26. a. 5; b. 10; c. 3; d. 1; e. 9; f. 2; g. 8; h. 7; i. 4; j. 6
27. a. 1 (0); b. 1 (1); c. 3 (101); d. 4 (1010); e. 5 (11001); f. 5 (11110); g. 6 (111111); h. 7 (1000000); i. 7 (1001011); j. 7 (1100100)
28. a. 3 (111); b. 4 (1111); c. 2 (11); d. 9 (111111111); e. 10 (1111111111); f. 6 (111111); g. 8 (11111111); h. 1 (1); i. 7 (1111111); j. 5 (11111)
29. a. 1 (0, 1); b. 2 (00, 01, 10, 11); c. 3 (000, 001, 010, 011, 100, 101, 110, 111); d. 4; e. 4; f. 5; g. 5; h. 6; i. 7; j. 7
30. Megahertz, 1000
31. 0.05, 50,000
32. 1.5, 1500, 150,000, 1,500,000
33. 0.5, 0.0005, 0.0000005
34. b
35. d
36. c
37.

Test Result	Disease	Nondiseased	Total
Positive	80	20	100
Negative	50	850	900
Total	130	870	1000

$$\text{SENS} = \frac{80}{130} = 0.62$$

$$\text{SPEC} = \frac{850}{870} = 0.98$$

$$\text{PPV} = \frac{80}{100} = 0.80$$

$$\text{NPV} = \frac{850}{900} = 0.94$$

$$\text{ACC} = \frac{(80 + 850)}{1000} = 0.93$$

38. $x = 1\frac{1}{2}$

 $y = -1/2$

1. Goldberg BB, Raichlen JS: Ultrasound contrast agents, London, 2001, Martin Dunitz.
2. Burns PN: Contrast agents for ultrasound. In Rumack CM, et al, editors: Diagnostic ultrasound, ed 4, St Louis, 2011, Elsevier/Mosby.
3. Sohn YM, Kim MJ, Kim EK, Kwak JY, Moon HJ, Kim SJ: Sonographic elastography combined with conventional sonography: How much is it helpful for diagnostic performance? J Ultrasound Med 28:413–420, 2009.
4. National Electrical Manufacturers Association: Digital Imaging and Communications in Medicine (DICOM) Set, Standards PS 3.1–3.16, Rosslyn, Va, 2003, The Association. http://medical.nema.org/dicom/
5. Nelson TR, et al: Sources and impact of artifacts on clinical three-dimensional ultrasound imaging. Ultrasound Obstet Gynecol 16:374–383, 2000.
6. Baker KG, Robertson VJ, Duck FA: A review of therapeutic ultrasound. Phys Ther 81:1339–1350, 2001.
7. Harris GR: Progress in medical ultrasound exposimetry. IEEE Trans Ultrason Ferroelectr Freq Control 52:717–736, 2005.
8. AIUM Bioeffects Consensus Report. J Ultrasound Med 27:499–644, 2008.
9. American Institute of Ultrasound in Medicine: Medical ultrasound safety, ed 2, Laurel, MD, 2009.
10. American Institute of Ultrasound in Medicine: Recommended ultrasound terminology, ed 3, Laurel, MD, 2008.

Index